D1273771

Men'sHealth.
Total-Body
Health & Fitness
Guide
2012

RODALE.

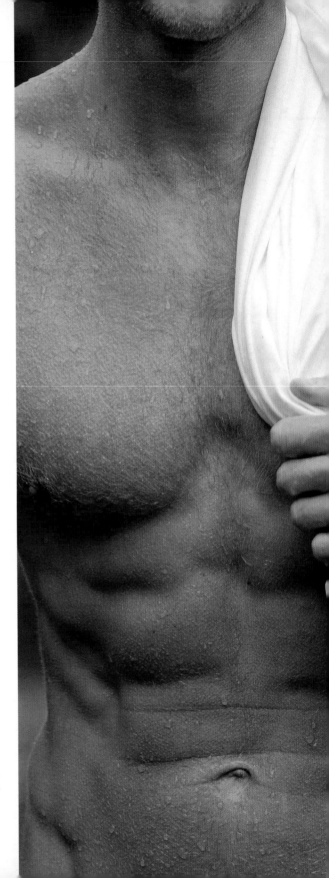

© 2011 by Rodale Inc.

Men's Health is a registered trademark of Rodale Inc.

Printed in the United States of America

Rodale Inc. makes every effort to use acid-free ∞, recycled paper ♲.

ISBN 978-1-60961-794-3   hardcover

2 4 6 8 10 9 7 5 3 1   hardcover

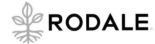

We inspire and enable people to improve their lives and the world around them.

For more of our products visit **rodalestore.com** or call 800-848-4735.

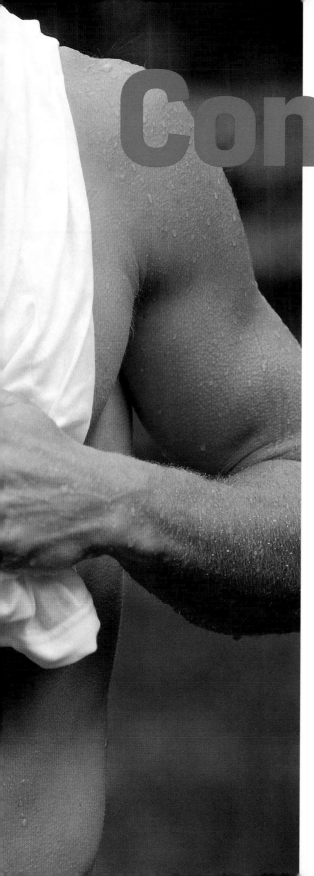

Contents

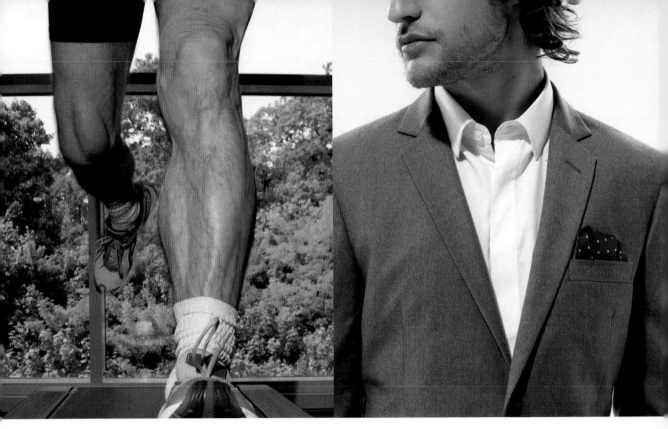

Part 3:

Muscle Up Fast

Part 4:

Look Better Instantly

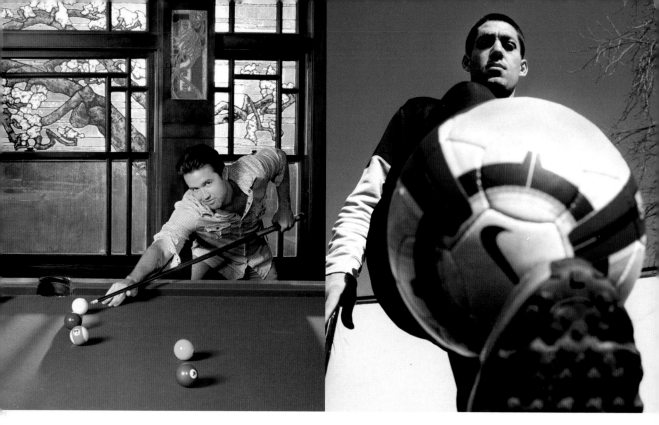

$2,646.

That's the annual cost of being obese for a man. Can you afford it? Probably not. Fitness has so many benefits, it's practically money in the bank.

We polled 2,399 men about their fitness, and resultant self-esteem, and here's what we discovered. How do you measure up?

1 Are you satisfied with the way you look shirtless?

YES	NO
32%	68%

2 Do you plan to whip yourself into shape before summer?

YES	NO
98%	2%

3 How many times do you expect to go to the beach this summer?

0: 9 percent
1 to 5: 50 percent
6 or more: 41 percent

4 Describe a time when you felt extremely self-conscious about the way you looked.

"I saw my wedding photo and thought it was someone else with my wife." —Keith, 34

"South Beach." —Jorge, 23

"Looking as pregnant as my wife as I held our newborn in the hospital." —Chris, 31

"When I'm driving. It's like my gut is sitting there reminding me to get rid of it." —Dwight, 22

5 When were you in the best shape of your life?

Right now: 43 percent

Less than 10 years ago: 47 percent

More than 10 years ago: 10 percent

6 Which is better for your self-confidence?

Lean physique: 67 percent
Large muscles: 18 percent
Good hair and skin: 15 percent

7 Would you rather have functional strength, like a construction worker, or a killer bod, like a lifeguard?

Functional strength: 32 percent
Killer bod: 68 percent

8 Which strategy would best transform the way you look?

Weights: 44 percent
Diet: 30 percent
Cardio: 26 percent

9 What's your best physical asset?

Eyes: 22 percent
Arms: 17 percent
Shoulders: 14 percent
Legs: 13 percent
Chest: 12 percent
Abs: 9 percent
Back: 7 percent
Hair: 6 percent

10 If you had a six-pack, would you go shirtless more often?

YES	NO
78%	22%

11 How often do you weigh yourself?

Daily: 20 percent
Weekly: 41 percent
Monthly: 21 percent
Rarely: 18 percent

12 Does your partner perceive your body differently than you do?

She likes it more than I do:
56 percent

She likes it less than I do:
12 percent

We like it the same:
32 percent

13 What's the best compliment a woman has ever given you about your looks?

"How are you always the best dressed man in the room?"
—Wade, 28

"I still find you attractive after all these years." —Brandon, 35

"I'm going to nickname you El Cuerpo—The Body." —Noel, 24

"If Brad Pitt and Hugh Jackman had a child, you'd be it."
—Randall, 41

14 Would you prefer to be taller or leaner?

Taller: 42 percent
Leaner: 58 percent

15 Which clothes do you feel most confident wearing?

Casual: 58 percent
Business: 42 percent

16 Does having a good scent improve your self-confidence?

YES	NO
82%	18%

17 Do most men who wear cologne overdo it?

YES	NO
68%	32%

18 What would you do if you had a lot of back hair?

Have it removed: 84 percent
Live with it: 16 percent

19 What's your opinion of barbershops versus salons?

"They're fine, if you're over 40. But not while you still have your hair."
—Andrew, 28

"A good barber is as important as a good bartender." —David, 31

"I recently went back to one after years away, and it was like finding my favorite jacket." —Stephen, 27

20 Would you rather go gray or go bald?

Gray: 92 percent
Bald: 8 percent

21 Do you groom "down there"?

YES	NO
84%	16%

22 Have you ever had six-pack abs?

YES	NO
46%	54%

23 If an attractive woman invited you to a nude beach, would you go?

YES	NO
68%	32%

Be Your Best

Now it's time to boost your appeal, and in your hands you hold the tools! In the *Men's Health Total-Body Health & Fitness Guide 2012,* you'll learn how to

PART **1**: **Lose Your Gut**

PART **2**: **Flat-Belly Foods**

PART **3**: **Muscle Up Fast**

PART **4**: **Look Better Instantly**

PART **5**: **Live Longer, Live Better**

PART **6**: **Improve Your Game**

Welcome to the best year of your life!

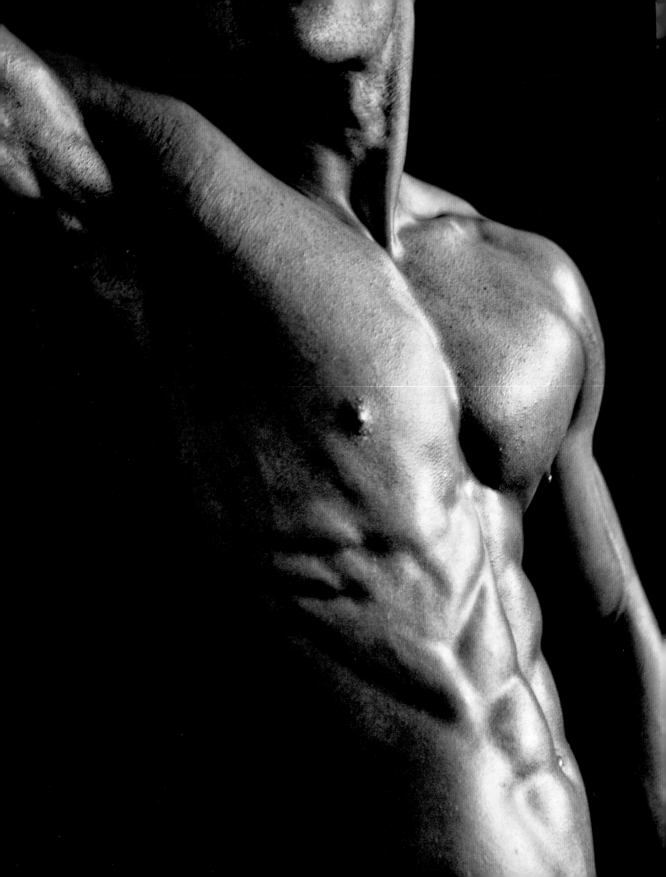

1

Lose Your Gut

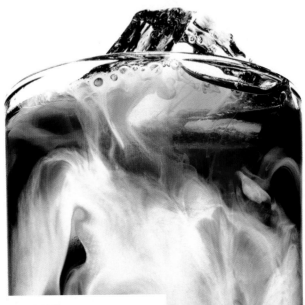

What to Drink

The quickest, most effective way to trim down and firm up is by changing your drinking habits. Here's the key to sipping your way thin.

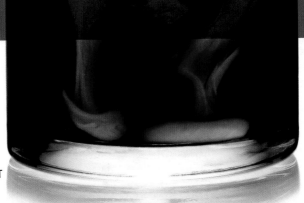

It's one of the most instantly gratifying pleasures known to man: that first cold, refreshing glug of your favorite icy beverage on a hot summer day. When it slips past your lips, bounces over your tongue, and hits that dry spot in the back of your throat, bam! You're happy. And when the weather turns cold? A steaming drink is the fastest way to crowd out the chill. Whether it's a time to celebrate (champagne, anyone?) or seek solace (with a misery-drowning martini), there's always the right beverage. What could be wrong with that?

As it turns out, plenty: Drinking the wrong beverages is the fastest way to blow out your waistline. A 2007 study in the journal *Obesity* showed that Americans were taking in 21 percent of their calories—about 460 a day—from drinks. Imagine tossing two slices of Domino's sausage pizza into a blender, pressing "puree," and guzzling it down. Disgusting, right? Yes, but beyond those sickening statistics is actually some terrific news: If you want to lose weight, simple drink swaps can shave pounds off your body at a remarkable pace.

A recent study at Johns Hopkins University found that people who cut liquid calories from their diets lost more weight—and kept it off longer—than people who cut food calories. Slashing your drink calories in half could mean dropping more than 23 pounds in just 1 year.

That's why we wrote our newest book, *Drink This, Not That!*—to uncover the hidden dangers of our drinking habits and provide thirsty guys with the strategies they need to sip off the pounds. From the first morning beverage to that last libation of the night, this is your blueprint for a lifetime of healthy drinking.

8:00 a.m. Breakfast

Choosing the right beverage is never more important than in those first moments after you roll out of bed. A hot cup of coffee? Excellent—it's loaded with antioxidants, and caffeine has been shown to speed metabolism. A cold glass of milk? Absolutely—protein and a bit of fat is a great idea first thing in the a.m. Some juice or a freshly blended smoothie? Well, not so fast. That juice in your fridge may just be a glorified (but well-disguised) glass of sugar water, ready to douse your fat-burning fire before the day even starts. And that smoothie you just grabbed on the go? The way drink purveyors have been exploiting the smoothie's healthy reputation, it could be closer to a milk shake than the fruit-driven, protein-packed ideal we hold dear.

The first and most vital rule of drinking is especially relevant in the morning hours: If you sacrifice your hard-earned calories on a liquid breakfast, then it had better deliver substantial benefits in return. If your beverage of choice doesn't fit the bill, then you shouldn't be drinking it.

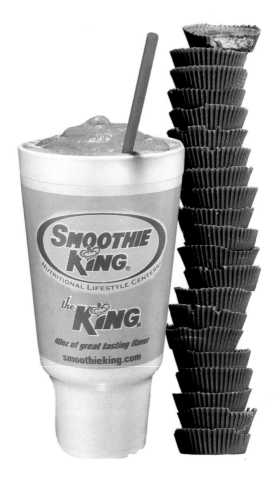

WORST BREAKFAST BEVERAGE
SMOOTHIE KING PEANUT POWER PLUS GRAPE (40 OUNCES)

1,498 calories, 44 grams fat, 214 grams sugar
Sugar equivalent: 21 REESE'S CUPS

Time to storm the castle and depose the monarch: Smoothie King serves up 16 different 40-ounce smoothies that come packed with more than 1,000 calories. Blame the obscene serving sizes and the shameless overdose of sugar. Among the worst is this freakish play on PB&J, which pollutes already sweet grape juice with sugar and honey. Drink one of these and you'll be slurping up more than 60 percent of your day's calories in mere minutes.

DRINK THIS INSTEAD!
SMOOTHIE KING HIGH PROTEIN BANANA (20 OUNCES)

322 calories, 9 grams fat, 23 grams sugar

This smart alternative is low in calories and sugar and packed with protein: Smoothie King's blend provides 27 grams of the muscle-building macronutrient in this 20-ounce serving.

WORST BOTTLED SMOOTHIE
STONYFIELD FARM ORGANIC STRAW-BERRY SMOOTHIE (10-OUNCE BOTTLE)

230 calories, 3 grams fat, 38 grams sugar

Stonyfield produces a few great products—its line of high-protein Greek yogurts, for example—but its smoothies don't make the grade. The first three ingredients in this one are milk, sugar, and strawberry juice, and the bottle contains more sugar than you'd ingest from three bowls of Froot Loops.

DRINK THIS INSTEAD!
BOLTHOUSE FARMS BERRY BOOST (15.2-OUNCE BOTTLE)

209 calories, 0 grams fat, 50 grams sugar

Not only is there more smoothie here for fewer calories, but this bottle also offers nearly 8 grams of fiber to help slow absorption of the sugar, 100 percent of which comes from fruit.

WORST JUICE
OCEAN SPRAY CRAN-APPLE (8 OUNCES)

130 calories, 0 grams fat, 32 grams sugar

Beware of the impostor juice drinks. This misleading bottle contains only 15 percent

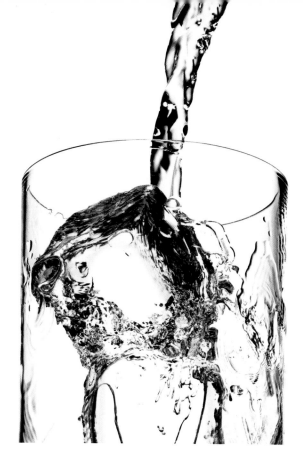

There's no use trying to improve on nature's already-perfect formula. Nothing will ever beat a glass of ice-cold water.

fruit juice; water and sugar are the first two ingredients.

DRINK THIS INSTEAD!
SIMPLY GRAPEFRUIT (8 OUNCES)

90 calories, 0 grams fat, 18 grams sugar

Orange juice might be king of the breakfast table, but grapefruit deserves the crown. It's lower in sugar, and it's also rich in lycopene. It's the most underrated juice in the cooler.

12:30 p.m. Lunch

Each year, about 3,000 U.S. companies in the bottled- and packaged-beverage industry reap $70 billion in profits—all in the name of quenching thirst. Maybe that's why we're drinking so little H_2O at mealtimes: We're too busy filling our bellies with soda, syrupy coffee drinks, and so-called functional beverages. Not only are these drinks adding inches to our waistlines, but they're just not working hard enough to keep us hydrated. Now that's a real drinking problem, and your hangover will come at the belt line.

While drinking more water is crucial, when you drink can be just as important. Thirty minutes before you belly up to the sandwich counter or the salad bar, chug a large glass of agua. In one study from Virginia Polytechnic Institute, 24 over-weight participants were served breakfast on two separate days. On the first day, they drank 17 ounces of water before eating; the next day, they skipped the water. They ended up consuming 9 percent fewer calories at that first breakfast than they did at the second. Over time, those differences add up.

If you need something sweet to wash down that turkey hero, make sure your drink of choice has fewer than 100 calories and provides some nutrition in return. Lightly sweetened iced tea and the emerging line of water-juice hybrids fit the bill. But really, nothing will ever beat a glass of ice-cold water.

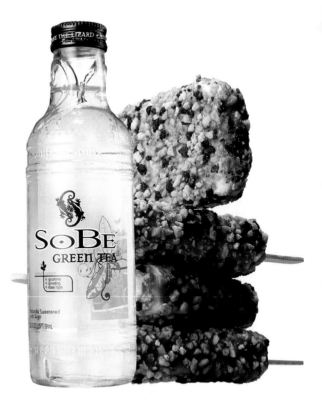

WORST LUNCH DRINK
SOBE GREEN TEA (20-OUNCE BOTTLE)

240 calories, 0 grams fat, 61 grams sugar

Sugar equivalent:
4 GOOD HUMOR CHOCOLATE ECLAIRS

Since the explosive green-tea craze, SoBe, Lipton, and Snapple have been doing their best to turn iced tea into a veritable soft drink. Let's be clear: When people talk about green tea fighting cancer, boosting metabolism, and extending life, they're not talking about the sugary sludge these companies are pumping out. In fact, ounce for ounce, this bottle has more calories than Coke.

DRINK THIS INSTEAD!
HONEST TEA ORGANIC HONEY GREEN TEA (16-OUNCE BOTTLE)

74 calories, 0 grams fat, 18 grams sugar

When *Men's Health* sent a crate of teas off to a nutrition lab to be analyzed for antioxidant content, we discovered that most brands failed to live up to the health claims posted on their labels. The one that actually did? The aptly named Honest Tea. With more metabolism-boosting, cancer-fighting catechins than its competitors, Organic Honey Green Tea delivers exactly what you want out of a cup of tea, with just enough sugar to make it go down easy.

WORST SINGLE-SERVING JUICE
ARIZONA KIWI STRAWBERRY (23.5-OUNCE CAN)

360 calories, 0 grams fat, 84 grams sugar

The twisted minds at the Arizona factory outdid themselves with a can the size of a mortar shell, loaded with enough sweet stuff to build a 34-cube sugar pyramid. The most disturbing part: This supersized serving costs just 99 cents, so it's temptingly cheap—until you consider the health costs.

DRINK THIS INSTEAD!
OCEAN SPRAY CRANERGY RASPBERRY CRANBERRY LIFT (12-OUNCE BOTTLE)

50 calories, 0 grams fat, 13 grams sugar

Ocean Spray may be a pusher of juice "cocktails" (read: not much juice), but its line of Cranergy drinks is a surprisingly decent hydration option. It combines 20 percent juice with filtered water and green-tea extract, along with a flurry of B vitamins. All told, you'll drink up 100 percent of your daily vitamin C needs, plus 70 percent of five other essential nutrients, all for the calorie cost of two gulps of the Arizona atrocity.

WORST SOFT DRINK
SUNKIST ORANGE SODA (20-OUNCE BOTTLE)

325 calories, 0 grams fat, 85 grams sugar

All sodas are terrible, but that doesn't mean there aren't degrees of awfulness. Fruity sodas tend to have more sugar than their cola counterparts, and no brand makes that more apparent than Sunkist, as nine out of 10 rich dentists would surely agree.

DRINK THIS INSTEAD!
IZZE ESQUE SPARKLING MANDARIN (12-OUNCE BOTTLE)

50 calories, 0 grams fat, 11 grams sugar

Izze's sparkling juice drinks make for perfect soda substitutes, and the new Esque line is its best stuff yet, with 25 percent juice (down from 70 percent in the regular Izzes), sparkling water, and little else.

3:00 p.m. Afternoon Slump

These days, afternoon pick-me-ups have morphed into afternoon fill-me-outs. Researchers in New York City who monitored people's afternoon coffee choices discovered that two-thirds of Starbucks customers and a quarter of Dunkin' Donuts patrons opted for blended coffee drinks over regular brewed coffee (or tea). The average caloric impact of the blended drinks? A whopping 239 calories, versus the average 63 calories in brewed coffee or tea even after you add cream and sugar. So even if you like your coffee sweet and light, you can strip away 176 calories every day by making this swap.

It's not just latte love that's helping to pack on midday pounds. The nearly $5 billion energy-drink industry promises a taurine-tinged solution to our collective torpor. Maybe marketers are betting that we're too exhausted to be skeptical, because most of these drinks offer little beyond nutraceutical hype, sugar overload, and a hefty price tag. So the next time your eyelids begin to droop, be careful about what you use to prop them open.

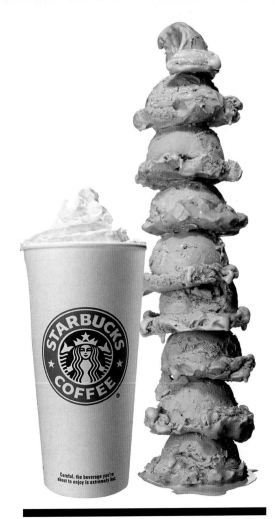

WORST COFFEE DRINK
STARBUCKS VENTI PEPPERMINT WHITE CHOCOLATE MOCHA WITH WHIPPED CREAM

660 calories, 22 grams fat, 95 grams sugar

Sugar equivalent: MORE THAN 2 PINTS OF EDY'S SLOW CHURNED LIGHT COFFEE ICE CREAM

A good rule of thumb at Starbucks: The more syllables a drink contains, the more damage it's likely to do. This 20-ounce tongue twister packs more than 25 percent of your day's calories and enough sugar to ensure a crash as soon as the caffeine wears off. You'd be better off (calorically, that is) eating four Fresco Grilled Steak Soft Tacos from Taco Bell.

DRINK THIS INSTEAD!
STARBUCKS VENTI CARAMEL CAPPUCCINO (VENTI CAPPUCCINO + 1 PUMP CARAMEL SYRUP)

170 calories, 6 grams fat, 18 grams sugar

The best thing about Starbucks is the control it gives you. Want less milk? More espresso? Sugar-free syrup? Just ask and the staff will make it happen. This is our current favorite customized drink: cappuccino (because it saves you 90 calories over the same size latte) with a single caramel shot (because the standard five sickly sweet pumps in the Venti Peppermint White Chocolate Mocha is the biggest waste of 190 calories you'll ever regret).

WORST CAFFEINATED DRINK
ARIZONA RASPBERRY ICED TEA (23-OUNCE CAN)

259 calories, 0 grams fat, 63 grams sugar

With more caffeine than what you'd find in green tea, black tea will definitely wake you up. But you'd have to be Rip Van Winkle to need a gargantuan can of iced tea with the equivalent of more than 13 teaspoons of sugar. In fact, you might just fall asleep after the resulting sugar crash.

DRINK THIS INSTEAD!
ILLY ISSIMO CAFFE (6.8-OUNCE CAN)

50 calories, 0 grams fat, 11 grams sugar

The Italian company Illy has long been a producer of top-quality espresso and coffee beans; it's now offering the best packaged coffee drinks on the market. This little can brings you all the lift you need, with less of the excess sugar you don't.

WORST ENERGY DRINK
ORIGINAL ROCKSTAR ENERGY DRINK (16-OUNCE CAN)

280 calories, 0 grams fat, 62 grams sugar

None of the full-sugar energy drinks provides enough of a boost to justify the hefty caloric load, but Rockstar's take is bloated to Kevin Smith proportions. Each can is packed with 80 more calories than a can of Monster.

DRINK THIS INSTEAD!
ROCKSTAR ROASTED LIGHT VANILLA (15-OUNCE CAN)

94 calories, 3 grams fat, 13 grams sugar

We prefer the coffee-tinged variety of energy drinks, and not just because they avoid the typical liquid-Smarties flavor. More important, coffee has something to offer you: a host of antioxidants and a ream of research supporting its role as a serious defender against a variety of diseases from dementia to diabetes. This can contains about twice the amount of caffeine that your average cup of joe has, and about 200 percent of your daily value for most B vitamins. Not a bad nutritional boost for a drink that clocks in under 100 calories.

A Belly-Filling Breakfast in a Glass

In a perfect world, smoothies would be short on sugar and long on whole fruit, fiber, and protein—traits that the Ultimate Power Smoothie encapsulates perfectly. Its onslaught of vital nutrients—protein from the peanut butter and the protein powder, fiber from the fruit and the psyllium, omega-3s from the flaxseed—fill your stomach, charge your metabolism, and keep your mind sharp all morning long.

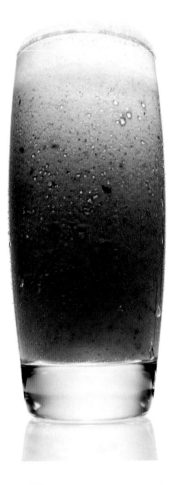

The Ultimate Power Smoothie

½ Tbsp peanut butter
1 banana
½ cup milk
¼ cup orange juice
½ cup Greek-style yogurt
1 Tbsp vanilla- or chocolate-flavored protein powder
1 Tbsp unflavored psyllium husk (fiber powder)
1 Tbsp ground flaxseed
3 or 4 ice cubes

Blend all ingredients until smooth.

Makes 1

Per serving:
397 calories, 18 g protein, 30 g carbohydrates, 24 g fat, 12 g saturated fat, 10 g fiber, 134 mg sodium

5:30 p.m. Postworkout

There's no better way to undo the benefits of a sturdy workout than to replace sweat with sugar. The aisles of supermarkets and pill palaces like GNC are awash in products that claim quick recovery and long-lasting muscle growth. But that's rarely the case. Here's what you need: protein, of course, to maximize muscle growth; carbohydrates to help replenish your depleted glycogen reserves, the fuel your body runs on; and potassium, which helps balance fluids and ensure rapid recovery. Which single beverage delivers these three nutrients best? You might be surprised.

WORST WATER
SOBE LIFEWATER ORANGE TANGERINE (20-OUNCE BOTTLE)

100 calories, 0 grams fat, 24 grams sugar

The bottled-beverage industry has even found a way to besmirch the sterling reputation of the most essential compound on Earth. Sure, you might down a few extra vitamins with this water, but those spoonfuls of sugar make the medicine beside the point.

DRINK THIS INSTEAD!
FILTERED TAP WATER

0 calories, 0 grams fat, 0 grams sugar

We've tasted our way through dozens of highfalutin "enhanced" waters, but there's no use in trying to improve on nature's perfect-already formula.

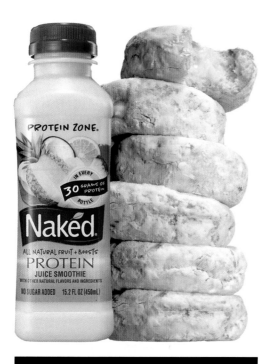

let you have an after-gym-class treat: British researchers found that the ratios of electrolytes and potassium in milk make it more effective than water or sports drinks at rehydrating the body. A study from Indiana University showed that people who drank chocolate milk between intense workouts could exercise longer and perform more total work than those who downed a carb-replacement drink.

WORST SPORTS DRINK
CYTOSPORT PERFORMANCE PLUS COOL CITRUS CYTOMAX (20-OUNCE BOTTLE)

130 calories, 0 grams fat, 7 grams sugar

Ending your workout by guzzling a typical sports drink only sets your weight-loss goals back. This one contains a cocktail of natural and artificial sweeteners, plus a laundry list of unpronounceable additives; and the jumbo-sized bottle gives you calories without the muscle-building protein payload of milk.

DRINK THIS INSTEAD!
ZICO PURE COCONUT WATER MANGO (11-OUNCE CONTAINER)

60 calories, 0 grams fat, 14 grams sugar

Although coconut water doesn't offer the protein you need after a workout, neither do any of the major sports drinks. But an 11-ounce serving packs more potassium than a banana (and a lot more than your average sports drink), and it does so with a modest calorie toll and just three ingredients.

WORST POSTWORKOUT DRINK
NAKED PROTEIN ZONE JUICE SMOOTHIE (15.2-OUNCE BOTTLE)

418 calories, 4 grams fat, 53 grams sugar

Sugar equivalent: 6 DUNKIN' DONUTS BAVARIAN KREME DOUGHNUTS

Naked makes some excellent bottled smoothies, but this postworkout option isn't one of them. The first four ingredients are tooth-rattlingly sweet: apple juice, banana puree, orange juice, and pineapple juice. Okay, it all comes from real fruit, but 53 grams of sugar is about twice as much as you want after a serious workout.

DRINK THIS INSTEAD!
HORIZON ORGANIC CHOCOLATE REDUCED FAT MILK (8-OUNCE BOX)

180 calories, 5 grams fat, 27 grams sugar

Banging out a few sets doesn't give you an excuse to skip straight to dessert. But we'll

9:00 p.m. Nightcap

Red wine isn't the only health hooch. Alcohol in moderation—one or two drinks a day—has been shown to raise HDL (good) cholesterol, boost blood flow, and improve sugar metabolism. It's even been linked to a reduced risk of dementia and heart disease.

It can also help you drop pounds: A recent study in the journal *BMC Public Health* showed that people who had a daily drink were 54 percent less likely to be obese than teetotalers were. Even two drinks a day resulted in a 41 percent risk reduction.

But when you ask for that third one, your risk of obesity starts to climb. In restaurants these days, a single "signature" cocktail can contain nearly half a day's calorie allowance and three or more servings of alcohol. It all proves that age-old adage: Think before you drink.

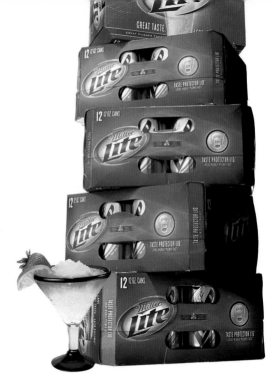

WORST COCKTAIL
RED LOBSTER TRADITIONAL LOBSTERITA

890 calories, 183 grams carbohydrates
Carbohydrate equivalent: 57 MILLER LITES

Of all the egregiously bad beverages we looked at in compiling this list, the Lobsterita surprised us the most. The reason? Even though Red Lobster, the nation's beloved fish purveyor, is one of the few big players in the restaurant biz to provide customers with a wide selection of truly healthy food options, its barkeeps are mixing up bad news in the back room. Drink one of these margaritas every Friday night and you'll put on more than a pound of flab each month. Downgrade to a regular margarita on the rocks and save the extra 640 calories for another day.

DRINK THIS INSTEAD!
RED LOBSTER CLASSIC MARTINI WITH GIN

140 calories, 0 grams carbohydrates

We like our booze as unadorned as possible. And not just for the 007-level sophistication, but because the sugar-spiked mixers might be more dangerous than the alcohol itself. Opt for a vodka martini if you like, but we like the herbal notes of the more traditional gin version. Bonus: The juniper berries used to make gin have been shown to have stabilizing effects on blood-glucose levels.

WORST BEER
SIERRA NEVADA BIGFOOT (12-OUNCE BOTTLE)

330 calories, 32 grams carbohydrates, 9.6% alcohol

Most beers carry fewer than 150 calories, and even your average extra-heady brew rarely eclipses 200. That makes Sierra's

Bigfoot the scariest beast in the beer jungle. Granted, the alcohol itself provides most of the calories, but it's the extra helping of carbohydrates (three times what you'd find in a can of Guinness) that stuffs almost 2,000 calories into each six-pack.

DRINK THIS INSTEAD!
ABITA AMBER
(12-OUNCE BOTTLE)

128 calories, 10 grams carbohydrates, 4.5% alcohol

This trusty Louisiana label has expanded production in recent years, and you can probably find it in a cooler near you. That's great news, because you'd be hard-pressed to drink a more robust, satisfying beer for fewer than 130 calories. Set it up next to a plate of tacos or a bowl of spicy gumbo.

WORST LIGHT BEER
SAM ADAMS LIGHT
(12-OUNCE BOTTLE)

119 calories, 9.3 grams carbohydrates, 4% alcohol

There are too many good light-beer options on the market these days to settle for one with more than 100 calories. In fact, this one's only 7 calories shy of the frothy-headed god of beers, Guinness.

DRINK THIS INSTEAD!
AMSTEL LIGHT
(12-OUNCE BOTTLE)

95 calories, 5.5 grams carbohydrates, 3.5% alcohol

Beery brinksmanship has broken out among major brewers like Miller, Beck's, and Budweiser, who are scrambling to outdo one another in the low-calorie suds arena. But we still think it's tough to beat the flavor-to-calories ratio of Amstel.

The Classic Margarita

In Mexico, the margarita is a simple, perfectly balanced cocktail. But as it traveled north of the border, the classic picked up a suitcaseful of calories. Ditch the bottle of neon mix and return the marg to its unadulterated self.

Coarse salt
1½ oz 100% agave silver tequila
1 oz Cointreau or triple sec (or a splash of OJ)
1½ oz lime juice (from one large lime)
1 tsp agave syrup
Lime slice for garnish

Pour enough salt onto a plate to cover it lightly. Rub the rim of a rocks glass with the cut side of a lime, and dip it into the salt to create a light salt rim. Add a few large ice cubes to the glass. Combine the tequila, Cointreau, lime juice, and agave syrup in a cocktail shaker and shake vigorously for 20 seconds. Pour, slurp, and pucker.

Makes 1

Per serving: 263 calories, 0g protein, 23 g carbohydrates, 0 g fat, 0 g saturated fat, 0 g fiber, 243 mg sodium

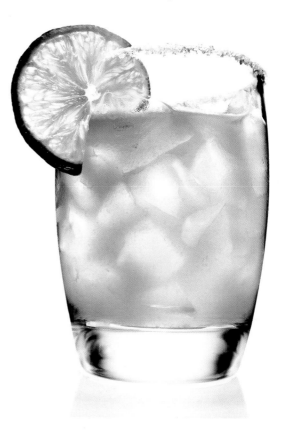

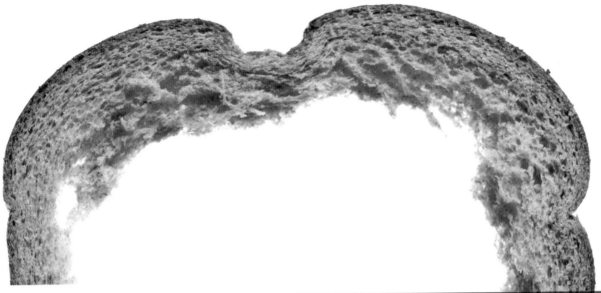

Part 1: LOSE YOUR GUT

The Gluten-Obesity Connection

The truth about gluten, the food industry, and your belly

Turkey and tomato on wheat. Whole-grain pasta. Healthy, right? Maybe. But more and more people believe that these foods are parts of a potentially disastrous trap. They claim that sluggishness and weight gain can be blamed on an insidious substance hiding in wheat and many other common grains: gluten.

Avoiding gluten has become big business. Sales of gluten-free products grew about 30 percent a year from 2006 to 2010, and they will hit $3.9 billion by next year, according to the market-research company Packaged Facts. Supermarket shelves are filled with gluten-free breads, soups, and cake mixes—even gluten-free ketchup and soy sauce.

NFL quarterback Drew Brees won a Super Bowl while on a gluten-free diet. Cyclist Tom Danielson, a record-breaking member of the Garmin-Cervélo team, says his training and racing have improved since he and his teammates went gluten-free more than a year ago.

Have most common whole grains been acting as insidious nutritional double agents all these years? Or are they essential components of a healthy diet? Let's separate the wheat from the chaff.

WHAT IS GLUTEN, ANYWAY?

Gluten is a protein found in wheat, barley, and rye, as well as in many common food additives. It's what gives dough its elasticity and baked goods their satisfying chewiness. But for people with celiac disease—a type of autoimmune disorder—eating foods that contain gluten can lead to a cascade of nasty reactions, including damage to the small intestine, poor nutrient absorption, diarrhea, abdominal pain, bloating, anemia, and fatigue.

Celiac disease is surprisingly common, affecting about one in every 133 people, according to an oft-cited 2003 study from the University of Maryland Center for Celiac Research. There is no cure for celiac disease and no drugs that can treat it. You can only manage the condition, by sticking to a gluten-free diet for life.

Even if you don't have celiac disease, gluten might still be bad for you, says Lara Field, MS, RD, a dietitian at the University of Chicago's Celiac Disease Center. Many people consider themselves "gluten sensitive." If you think you might have symptoms of a gluten intolerance, ask your doctor about scheduling a blood test to find out for sure. Gluten is also shunned by another group: people who simply think gluten encourages weight gain and who claim to feel more energetic when they don't consume it. They say humans didn't evolve the ability to digest certain grains containing gluten, and that avoiding gluten leads to more energy, better absorption of nutrients, and weight loss.

Allen Lim, PhD, who was an exercise physiologist for the Garmin team, believes going gluten-free helped his team perform at a higher level. So does Danielson, who, like any competitive cyclist, burns (and eats) a huge number of calories.

"After I started the diet, I had better results. I didn't feel as fatigued, and my recovery period was quicker," says Danielson, who puts in 6-plus hours during a typical training session.

But this is anecdotal evidence; mainstream research still hasn't substantiated the claims of those who believe gluten is bad for everyone.

"There is no strong scientific evidence to support the claim that avoiding gluten leads to benefits for the general population," says Tricia Thompson, MS, RD,

Avoid gluten and you avoid refined carbs. Is that the weight-loss secret?

author of *The Gluten-Free Nutrition Guide*.

Still, cutting out gluten can lead to weight loss—but not for the reason gluten-free advocates think. A strict gluten-free diet forces you to avoid some refined carbs that can lead to weight gain, Field says. And that is a key to losing weight.

Gluten is found in many of the familiar weight-gain culprits: pizza, beer, burgers, pancakes. "Gluten itself probably isn't the reason you've packed on pounds," says Field. "Eating too many refined carbohydrates is what expands your waistline."

Commit to staying gluten-free and your food choices can become a snapshot of healthy eating—fruits, vegetables,

brown rice, seeds and nuts, along with meat, fish, eggs, and milk products.

Avoiding gluten also means you're likely to adopt other whole grains and flours, such as buckwheat, quinoa, millet, teff, sorghum, and wild rice (which is not related to brown rice and white rice). These aren't necessarily healthier options than gluten-rich wheat, barley, or rye, but a wider range of grains gives your diet nutritional variety. That's another good thing.

GO GLUTEN-FREE FOR WEIGHT LOSS?

A gluten-free diet can work, but dealing with the diet's restrictions can be daunting.

"You have to commit to a true lifestyle change, and that can be tough," says Edward Abramson, PhD, a professor emeritus at California State University at Chico and the author of *Emotional Eating*. "Men might be able to follow gluten-free for a short time," he says, "but without a real medical need, they might have a rough time sticking to it."

But the notion of a panacea for excess weight remains seductive, and that may be part of the appeal of the gluten-free movement, says Michael R. Lowe, PhD, a professor of psychology at Drexel University who specializes in nutritional approaches to weight loss. It sounds simple: If I do this one thing, then I will see the results I'm after. "That's the driving appeal of elimination diets," Dr. Lowe says.

Ironically, the boom in gluten-free products isn't necessarily conducive to weight loss. "You can buy gluten-free versions of practically every type of wheat-based food—pizza, pasta, cookies, you name it,"

Thompson says. But here's the catch: Healthy-sounding gluten-free items often have just as many calories as the originals. "People see 'gluten-free' and think they can down an entire box of gluten-free cookies with no repercussions" says Field.

So even if you stick to a gluten-free diet, you can put on pounds. A 2006 study in the *American Journal of Gastroenterology* followed 188 people with celiac disease on a gluten-free diet for 2 years and found that 81 percent of them gained weight.

If you do give up gluten, use your new eating plan as a lens to reexamine your diet—and your life. Cyclist Danielson says, "I don't know if it was directly tied to the food, but I found that by having to pay more attention to my daily diet, I became more focused on my cycling."

Avoiding gluten takes constant monitoring—the same attention to detail you need to excel in your workouts.

"I became more dedicated and took a more professional approach to my training when I went gluten-free," Danielson says. "I couldn't get lazy and down whole pizzas and bowls of pasta. I had to focus on putting better food in my body, and this made me realize how much my eating habits off the bike affected my performance on it."

Mindful eating is key. After all, "you don't need to go gluten-free to avoid refined processed carbs," says Thompson.

The New Power Grains

Even if you don't need to avoid gluten, it's a good idea to explore the world of gluten-free grains. All of them are rich in belly-filling fiber, and each offers unique benefits.

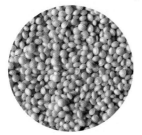

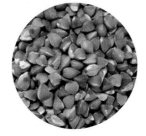

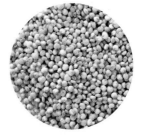

Amaranth
A grain the size of a poppy seed, amaranth has more protein than wheat and twice that of white rice. Initial studies in rodents suggest that amaranth's high protein content can help lower cholesterol.

Buckwheat
Buckwheat is rich in rutin, a flavonoid that has potent antioxidant properties. It's also rich in heart-healthy magnesium.

Quinoa
Once an energy booster for Inca warriors, this superfood of the Andes provides complete protein, with all nine essential amino acids. It's also low on the glycemic index, so it won't spike your blood sugar.

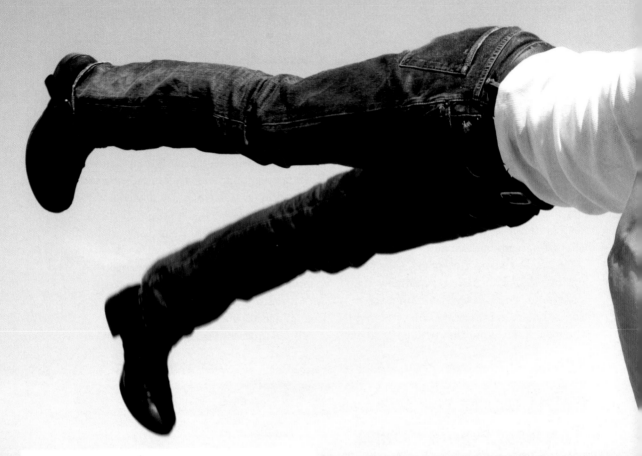

Part 1: LOSE YOUR GUT

The Body You Want,

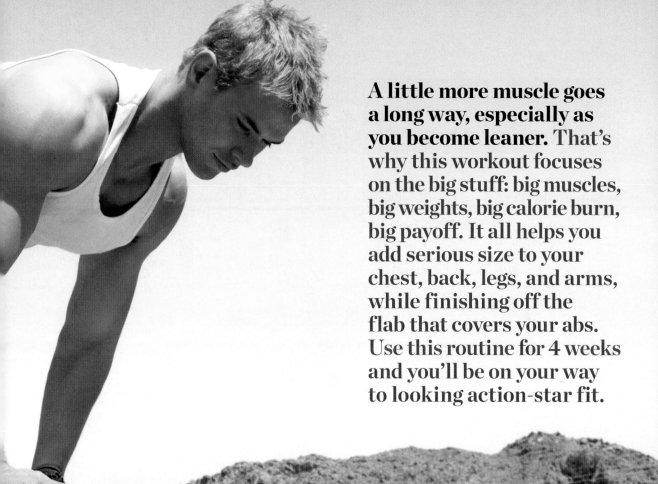

A little more muscle goes a long way, especially as you become leaner. That's why this workout focuses on the big stuff: big muscles, big weights, big calorie burn, big payoff. It all helps you add serious size to your chest, back, legs, and arms, while finishing off the flab that covers your abs. Use this routine for 4 weeks and you'll be on your way to looking action-star fit.

Sculpt your body from every angle with this muscle–building, fat–melting workout

in 28 Days

WORKOUT A

Do three workouts a week, alternating between WORKOUT A and WORKOUT B. (You'll do each workout six times in 4 weeks.) In each workout, do alternating sets of each exercise pair (1A/1B, 2A/2B, and 3A/3B). That is, do 1 set of the first exercise and rest 1½ to 2 minutes. Then do 1 set of the second exercise and rest again for 1½ to 2 minutes. Repeat until you've done 3 sets of each exercise pair.

1A
Barbell Deadlift
5 reps

Bend at your hips and knees and grab the bar using an overhand grip. Your lower back should be slightly arched and your arms straight (**A**). Without allowing your lower back to round, stand up with the barbell (**B**). Pause momentarily, then lower the bar to the floor.

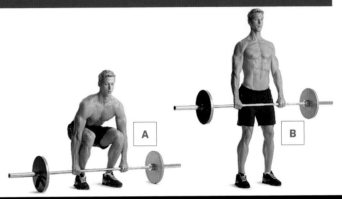

2A
Barbell Split Squat
6 to 8 reps each leg

Hold a barbell across your upper back and stand in a staggered stance, your left foot in front of your right (**A**). Keeping your torso upright, lower your body until your front knee is bent 90 degrees (**B**). Then push yourself back to the starting position. That's 1 rep.

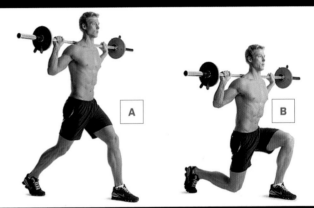

3A
Cable Face Pull
8 to 10 reps

Attach a rope to the high pulley of a cable station and grab an end with each hand. Back a few steps away until your arms are extended in front of you (**A**). Pull the middle of the rope toward your face (**B**). Pause, and reverse the movement back to the starting position.

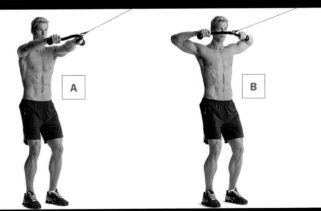

1B
Chinup
6 to 8 reps

Grab a chinup bar using a shoulder-width, underhand grip, and hang at arm's length (**A**). Now squeeze your shoulder blades down and back, bend your elbows, and pull the top of your chest to the bar (**B**). Pause, slowly lower your body back to the starting position, and repeat.

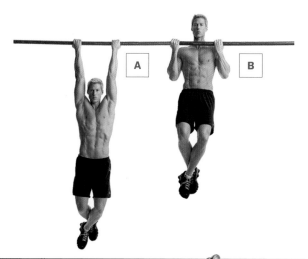

2B
Single-Arm Overhead Dumbbell Press
6 to 8 reps each arm

Stand holding a dumbbell with your right hand just above and outside your right shoulder. Your palm should be turned toward your head (**A**). Push the weight straight up over your shoulder (**B**). Then lower it, and repeat without pausing.

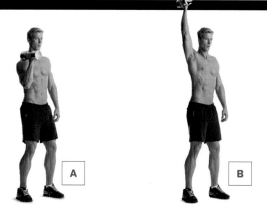

3B
Barbell Rollout
8 to 12 reps

Load a bar with 10-pound plates and kneel on the floor. Grab the bar with an overhand, shoulder-width grip. Keep your lower back naturally arched and your core stiff (**A**). Roll the bar forward as far as you can without letting your hips or back sag (**B**). Pause, and return to the starting position.

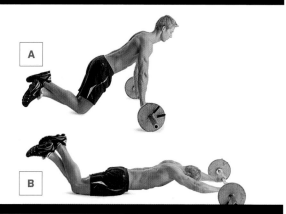

WORKOUT B

1A
Barbell Squat

6 reps

Hold a bar across your upper back with an overhand grip, and stand with your feet set shoulder-width apart (**A**). Push your hips back, bend your knees, and lower your body until the tops of your thighs are at least parallel to the floor (**B**). Pause, and return to the starting position.

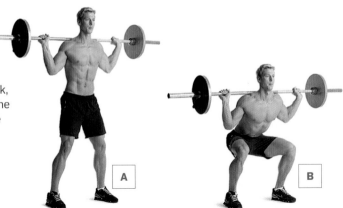

2A
Barbell Straight-Leg Deadlift

6 to 8 reps

Grab the bar with an overhand grip, and hold it at arm's length in front of your thighs, your knees slightly bent (**A**). Without allowing your back to round, bend at your hips and lower your torso until it's almost parallel to the floor (**B**). Pause, and rise back to the starting position.

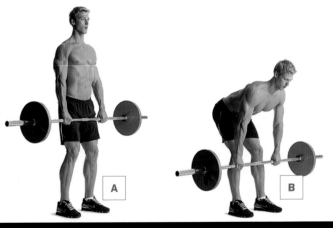

3A
Barbell Curl

8 to 10 reps

Grab a barbell with an underhand, shoulder-width grip, and let it hang at arm's length in front of your hips (**A**). Without moving your upper arms, bend your elbows to curl the bar as close to your shoulders as you can (**B**). Pause, and lower it back to the starting position.

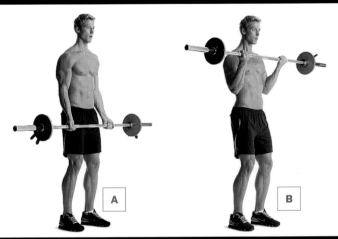

1B
Chest-Supported Row
6 to 8 reps

Grab a pair of dumbbells and lie chest down on an adjustable bench set to a low incline. Let the dumbbells hang at arm's length from your shoulders, your palms facing each other (**A**). Without moving your torso, pull the weights to your sides (**B**). Pause, lower, and repeat.

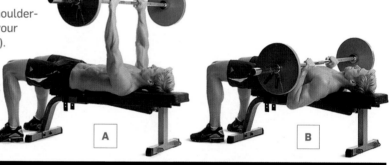

2B
Close-Grip Bench Press
6 to 8 reps

Grab a barbell with an overhand, shoulder-width grip, and hold the bar above your sternum with your arms straight (**A**). Lower the bar straight down as you tuck your elbows close to your sides (**B**). Pause, press the bar back to the starting position, and repeat.

3B
Swiss-Ball Jackknife
8 to 10 reps

Start in pushup position, but with your shins on a Swiss ball. Your body should form a straight line from ankles to head (**A**). Without rounding your lower back, contract your abs and use your feet to pull the ball toward your chest by bending your knees (**B**). Pause, and return to the starting position.

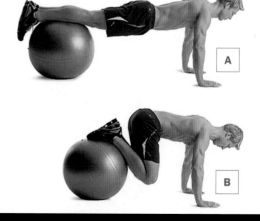

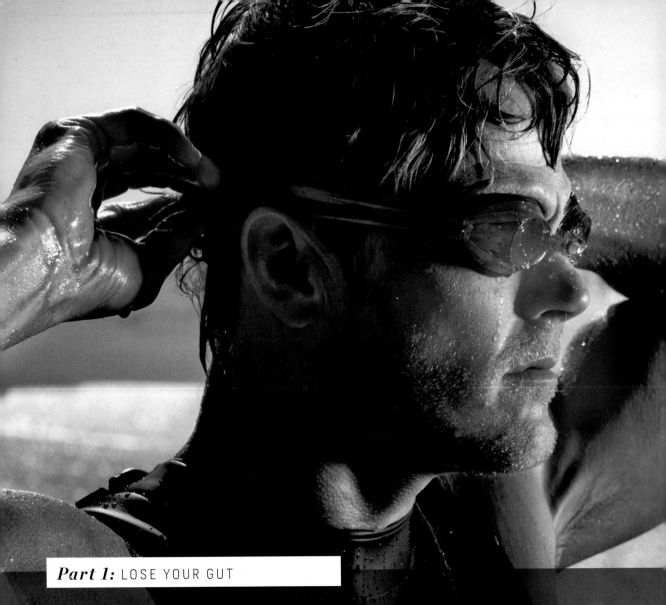

The Blubb

Use these body-building routines to strip away belly flab

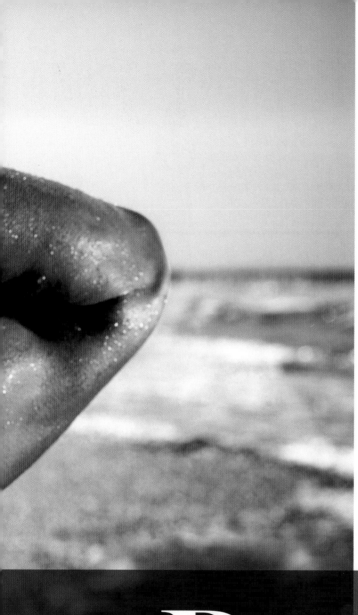

Has time gotten away from you? Even if you've let your workouts—and your body—go for a while, these workouts can reverse months of neglect—in just 30 days. They employ density training, a technique that allows you to do more work in less time. You'll sweat like crazy while you burnish your muscles and torch fat.

er Buster

WORKOUT A

For each exercise pairing (1A and 1B, for example), alternate back and forth between sets of the two exercises, completing as many sets as possible in 10 minutes and resting only as needed. After you finish, rest for 2 to 3 minutes and then move on to the next pair of exercises. On each exercise, perform only 5 reps per set, but use a weight you can lift 10 times. Increase your rest, if needed, to complete all 5 reps.

WORKOUT B

Perform these six exercises as a circuit, doing one after another until all the exercises have been completed. That's 1 round. Do 10 repetitions of each exercise and rest 30 seconds before moving to the next one. Try to increase the weight you use each week. Complete a total of 3 rounds.

WORKOUT A

1A
Goblet Squat

Your elbows should point toward the floor.
Hold a dumbbell vertically next to your chest, with both hands cupping the dumbbell head (**A**). Brace your abs, and lower your body as far as you can by pushing your hips back and bending your knees (**B**). Pause, then push through your heels to return to the starting position.

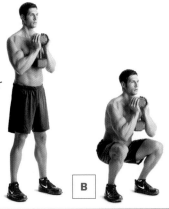

2A
Push Press

Keep your upper arms in line with your head as you raise the dumbbells.
Stand holding a pair of dumbbells next to your shoulders with your elbows bent and your palms facing each other (**A**).Dip your knees, and push up with your legs as you press the dumbbells over your head (**B**). Lower the dumbbells back to the starting position.

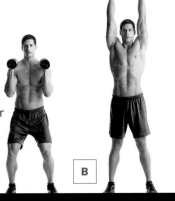

3A
Alternating Dumbbell Bench Press

Push the dumbbell straight up from your chest.
Grab a pair of dumbbells and lie on your back on a flat bench, holding the dumbbells over your chest with arms straight (**A**). Lower one dumbbell to the side of your chest, then press the weight back to the starting position (**B**). Switch arms and repeat. That's 1 rep.

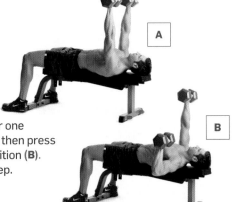

1B
Chinup

Don't allow your body to swing as you pull your weight up.

Grab a chinup bar with a shoulder-width, underhand grip, and hang at arm's length (**A**). Then pull your chest to the bar (**B**). Once the top of your chest touches the bar, pause, then slowly lower your body back to the starting position.

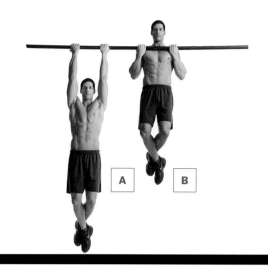

2B
Single-Arm Dumbbell Row

Keep your torso parallel to the floor and your back naturally arched.

Place your left hand and knee on a bench, and hold a dumbbell in your right hand. Let the dumbbell hang straight down from your shoulder (**A**). Row the weight by raising your elbow straight up (**B**). Lower to the starting position. Do 5 reps, switch sides, and repeat.

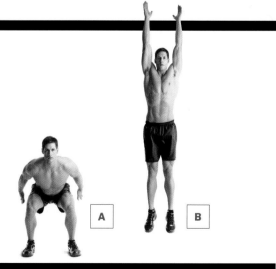

3B
Jump Squat

Throw your hands into the air explosively to help you jump higher.

Stand as tall as you can with your feet shoulder width apart, then lower your body as far as you can by pushing your hips and arms back (**A**). Pause, and jump as high as you can (**B**). When you land, immediately squat down and jump again.

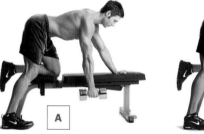

WORKOUT B

1
Dumbbell Hang Pull

Keep your lower back slightly arched, and don't round it.
Hold a pair of dumbbells just below your knees, with your hips pushed back and knees slightly bent (**A**). Pull both dumbbells to shoulder height by thrusting your hips forward and standing up on your toes (**B**). Return to the starting position, pause, and repeat.

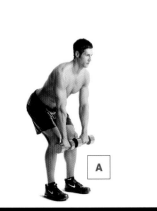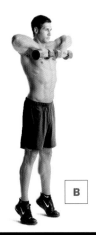

3
Reverse Lunge and Swing

Rotate your shoulders to bring the dumbbell to your hip and "throw" the dumbbell up.
Hold a dumbbell in front of your chest (**A**). Lunge back with your right leg as you rotate to your right and swing the dumbbell to your right hip (**B**). Then push back to a standing position as you swing the dumbbell to eye level (**C**). Repeat to the left. That's 1 rep.

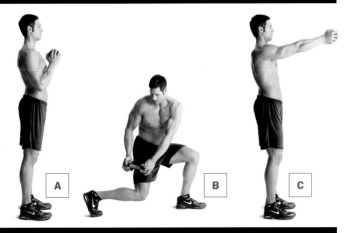

5
Dumbbell Swing

Lower your torso until it forms a 45-degree angle to the floor.
Hold a dumbbell with both hands at arm's length, bend at your hips and knees, and swing the dumbbell between your legs (**A**). Then thrust your hips forward and swing the dumbbell to chest level (**B**). That's 1 rep. Continue to swing back and forth.

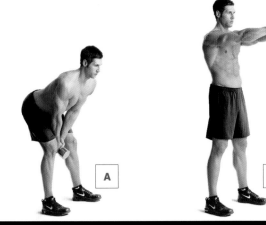

2
Dumbbell Pushup and Row

Position your feet about shoulder-width apart wto help stabilize your body as you row the dumbbell.

Place a pair of hex dumbbells on the floor, shoulder width apart. Grab the handles and set yourself in pushup position (**A**). Do a pushup (**B**). then row one dumbbell to the right side of your chest (**C**). Return to the starting position and repeat on the left side. That's 1 rep.

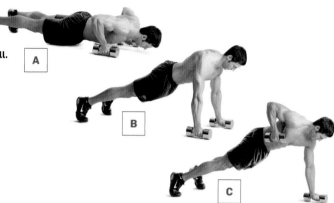
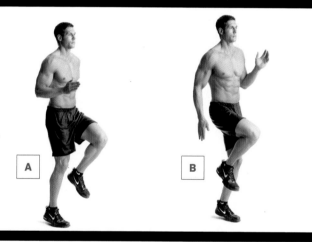

4
High-Knee Run

Keep your chest up and swing your arms quickly with each step.

Stand tall and run in place as fast as you can. Drive through the balls of your feet and try to bring your heels up under your backside so that your knees go high (**A**). Keep your hands relaxed, elbows bent, and shoulders down, and swing your arms back and forth (**B**).

6
Cross-Body Mountain Climber

Tighten your abs and glutes to help prevent your hips from sagging.

Assume a pushup position with your arms straight (**A**). Lift your left foot off the floor and raise your left knee toward your right elbow (**B**). Return to the starting position and raise your right knee to your left elbow. That's 1 rep. Keep your hips level and don't pause during the motion.

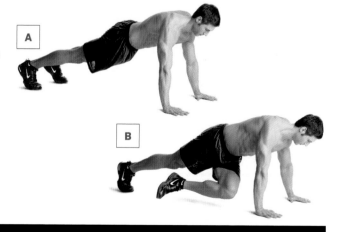

Six Ways to Silence a Grumbling Gut

Harness your hunger today

Try this experiment: On Monday, eat two doughnuts for breakfast. Make a mental note of when your gut starts grumbling. On Tuesday, eat an egg-and-cheese sandwich on whole-wheat toast. Now when did you get hungry?

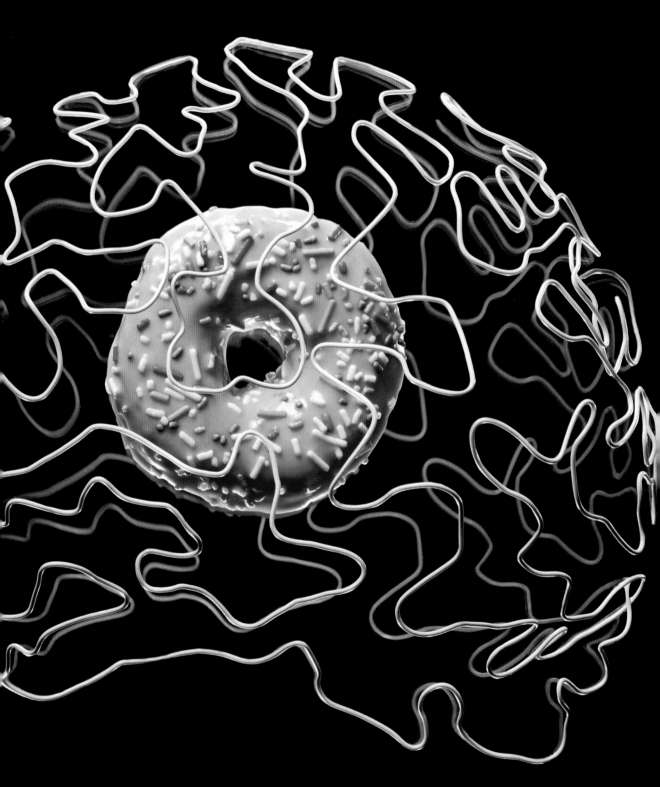

Both breakfasts are satisfying—at the time. But it's a good bet the egg-cheese-and-toast breakfast kept you feeling fuller longer. What was the difference? The answer, fellow hungry men, lies in your brain's dual perceptions of fullness. "Satiation" is the feeling of fullness at the end of a meal. "Satiety," on the other hand, is a measure of how long it takes before you're hungry again. Of course, food companies don't want you to stay satisfied. Fifteen years ago, Susanna Holt, PhD, an Australian researcher who ranked foods according to their satiety power, approached a number of food companies for funding to continue her work. She's still waiting: The companies were motivated to decrease the satiety of their foods—so people would buy more. Take control. Master satiation and you can keep portion sizes in check; boost satiety and you can prevent needless snacking. Read on and you'll be able to fill your gut—and then lose it.

SATIETY SECRET #1
Know what (and when) to drink.

Think of your stomach as a balloon. As you eat, it stretches. And once it expands to its maximum capacity, the sensors throughout your digestive system tell your brain's amygdala that it's time to stop chowing down—regardless of what you've filled your belly with. As Alan Aragon, MS, *Men's Health* nutrition advisor, puts it, "Eating half a roll of toilet paper would make you feel full."

To stretch your stomach without stuffing it with calories (or paper products),

you need water. Aragon recommends drinking a glass 30 minutes before a meal and sipping frequently while eating. Water-rich foods—soup, salad, fruit, and vegetables—will also fill your belly without contributing excessive calories.

SATIETY SECRET #2
Fill up with fiber.

Fiber draws water from your body and from the food you've eaten, and transports it to your intestinal tract, helping to deliver that meal-ending satiation, according to a 2009 study by researchers at the University of Washington.

Fiber may boost satiety, too. Because it passes through the body undigested, fiber slows the absorption of nutrients and makes you feel fuller longer, according to a 2008 study by researchers at the University of Minnesota. To reap the satiating benefits of fiber, aim for 25 to 35 grams daily.

SATIETY SECRET #3
Pack in the protein.

Protein, your muscle-growing fuel, also has the power to raise levels of peptides in your stomach. "These peptides initiate cross-talk with the brain on a molecular level to send out satiety signals," says Aragon. He recommends aiming for 20 to 40 grams of protein at each meal.

SATIETY SECRET #4
Savor the flavors.

Your belly is rumbling, and a waiter sets a juicy burger in front of you. Resist the urge to unhinge your jaws and swallow it whole. Thoroughly chewing your food increases what researchers call "oro-sensory factors," which send satiation signals to your brain, helping you feel full on less food, according to a 2009 study by Dutch researchers. Study participants who chewed each bite for an extra 3 seconds consumed less.

SATIETY SECRET #5

Trick your belly full.

You can't trust your gut. Maybe you've heard about the Cornell University study with the trick bowls: People who ate soup from bowls that continuously refilled ate 73 percent more than those who ate from ordinary bowls. The kicker: They rated themselves as feeling no more full. Scientists call this use of sensory cues to assess fullness "learned satiation."

Try this: Dole out a portion of food onto a smaller plate and immediately place the rest in the refrigerator. Once you eat, the visual cue of a clean plate will signal that you've had enough, and the leftovers will stay out of sight and out of mind, in the fridge.

SATIETY SECRET #6

Avoid distraction at dinner.

What you're doing while you eat might be as important as what you're eating. You're likely to consume much more food and eat for longer periods of time when you're distracted by television, music, or a computer, according to a 2009 review of studies published in *Trends in Food Science & Technology.*

Block That Binge

Eat these satiating foods at mealtimes—and two sane snacks in between—to stay satisfied all day long.

BREAKFAST
A glass of milk (8 oz), 3 large scrambled eggs, a slice of Cheddar, and a medium apple

Pour tall: There's a gram of protein in every ounce. And the fluid aids satiation.

One egg contains about 7 grams of filling protein.

This on-the-go breakfast finale has 4 grams of fiber.

LUNCH
Chicken salad (½ cup) on whole-wheat bread and a glass of iced tea (8 oz)

It's an easy way to pack in 22 grams of protein per serving.

Always pick whole-wheat over white for the extra fiber. Look for at least 3 grams in each slice.

Drink the real, unsweetened stuff, not the sugar-water posers.

DINNER
Seared meat or fish (8 oz), some steamed broccoli (½ cup), a medium baked sweet potato, and a glass of water (12 oz)

It's loaded with enough protein to fend off a midnight snack attack.

Vegetables are a low-calorie way to eat more fiber.

H_2O may help stop you from scrambling for seconds.

Your Sentence: The Chair

Regardless of how often or how hard you work out, there's still a good chance that you're sitting your life away

Do you lead an active lifestyle or a sedentary one? The question is simple, but the answer may not be. Let's say you're a busy guy who works 60 hours a week at a desk job but finds time for five 45-minute bouts of exercise. Most experts would label you as active. But Marc Hamilton, PhD, has another name for you: couch potato. Perhaps "exercising couch potato" would be more accurate, but Dr. Hamilton would still classify you as sedentary.

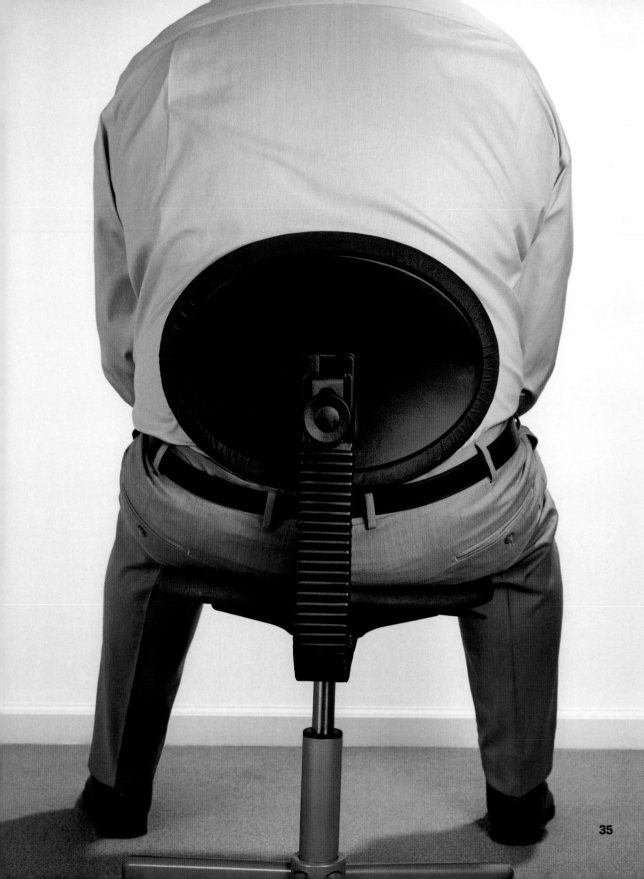

"People tend to view physical activity on a single continuum," Dr. Hamilton, a physiologist and professor of the Pennington Biomedical Research Center in Baton Rouge, Louisiana, says. "On the far side, you have a person who exercises a lot; on the other, a person who doesn't exercise at all. However, they're not necessarily polar opposites."

Dr. Hamilton's take, which is supported by a growing body of research, is that the amount of time you exercise and the amount of time you spend on your butt are completely separate factors for heart-disease risk. New evidence suggests, in fact, that the more hours a day you sit, the greater your likelihood of dying an earlier death regardless of how much you exercise or how lean you are. That's right: Even a sculpted six-pack can't protect you from your chair.

But it's not just your heart that's at risk from too much sitting; your hips, spine, and shoulders could also suffer. In fact, it's not a leap to say that a chair-potato lifestyle can ruin you from head to toe.

Statistically speaking, we're working out as much as we were 30 years ago. It's just that we're leading more sedentary lives overall. A 2006 University of Minnesota study found that from 1980 to 2000, the percentage of people who reported exercising regularly remained the same, but the amount of time people spent sitting rose by 8 percent.

Now consider how much we sit today compared with, say, 160 years ago. In a clever study, Dutch researchers created a sort of historical theme park and recruited actors to play 1850s Australian settlers for a week. The men did everything from chop wood to forage for food, and the scientists compared their activity levels with those of modern office workers. The result: The actors did the equivalent of walking 3 to 8 miles more a day than the deskbound men. That kind of activity is perhaps even more needed in today's fast-food nation than it was in the 1800s, but not just because it boosts calorie burn.

A 2010 study in the *Journal of Applied Physiology* found that when healthy men limited their number of footsteps by 85 percent for 2 weeks, they experienced a 17 percent decrease in insulin sensitivity, raising their diabetes risk.

"We've done a lot to keep people alive longer, but that doesn't mean we're healthier," says Dr. Hamilton.

Today's death rate is about 43 percent lower than it was in 1960, but back then, less than 1 percent of Americans had diabetes and only 13 percent were obese. Compare that with now, when 6 percent are diagnosed with diabetes and 35 percent are obese.

Make no mistake: "Regularly exercising is not the same as being active," says Peter Katzmarzyk, PhD, Hamilton's colleague at Pennington, the nation's leading obesity research center. Dr. Katzmarzyk is referring to the difference between official exercise activity, such as running, biking, or lifting weights, and so-called nonexercise activity, like walking to your car, mowing the lawn, or simply standing. "A person may hit the gym every day, but if he's sitting a good deal of the rest of the time, he's probably not leading an overall active life," says Dr. Katzmarzyk.

You might dismiss this as scientific semantics, but energy expenditure statistics support Dr. Katzmarzyk's notion. In a 2007 report, University of Missouri scientists said that people with the highest levels of nonexercise activity (but little to no actual "exercise") burned significantly more calories a week than those who ran 35 miles a week but accumulated only a moderate amount of nonexercise activity. "It can be as simple as standing more," Dr. Katzmarzyk says. For instance, a "standing" worker—say, a sales clerk at a Banana Republic store—burns about 1,500 calories while on the job; a person behind a desk might expend roughly 1,000 calories. That goes a long way toward explaining why people gain 16 pounds, on average, within 8 months of starting sedentary office work, according to a study from the University of North Carolina at Wilmington.

But calories aren't the only problem. In 2009, Dr. Katzmarzyk studied the lifestyle habits of more than 17,000 men and women and found that the people who sat for almost the entire day were 54 percent more likely to end up clutching their chests than those who sat for almost none of the time. That's no surprise, of course, except that it didn't matter how much the sitters weighed or how often they exercised.

"The evidence that sitting is associated with heart disease is very strong," says Dr. Katzmarzyk. "We see it in people who smoke and people who don't. We see it in people who are regular exercisers and those who aren't. Sitting is an independent risk factor."

This isn't actually a new discovery. In a

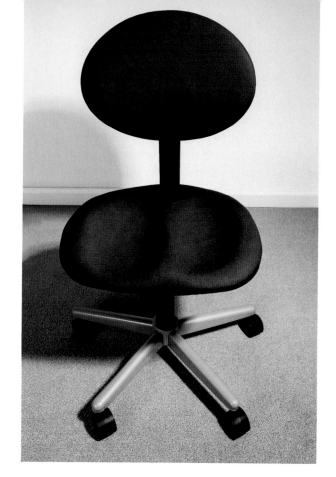

Your chair might be
as lethal as the
one in the state pen.

British study published in 1953, scientists examined two groups of workers: bus drivers and trolley conductors. At first glance, the two occupations appeared to be pretty similar. But while the bus drivers were more likely to sit down for their entire day, the trolley conductors were running up and down the stairs and aisles of the double-decker trolleys. As it turned out, the bus drivers were nearly twice as likely to die of heart disease as the conductors were.

A more recent interpretation of that study, published in 2004, found that none of the participants ever exercised. But the two groups did sit for different amounts of time. The analysis revealed that even after the scientists accounted for differences in waist size—an indicator of belly fat—the bus drivers were still more likely to die before the conductors did. So the bus drivers were at higher risk not simply because their sedentary jobs made them resemble Ralph Kramden, but also because all that sitting truly was making them unhealthy.

Dr. Hamilton came to call this area of science "inactivity physiology" while he

One study found that the people who sat for almost the entire day were 54 percent more likely to have a heart attack.

was conducting studies to determine how exercise affects an enzyme called lipoprotein lipase (LPL). Found in humans as well as mice, LPL's main responsibility is to break down fat in the bloodstream to use as energy. If a mouse (or a man) doesn't have this enzyme, or if the enzyme doesn't work in their leg muscles, the fat is stored instead of burned as fuel.

Dr. Hamilton discovered that when the rodents were forced to lie down for most of their waking hours, LPL activity in their leg muscles plummeted. But when they

simply stood around most of the time, the gene was 10 times more active. That's when he added an exercise session to the lab-rat routine and found that exercise had no effect on LPL. He believes the finding also applies to people.

"Humans sit too much, so you have to treat the problem specifically," says Dr. Hamilton. "The cure for too much sitting isn't more exercise. Exercise is good, of course, but the average person could never do enough to counteract the effect of hours and hours of chair time.

"We know there's a gene in the body that causes heart disease, but it doesn't respond to exercise no matter how often or how hard you work out," he says. "And yet the activity of the gene becomes worse from sitting—or rather, the complete and utter lack of contractile activity in your muscles. So the more nonexercise activity you do, the more total time you spend on your feet and out of your chair. That's the real cure."

"Your body adapts to what you do most often," says Bill Hartman, PT, CSCS, a *Men's Health* advisor and physical therapist in Indianapolis. "So if you sit in a chair all day, you'll essentially become better adapted to sitting in a chair." The trouble is, that makes you less adept at standing, walking, running, and jumping, all of which a truly healthy human should be able to do with proficiency. "Older folks have a harder time moving around than younger people do," says Hartman. "That's not simply because of age; it's because what you do consistently from day to day manifests itself over time, for both good and bad."

Do you sit all day at a desk? You're courting muscle stiffness, poor balance and mobility, and lower-back, neck, and hip pain. But to understand why, you'll need a quick primer on fascia, which is a tough connective tissue that covers all your muscles. While fascia is pliable, it tends to "set" in the position your muscles are in most often. So if you sit most of the time, your fascia adapts to that specific position.

"The changes to your muscles and posture from sitting are so small that you won't notice them at first. But as you reach your 30s, 40s, 50s, and beyond, they'll gradually become worse," says Hartman, "and a lot harder to fix."

So what's a desk jockey to do? Here's Dr. Hamilton's advice: Think in terms of two spectrums of activity. One represents the activities that you do that are considered regular exercise. But another denotes the amount of time you spend sitting versus the time you spend on your feet. "Then every day, make the small choices that will help move you in the right direction on that sitting-versus-standing spectrum," says Hamilton. "Stand while you're talking on the phone. It all adds up, and it all matters."

Of course, there's a problem with all of this: It kills all of our lame excuses for not exercising—no time for the gym, fungus on the shower-room floor, a rerun of *The Office* you haven't seen. Now we have to redefine "workout" to include every waking moment of our days. But there's a big payoff: more of those days to enjoy in the future. So get up off your chair and start nonexercising.

The Desk Jockey Workout

"Your body isn't meant to be seated 8 hours a day," says Bill Hartman, PT, CSCS. "But you can offset some of the damage." Perform this circuit three times a day to beat bad posture before it starts.

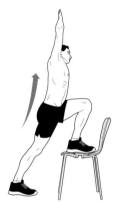

Standing Hip-Extension Stretch

Why it's good: Loosens your hip flexors and strengthens your glutes

How to do it: Stand and place your left foot on a chair with your knee bent 90 degrees. Tighten your right buttock and reach overhead as high as you can with your right arm. Side-bend slightly to the left. Hold 30 seconds; repeat on the other side.

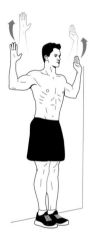

Scapular Wall Slide

Why it's good: Prevents rounded shoulders

How to do it: Stand with your back and head against a wall. Place your arms against the wall so they form a W. Slide your arms upward into a Y. Hold for a count of 3, then lower them. Do this 12 times.

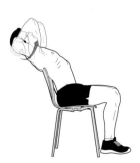

Chair Mobilization

Why it's good: Prevents the hunchback look

How to do it: Sit so the back of your chair is just below shoulder blade level. Place your hands behind your head and bring your elbows toward each other. Arch back and push your elbows upward as you exhale. Hold for a count of 3; do this 12 times.

PROVE IT

KNOW YOUR MAX

A new formula called Maximum Weight Limit (MWL) sets one weight that you should not exceed to minimize your health risks. Based on the body mass index, the MWL is a good guideline for couch potatoes, but it might not be for more muscular guys who lift weights regularly. If that describes you, don't worry if you exceed these weights.

Height	Max weight
5'11"	185
5'10"	180
5'9"	175

For other heights, add or subtract 5 pounds for every inch.

SHOP TILL YOU DROP (POUNDS)

When you're food shopping, be selfish: You're more likely to bring home junk if you're buying for your family or friends, a new University of Miami study reveals. The scientists found that people stocking up for themselves made healthier choices than those shopping for others.

We buy healthy foods for ourselves in an effort to avoid eating junk, the scientists say. When we shop for others, this discipline erodes. Ask your family for a list of what they want—and stick to it.

SLICE YOUR HUNGER PANGS

Eat protein at breakfast to stay full, and make your toast rye. In a study comparing breakfasts that were identical except for bread

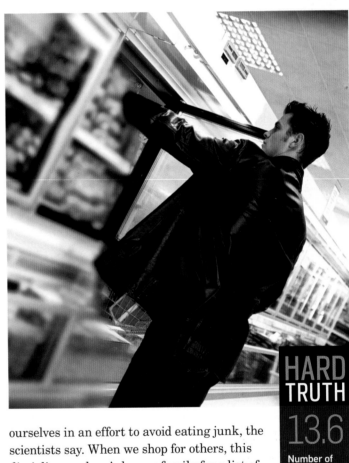

HARD TRUTH

13.6

Number of pounds gained in 3.5 years by people who consumed 15 percent of calories between 11 P.M. and 5 A.M.

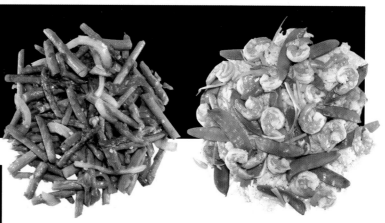

**P.F. Chang's
Sichuan-style Asparagus**
+115 percent
In the study, this dish had more than double the calories the restaurant claimed it had.

**P.F. Chang's
Cantonese Shrimp**
-31 percent
On the other hand, this dish had one-third fewer calories than the restaurant claimed it had.

choices, Swedish researchers found that rye eaters were less hungry after 8 hours than wheat eaters were. The researchers think compounds created when rye's fiber ferments in your colon may help you feel fuller. Look for bread that includes rye bran, which boosts fiber content.

CUT CARBS

A worldwide consensus has formed: Eating a diet that's low in carbs, not fats, is the best way to lose weight. In a recent United Arab Emirates study, people who followed a low-carb diet had lower body weights, insulin levels, and triglyceride levels than those who went with a low-fat diet. And a European study that tracked nearly 90,000 people for several years found that participants with a low fat intake had the same risk of being overweight as those who ate higher amounts of fat. Still, if you boost your fat intake, make sure you adjust your calories and physical activity accordingly.

DISTRUST THE MENU

Can you trust the calorie postings at restaurants? Not always, say researchers at Tufts University. They tested 15 meals or side dishes and 14 individual items (such as pizzas and sandwiches) from chain restaurants. The researchers found that, on average, actual calorie counts were 18 percent higher than what the chains stated. More important, the range of mistakes was huge. Some dishes had 36 percent fewer calories than what the restaurant claimed; other foods had about 200 percent more calories. The most likely reason for the mistakes was flawed portion sizes, researchers say.

LOSE WEIGHT THE FUN WAY

It's your choice: Go for a trudging run, or play a game. Playing soccer is just as effective as running for helping you lose weight, say researchers in Switzerland. In the study, men who played in an hour-long soccer session two or three times a week were able to lose, on average, 4.5 pounds of fat and 1.3 inches from their waists in 3 months. That was just as good as the group that ran for the same time period. Playing soccer is similar to interval training, say the scientists. Find a beginners' league, or (actively) coach kids.

YOU ASKED

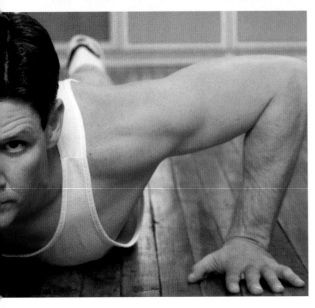

intake by up to 20 percent, because it makes you feel full. To avoid having to pound two glasses of H_2O, try this: Drink one glass and start with a broth-based soup, like miso, minestrone, or chicken noodle, says Alan Aragon, MS, a *Men's Health* nutrition adviser.

Q: I would love to work out, but I can't find the time. Any ideas?

A: People who halved their daily TV time burned an extra 120 calories a day, a recent Stanford study found. Doing this could help you lose 12 pounds in a year, says Travis Stork, MD, a faculty physician at Vanderbilt University Medical Center and the author of *The Lean Belly Prescription*.

Q: What one simple change can I make to jump-start my weight loss?

A: Consuming a liquid—whether it's two glasses of water or a cup of soup—to begin a meal can reduce your total calorie

Q: What's an easy, accurate way to calculate how many calories I should take in if I want to drop 10 pounds?

A: For a good estimate, you'll need a calculator and an honest accounting of your exercise habits, Aragon says. He uses this simple two-step process with clients who want to shed pounds: Take your total weekly exercise hours, add 10, and multiply that number by your target weight. The result will be your daily calorie intake. For example, if your target weight is 180 pounds and your weekly training includes 3 hours of weights and 1 hour of hoops, the math would work out to 2,520 calories a day. Missed a workout? Just reduce your intake by 350 to 750 calories, depending on how long or hard you typically train, says Aragon.

Q: If I keep my thermostat low, will I drop weight?

A: "Setting your thermostat in the 60-to-65-degree range will force your body to work harder to maintain its normal temperature, which will burn calories but not a significant amount. Plus, revving your interior thermostat to cope with the chill may spark your appetite," says David Katz, MD, MPH, the director of the prevention research center at Yale University and the author of *The Way We Eat.*

Q: **My family loves to eat at buffet restaurants. How can I join them, without sabotaging my diet?**

A: When you load your plate at a buffet, leave spaces between the foods you select, says Dr. Stork. You could consume up to 20 percent fewer calories than you would if your plate were packed.

Q: **What can I do to not cave to a crave?**

A: Before you succumb to a snack craving, picture your previous meal, Aragon says. In a British study, people who used this strategy ate a smaller snack than those who didn't stop to think about what they'd put into their mouths recently.

Q: **I shed 40 pounds, but now the skin around my belly sags. Can I lose it without surgery?**

A: It depends how heavy you were and for how long, says Galen Perdikis, MD, FACS, an associate professor of plastic surgery at the Mayo Clinic College of Medicine. "The issue is elasticity of your skin," he explains.

"When you stretch it beyond a certain point, and maintain that stretch, you exceed its ability to snap back."

The general rule is that if you weighed 30 percent more than you do now for 5 years or longer, then surgery is probably the best option. If you're not in that category, then your skin may tighten naturally over 6 to 12 months,

Exercise alters hormones so that fat is stored away from organs.

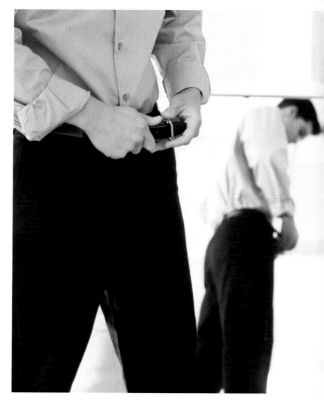

and exercising three times a week may help speed the process. Even if you are a surgery candidate, don't have it done if you want to lose more weight; dropping pounds post-op will just create more loose skin. When you're ready, choose a board-certified plastic surgeon (find one at plasticsurgery.org) who specializes in abdominoplasty (tummy tuck) and completes at least two procedures a month. Most saggy-skin cases are corrected by either this procedure (in which the surgeon removes the skin between your hip bones and belly button and tightens your abdominal muscles) or a "mini-tuck," which involves removing only your skin.

Q: Can playing video games on the Wii help me lose weight?

A: It depends whether you want to use Wii Tennis as your go-to workout or as a bonus calorie burner. "Video games can play a role in your weekly regimen, but they aren't enough by themselves to cause significant weight loss," says Kevin Short, PhD, an assistant professor of pediatrics at the University of Oklahoma Health Sciences Center. In his studies with children, he found that those who played Wii Sports games, including boxing and bowling, at high intensity burned 3 calories a minute—the equivalent of walking 2.6 miles an hour on a treadmill. (Dr. Short says these results would probably be similar in adults.) In other words, don't count on virtual sports for real-world weight loss.

Q: Do TV fitness gadgets work?

A: Maybe. But probably not. We took a look at the science behind some of the most recognizable ones.

1 SHAKE WEIGHT FOR MEN

$30 + $10 S&H
You hold. And shake. Ads say it causes up to 240 muscle contractions per minute and gives you a complete upper-body workout in 6 minutes.
What's the science say?
Muscles don't grow just because you contract them; they need the challenge of added weight, says Mark Peterson, PhD, a University of Michigan exercise physiologist.
Gym alternative: Moves that target multiple areas, such as the bench press or the bent-over row, grow muscle faster, Dr. Peterson says. Start your workout with a weight you can lift only 6 to 8 times, and do 3 or 4 sets of each exercise. As you become stronger, add weight.

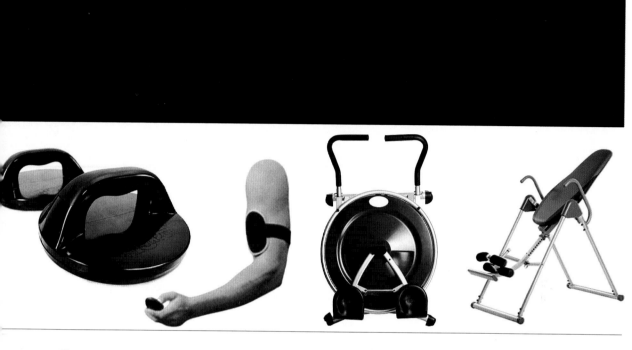

2 PUSH UP PRO

$10 + $6 S&H

These disks allow wrist rotation during pushups, which the ads say means less wrist stress, natural shoulder movement, and extra power.

What's the science say?
Rotating your wrists eases some strain, but that doesn't improve the effect of the pushup, says Eric Cressey, MS, co-owner of Cressey Performance.

Gym alternative: Place a pair of dumbbells on the floor and perform pushups while gripping the handles. When you do pushups this way, your wrists won't fold and strain under your body weight, Cressey says. Once you master the technique, place your feet on a bench to increase the difficulty.

3 THE FLEX ARMS

$200 + $16 S&H

Strap this device to your upper arms and electric shocks will "tone, tighten, firm, and strengthen" your muscles in 4 to 8 weeks.

What's the science say?
Your muscles grow when you stress them just enough to cause microtears in the fibers. Lifting weights does this, but small electric jolts probably won't, says Cressey.

Gym alternative: Bodyweight exercises can challenge your arm muscles with more weight than curls or bench presses ever will—and you need that extra weight in order to grow muscle. Add 2 or 3 sets of pushups and pullups at the end of your workout, says Martin Rooney, PT, CSCS.

4 AB CIRCLE PRO

$200 + $35 S&H

You kneel on it, grab on to both handles, and rotate your body from side to side, strengthening your core, according to the ads.

What's the science say?
The extreme rotation from the Ab Circle Pro may put dangerous torque on your spine, and its effectiveness as a cardio workout is questionable, Peterson says.

Gym alternative: Kettlebell swings combine cardio and resistance training, which allows you to safely lose weight and build core muscles, says Mike Robertson, CSCS.

5 BROOKSTONE INVERSION TABLE

$300 + $65 S&H

It flips you over, which the maker says stretches muscles, improves posture, and eliminates back pain.

What's the science say?
Temporary pain relief may come, but other benefits aren't backed by science. "Your muscles aren't working, which is what you need for a long-term fix," Cressey says.

Gym alternative: To improve your posture and ease back pain, build the muscles that support your spine, says Dr. Peterson. Activate your abs, hip flexors, glutes, and lower back with planks, side planks, and hip-extension holds. Do 3 sets apiece, holding each for 30 to 60 seconds.

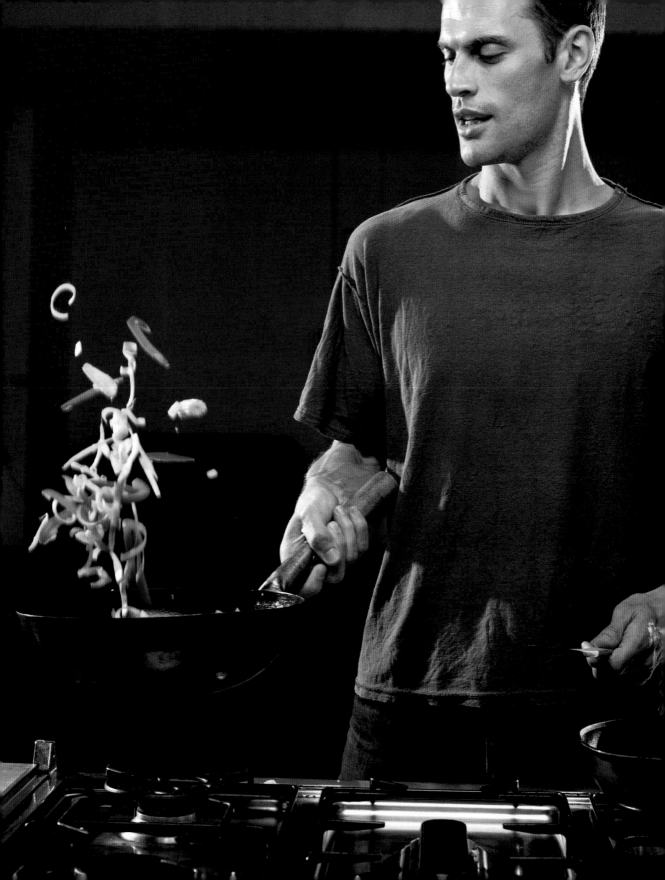

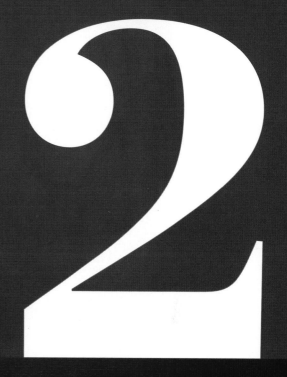

PART

2

Flat-Belly Foods

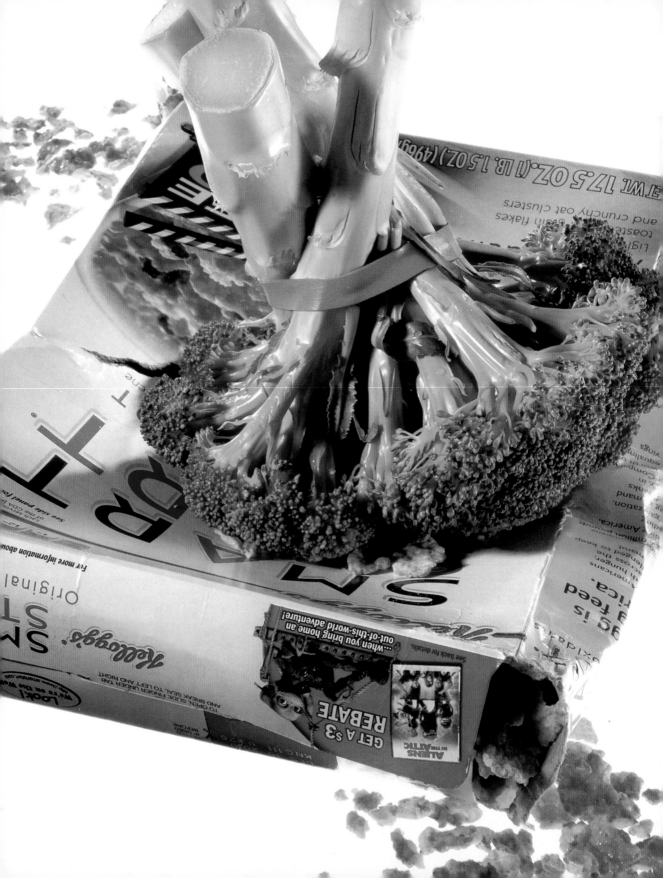

The Truth About Antioxidants

Miraculous disease-fighting nutrients or overhyped marketing gimmick? Here are the facts and the fiction—and what you need to know.

It's an epic story of good versus evil. The villains: free radicals, those nefarious DNA-attacking poisons of modern life. Our fearless defenders: antioxidants, poised to protect us from— well, everything. You've heard the claims:

They cure cancer! Prevent aging! Supercharge immunity! But while we think we know what antioxidants do, few know what antioxidants actually are. And food manufacturers are fine with that; the less you know, the more likely you are to swallow the hype. "Antioxidants have a health aura around them," says Marion Nestle, PhD, MPH, a professor of nutrition, food studies, and public health at New York University. "They are supposed to fight something bad in your body. Who wouldn't want to consume more of a helper like that?"

No doubt antioxidants can be good for you. But to maximize their benefit, we first have to strip away some assumptions.

49

MYTH #1

Free radicals must be destroyed.

NOT SO FAST.

The basics: Antioxidants fight free radicals, which are unstable molecules in the body that can cause DNA mutation. Even though free radicals have been linked to serious conditions like heart disease, Parkinson's, and cancer, they aren't necessarily villains. They're byproducts of a basic metabolic process called oxidation. "They're absolutely essential to life," says Jeffrey Blumberg, PhD, director of the antioxidants lab at Tufts University. "For example, immune cells will shoot free radicals onto invading bacteria in order to kill them. They're an important part of the body's defenses."

Too many free radicals, on the other hand, are harmful. Pollutants, cigarette smoke, and sun overexposure can generate so many free radicals that your normal antioxidant defenses become overwhelmed, leaving you vulnerable to cell damage and disease. Some researchers also link free-radical oxidation with aging.

That's where antioxidants come in. "We need to make sure we have adequate antioxidant defenses to combat all the excess free radicals," says Dr. Blumberg.

Do this: Assuming you've curbed bad habits such as smoking and excessive tanning, turn to your diet. If you eat a wide variety of fruits and vegetables, your diet is naturally rich in thousands of antioxidants. Studies suggest eating at least five servings of fruits and vegetables a day to reap the most health benefits.

MYTH #2

All antioxidants are created equal.

NOT EVEN CLOSE.

The basics: Any molecule that protects your cells against oxidation is technically an antioxidant, says Joe Vinson, PhD, a professor of chemistry at the University of Scranton, in Pennsylvania. "They're anti-oxidation." This includes familiar nutrients, like vitamins, as well as more unfamiliar types of antioxidants, like flavonoids and polyphenols—about 8,000 varieties in all.

But don't assume that all antioxidants operate the same way, Dr. Blumberg warns. "You can't say, 'Well, I'm not going to worry about taking in enough vitamin E, because I take lots of vitamin C.' All

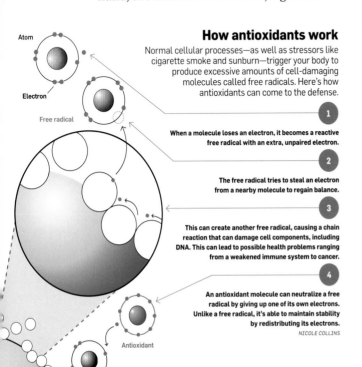

How antioxidants work

Normal cellular processes—as well as stressors like cigarette smoke and sunburn—trigger your body to produce excessive amounts of cell-damaging molecules called free radicals. Here's how antioxidants can come to the defense.

Atom

Electron

Free radical

1
When a molecule loses an electron, it becomes a reactive free radical with an extra, unpaired electron.

2
The free radical tries to steal an electron from a nearby molecule to regain balance.

3
This can create another free radical, causing a chain reaction that can damage cell components, including DNA. This can lead to possible health problems ranging from a weakened immune system to cancer.

4
An antioxidant molecule can neutralize a free radical by giving up one of its own electrons. Unlike a free radical, it's able to maintain stability by redistributing its electrons.

NICOLE COLLINS

Antioxidant

the vitamin C in the world won't substitute for vitamin E," says Dr. Blumberg. Some antioxidants excel at fighting certain types of free radicals while others are effective only in specific parts of a cell. Still others can battle free radicals only under the right conditions.

How do you create an effective defense system in the battle for your life? By building a multipronged counteroffensive—er, diet.

Do this: Branch out and try something new in the produce aisle. In a 2006 study, researchers at Colorado State University found that people who ate the widest variety of fruits and vegetables had the most DNA protection.

MYTH #3

All antioxidants come from fruits and vegetables.

NOPE.

The basics: The entire plant kingdom—including beans, nuts, seeds, and grains—is awash in antioxidants, according to a recent study from the University of Scranton. That's because all plants produce antioxidants to fight against predators and UV rays, says Dr. Vinson. It's important to steer clear of refined grains, though; they've been stripped of most of their antioxidant benefits.

Even meat, dairy products, and eggs contain some antioxidants, which come mainly from the nutrient-rich plants the animals fed on.

Do this: Eat whole-grain foods, beans, nuts, and seeds regularly. When animals are on the menu, make sure that they've been grass-fed; meat and dairy products from these better-fed beasts have been shown to contain higher levels of antioxidants. Eggs from pastured hens also rank higher in antioxidants. Look for them at farmers' markets.

MYTH #4

Antioxidant-fortified foods are healthier.

NOT REALLY.

The basics: The ink was barely dry on early antioxidant studies when food companies started slapping the A-word on their packaging. You can even chug an antioxidant-fortified version of Cherry 7UP. The FDA requires food manufacturers to list the variety of antioxidant in a product; that part is often in fine print. Look closely and the label reveals that you're receiving a tiny helping of vitamin E. Perhaps "Cherry 7UP Vitamin E" didn't sound as impressive.

If you're relying on processed foods to supplement your antioxidant intake, you might be surprised to find that many processed foods have relatively small amounts of just one or two kinds. Because variety is critical, you probably aren't making up for lost ground.

Do this: Ignore the hype. There's no research to prove that packaged products provide the same health benefits that whole foods do. Instead, focus on the ingredient list. If a food product contains mostly plant foods, it's likely to be rich in antioxidants.

HARD TRUTH

80

Percentage increase worldwide from 2005 to 2009 of products advertising antioxidant content on their labels, according to the Mintel Global New Products Database

Salt of the Earth

Insidious health threat or innocent flavor enhancer?
Take a closer look at the planet's tastiest mineral.

America has declared war on salt. The nutrition militia, claiming that the enemy is attacking you and your buddies, points to hypertension stats: More than 20 percent of American men between 35 and 44 have high blood pressure. Even the Institute of Medicine is leaning on the government to set standards for sodium content in foods. So should you enlist? It's a tough battle.

"If people want to avoid salt, they really can't—not unless they skip processed, prepared, and restaurant foods," says Marion Nestle, PhD, MPH, a professor of nutrition, food studies, and public health at New York University. What's more, salt may not even be the true enemy. Before you sign up to fight, tune out the hysteria and plunge into the latest nutrition intel.

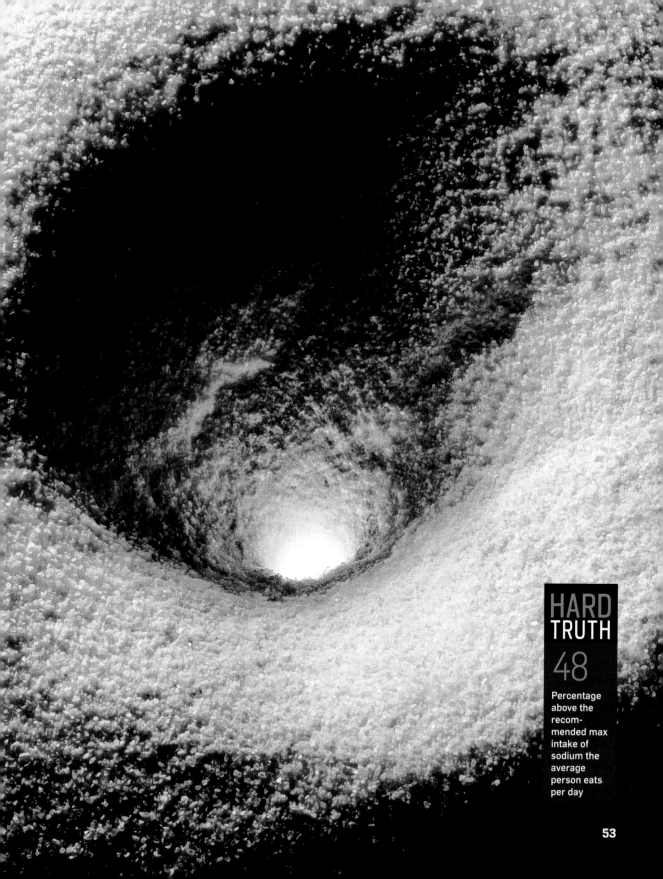

Can I Live Without Salt?
NOPE.

Salt is essential to health. Your body can't make it, and your cells need it to function, says Aryan Aiyer, MD, director of the Heart Center at Magee-Womens Hospital at the University of Pittsburgh Medical Center. In fact, the Institute of Medicine recommends consuming at least 3.8 grams of salt a day (just over ½ teaspoon), mainly for the sodium.

Sodium is an electrolyte, a humble member of that hyped class of minerals that help maintain muscle function and hydration. That's why sport drinks contain sodium. You're constantly losing sodium through sweat and urine, and if you don't replenish that sodium and water, your blood pressure may drop far enough to make you dizzy and light-headed.

"Sodium acts like a sponge to help hold fluids in your blood," says Rikki Keen, RD, an adjunct instructor of dietetics and nutrition at the University of Alaska.

However, people who chug too much water can lower their sodium levels so far that they develop hyponatremia, a potentially deadly condition more common in recreational exercisers than pro athletes, says Marie Spano, RD, a sports nutritionist in Atlanta. Salt does more than make our food taste good; without it, we'd die.

Do I Need to Watch My Salt Intake like a Hawk?
NOT NECESSARILY.

If you have high blood pressure, you've probably been advised to cut back on salt. The mechanism seems clear: Sodium causes your blood to hold more water, so your heart has to pump harder, making your blood pressure rise. If your blood pressure is already high, that's a problem. (A high intake of salt can also be dangerous for people who are salt-sensitive—that is, who have trouble excreting excess salt.)

What if you're a healthy guy? The Institute of Medicine is adamant in recommending that people ages 14 and over consume no more than 2,300 milligrams of sodium a day—about a teaspoon of salt. The institute sets a lower limit (1,500 milligrams, or slightly more than ½ teaspoon) for middle-age and older adults, African Americans, and people with kidney disease, hypertension, or diabetes.

But even though the average American blows past both limits, consuming an average of 3,400 milligrams of sodium a day, some experts say that's not a problem for most men.

"I don't know of any evidence that suggests that healthy men with normal blood pressure should reduce their sodium intake," says Michael Alderman, MD, a professor of medicine at Yeshiva University.

For starters, reducing the salt content of your diet could adversely affect your health, Dr. Alderman says.

And let's not forget that sodium isn't the only blood pressure booster. "The huge message everyone overlooks is that being overweight also contributes to high blood pressure," says Spano.

Can Food Counteract the Effect of Salt on My BP?
YES.

Quick biology lesson: Your body is constantly balancing the sodium on the outside of each cell and the potassium on the inside. A 2006 statement from the American Heart Association in the journal *Hypertension* revealed that an increase in potassium can lower blood pressure just as much as a decrease in sodium can. Even the Institute of Medicine doesn't deny this: "The sodium–potassium ratio is typically more closely associated with blood pressure than with intake of either substance alone."

Unfortunately, supersalty processed meals tend to crowd out our main dietary sources of potassium—fresh fruits and vegetables. Nutrition surveys reveal that younger men consume only about 60 percent to 70 percent of the recommended daily intake: 4,700 milligrams of potassium. Imagine the positive effect on our blood pressure levels if fast-food cashiers always asked, "You want broccoli with that?"

Should I Cut Back on Salt When I Cook?
DON'T BOTHER.

Tossing some salt into your pasta water isn't likely to send your blood pressure soaring. That's because 77 percent of the sodium in the average diet comes from processed and restaurant foods, according to the Centers for Disease Control and Prevention. Only 12 percent of sodium is naturally occurring in foods, and just 5 percent comes from home cooking.

Stick with kosher salt for cooking and try flaky sea salt for finishing a dish; both types are free of additives.

America's Five Saltiest Foods

The following meals contain at least a day's worth of sodium—along with gobs of fat and calories. Proceed with caution.

SALTIEST FOOD IN AMERICA

P.F. Chang's Double Pan-Fried Noodles with Pork
7,900 milligrams sodium
1,652 calories
84 grams fat

This abomination packs more than 3 days' worth of sodium into one pile of noodles.

SALTIEST BURGER

Chili's Jalapeño Smokehouse Bacon Burger
6,710 milligrams sodium
2,140 calories
139 grams fat

Bacon, Cheddar, and tortilla strips create a trio of saltiness.

SALTIEST BREAKFAST

Perkins Southern Fried Chicken Biscuit Platter
6,680 milligrams sodium
1,860 calories
86 grams fat

Call it the inflated-portion effect: This meal consists of two fried-chicken breakfast sandwiches, with eggs, bacon, and hash browns on the side.

SALTIEST STEAK MEAL

Claim Jumper Country Fried Steak
6,157 milligrams sodium
2,288 calories
66 grams fat

Southern staples like these have enough salt in the batter to de-ice your driveway.

SALTIEST NACHOS

On the Border Grande Fajita Chicken Nachos (appetizer)
5,180 milligrams sodium
1,540 calories
85 grams fat

Even if you share this appetizer with a friend, you'll have eaten an entire day's worth of sodium before the entrees arrive.

The New Rules of Barbecue

Step away from the gas grill and grab your aprons, men.
It's time you cooked up the real deal: slow–smoked barbecue.

It's 9 a.m. in downtown Memphis.

At first glance, you might mistake the tent- and trailer-filled Tom Lee Park, on the banks of the mighty, muddy Mississippi, for a shantytown. Last night's parties ended late, and crushed cups and over-turned kegs litter the ground. Then you notice the in-your-face signage: Ribbed for Your Pleasure, South Pork, Reservoir Hogs. Not to mention the machinery—massive slow cookers, including one fabricated from a vintage Greyhound bus and another built into a 1940s Ford. The fires in those giant cookers are already at full bore, and the air hangs heavy and delicious with smoky sweetness.

This is the Memphis in May World Championship Barbecue Cooking Contest, one of the largest competitions of its type in the world. Over the next 3 days, hundreds of teams from across the nation will compete for a $100,000 kitty, several human-size

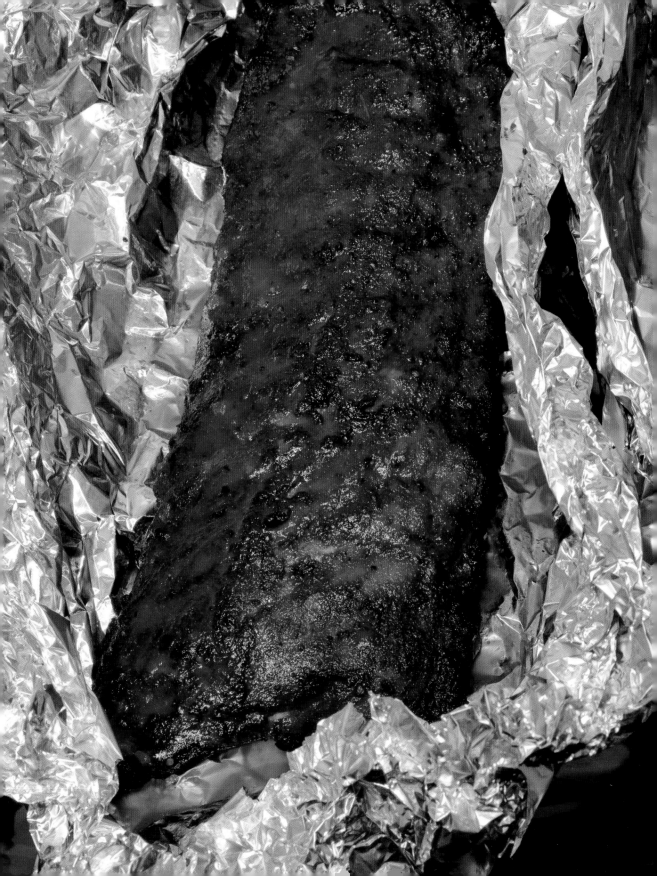

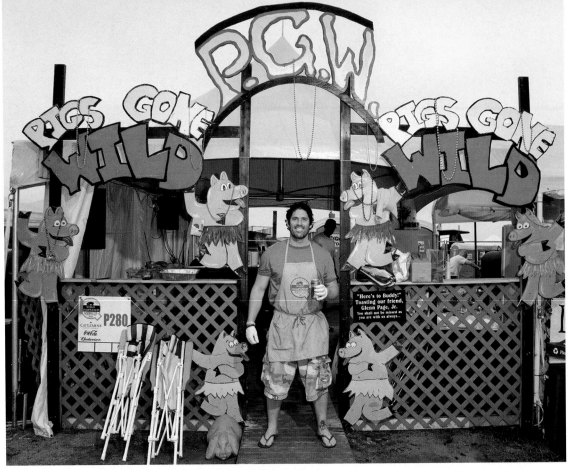

One of the many team tents at Memphis in May that pay tribute to the pig.

trophies, and the bragging rights that come with a victory here. Behind a bare-bones tent in an alley of grass, competitor Craig Samuel, chef and owner of Smoke Joint, in Brooklyn, sets a spice-rubbed 8-pound prime rib on the grill. From a nearby tent, Todd Hamilton, a pitmaster from the Memphis-based team known as Swine-O-Mite, can't help speaking up.

"Prime rib? Cooked in a kettle grill? This beef's gonna kill," Samuel says as he closes the lid on the cooker. "We're going all the way." Hamilton smiles and tosses wood chips into a pan of water. "Ah, no. You're not."

Do you barbecue?

Probably not. You grill. And slap on barbecue sauce. That's about as close to real barbecue as arena football is to the NFL. But slow-cooked meat, smoked to melting tenderness, is every man's birthright. You just need to know how to make it at home.

So the editors of *Men's Health* rounded up a crack team of New York barbecue chefs to compete in Memphis—and prove that the average guy can cook real barbecue. Hold on, you're thinking. Barbecue chefs from New York? That's right: Barbecue has become big in the Big Apple. And Samuel, along with Kenny Callaghan of Manhattan's Blue Smoke, John Stage of Harlem's Dinosaur Bar-B-Que, and Joe Carroll from Brooklyn's

Fette Sau, practice the art of barbecue with single-minded devotion.

Besides, as complete underdogs, the chefs' New York swagger might actually come in handy. While other competitors will be using 2-ton smokers (some spend tens of thousands building their rigs), the *Men's Health* 'Cue Crew will make do with run-of-the-mill rigs: charcoal-fueled kettle grills and low-tech bullet smokers.

Fact is, if these guys can make authentic barbecue with the same kind of equipment that's already sitting on your backyard patio, so can you. As long as you follow their lead—and their rules.

RULE NUMBER 1

When it comes to the grill, basic is beautiful.

Once we roll into steamy Memphis, the guys are all business, surveying the equipment behind their tent and unpacking the sauces and spice rubs. The kettle grills are a far cry from the rigs the 'Cue Crew chefs cook on back home, but they'll do the job. Unlike gas grills, kettle grills excel at both low-heat barbecuing and high-heat grilling; you just need to push the hot coals to the edges of the grill, creating an indirect-heat zone in the center. Carroll is pleased that the kettle grills are 26 inches wide.

"Plenty of room for meat in that center zone," Carroll says.

Meanwhile, Samuel is checking out the team's bullet smokers. Another easy option for backyard barbecuers, these oblong, vertical grills hold charcoal in a separate lower chamber, so there's no need

to create an indirect-heat area. You just throw in the lit charcoal and go. Samuel taps the built-in thermometer on the lid of one of the smokers and nods.

"It's all about keeping that heat under control," Samuel says.

But before the guys can start cooking tomorrow, they'll need to procure the last of their supplies: hardwood charcoal. Sure, bags of briquettes line the tent, but Carroll hates the way the chemicals they contain contaminate the flavor of the food. So the team hikes across the park to bum a bag from Jimmy Hagood, a buddy of Kenny's and the leader of the BlackJack barbecue team.

As the strains of "Love Me Tender" blare, the chefs ask J.B. McCarty, another BlackJack team member, about his rigs. He shows off his enormous Jedmaster box cooker, capable of cooking 50 pork shoulders at a time.

The *Men's Health* team whistles approval, but McCarty is unfazed and pragmatic.

"Look, I've been doing this long enough to know that anything can happen," he says. "Heat is heat, whether it's a Jedmaster or a Weber. It's not the arrow. It's the Indian."

RULE NUMBER 2

Good BBQ is about infusing flavor, not just slapping it on.

As evening falls, Carroll and Samuel start to prep the chicken and beef for tomorrow. "You want to give the seasonings time to penetrate," Carroll says. He adds flavor with a method not often used by pitmas-

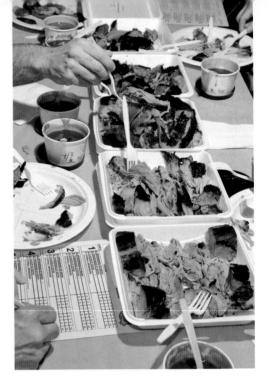

ters: brining. He combines water, brown sugar, and kosher salt, and adds ground espresso, cumin, and cinnamon. Then he submerges his heritage-breed birds in the muddy liquid and packs them in the cooler for an overnight soak.

Samuel, meanwhile, makes his classic Smoke Joint rub for his beef, mixing brown sugar with spices that include paprika, cayenne, and mustard powder.

"Prime rib is a tender cut, so it'll cook up way faster than brisket, and the rub will make it taste just as nuanced and rich," he says.

RULE NUMBER 3

Low, steady heat yields fall-off-the-bone meat.

The first day of competition dawns, and after a night in the cooler, both the chicken and the prime rib are ready to hit the grill. But neither of these hefty hunks of meat will turn tender and juicy if the chefs approach the job the way the average backyard bandit does—by cranking the heat, letting the flames engulf the meat, and then dousing the inevitable flare-ups with a bottle of beer. These hearty cuts need the gentle heat that only indirect cooking provides, and they need

that heat to stay steady for hours.

The chefs start by pouring hot, ash-covered coals from a chimney starter into the grills and pushing the coals to the sides.

"Some guys say keeping the temperature at the sweet spot of 225°F is a pain," Carroll says. "But it doesn't have to be." He uses a simple formula: One chimney starter's worth of charcoal brings the temperature in the smoker to between 225°F and 250°F. Then he checks the heat every half hour, adding coals one by one through an opening in the grate as needed to maintain the status quo.

Of course, where there's fire, there must

"Apply a light coat of mustard to your meat before adding any dry rub. It'll help adhere the rub to the meat, and the vinegar in the mustard will tenderize the meat."
—John Wheeler, team member, Natural Born Grillers, 2010 Memphis in May ribs champion and a 2008 world champion

Go Low and Slow

These three steps are the keys to perfectly cooked barbecue.

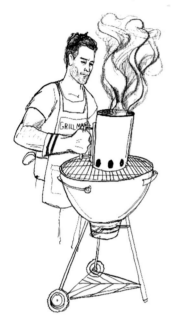
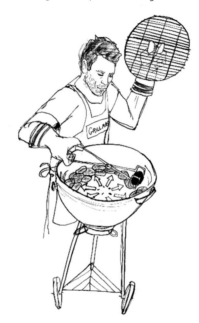
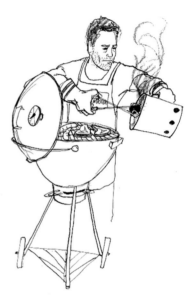

1 LIGHT YOUR CHARCOAL

"Skip the lighter fluid—it gives your food a funky smell and taste," says Joe Carroll. Instead, use a chimney starter, available at any hardware or kitchen store for about $15. Stuff a sheet or two of newspaper into the bottom of the chimney, set the chimney on the grill grates, and fill it with charcoal. Light the newspaper and watch for smoke to emerge from the top of the chimney. In about 15 minutes, your coals will be lightly covered with ash—a sign that they're ready to go. Hold the chimney in a heatproof glove or with a heavy dish towel and shake out the coals into your grill.

2 CREATE A COOKING ZONE

If you're cooking with a kettle grill, you'll need to create an indirect heat zone in the center of your grill using a technique called "banking." With a grill hoe or a pair of long metal tongs, push the coals to the edges of your grill, leaving an open space in the center. If you're using a bullet smoker, just add the hot coals to the bottom of the cooker. To add smoke, wrap your presoaked wood chunks or chips in foil, poke some large holes in the package, and toss directly onto the hot coals.

3 REGULATE THE HEAT

The sweet spot for barbecue is between 225°F and 250°F. "A low, even heat will help break down the collagen in the muscles and create tender meat," says Carroll. But it's important to monitor the temperature closely. "If the heat is below 140°F, it encourages bacteria to form. If it's too high, you're baking, not barbecuing." To lower the heat, vent the grill or open the lid for a minute or two. To raise the heat, add 4 to 6 more lit coals, one at a time. (Keep a supply on hand in the chimney starter.)

also be smoke. Samuel soaks hickory wood chips in water and then tosses them onto the coals, where they can release their sweet smoke into the meat as it cooks.

Within a few hours, the spice-rubbed prime rib has turned a gorgeous brick-red color, and the chickens are a burnished brown. Carroll cuts off a wing, bites into it, and nods. It's tender and juicy, perfumed with woodsmoke and spice. The only problem? The thigh meat is looking a bit pink at the bone, and there's no time to keep cooking it before the mandatory call time. Callaghan shakes his head and carves up the meat

for the "blind box" that Carroll carries to the judges' tent, hoping for the best.

Next, Samuel slices into his prime rib. He's stoked: The beef is perfectly cooked, right on time.

"Beautiful! Look at that smoke ring," he says, referring to the red coloring about half an inch into the meat's surface that indicates how deeply the smoke has penetrated. The humble Webers have done the trick.

Samuel cuts a few pieces for the crew; the beef meets with rapturous approval. For extra succulence, he quickly dunks them into a mixture of cooking juices and

Seven Must-Try Asian Condiments

Transform meals with these exotic flavor boosters suggested by Zakary Pelaccio, creative director of the Fatty Crab restaurants in New York.

THAILAND	**MALAYSIA**	**CHINA**	**KOREA**	**JAPAN**	**VIETNAM**	**INDONESIA**
Red curry paste	Satay sauce	Oyster sauce	Hot pepper paste	Ponzu	Fish sauce	Sambal
This paste infuses Thai curries and soups with citrusy heat. Slather it on chicken wings before grilling.	Satay sauce is crushed peanuts punched up with soy sauce and spices. It's delicious with kebabs, but try it over wok-fried vegetables or shrimp, too.	This condiment is a pleasant mix of salty and sweet. Drizzle it over sautéed spinach.	This slightly spicy bean paste is great as a condiment for Korean BBQ or as a marinade for fish.	This light citrus sauce, often made with soy sauce, enhances seared tuna or grilled chicken.	Sub it in for soy sauce and/or salt in stews and noodle dishes to add a savory (not fishy) note.	Usually made from crushed chilies and salt, sambal adds an instant kick to fried rice or scrambled eggs.

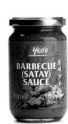
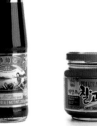
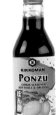
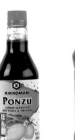
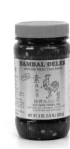

"Everyone should have their own personal rub. Start with chili-pepper powder, kosher salt, cumin, oregano, black pepper, and paprika. Then add your own secret ingredients, but keep it simple."

—Jim Butler, member of the PartyQ team, the 2009 Whole Hog Memphis in May champion

brown sugar before tucking them into the box bound for the judges' tent.

RULE NUMBER 4

Always have a secret weapon.

As the judges taste and deliberate, Stage and Callaghan prepare a trial run of baby back ribs for the big pork battle tomorrow. They start with the typical pitmaster's approach to ribs, coating them in a spice rub and barbecuing them for 3 hours. But then Callaghan goes rogue. He nestles each rib rack into a foil packet. Then he cracks open a can of pineapple juice and pours it over the pork before sealing the packets and returning them to the grill.

"Now the ribs will steam in sweetness," he says. The glaze is their next trick. While most of the competitors at Memphis in May merely tweak store-bought barbecue sauces, Callaghan and Stage create their own concoction, a combination of vinegar, honey, Asian chili sauce for garlicky heat, and Worcestershire for umami depth. Then they brush it on the ribs and return them to the grill. When the ribs come off the grill, it's clear the extra moves have paid off. The team members rave about the trifecta of intense

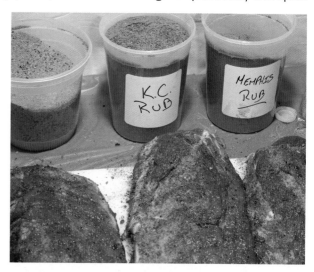

flavor, great smoke, and tenderness.

By noon on the day of competition, Callaghan and Stage have 10 gorgeous racks ready to eat. They'll need plenty for the blind box, plus at least three perfect racks for the three on-site judges who will be visiting their tent. Callaghan's mentor Mike Mills, a barbecue legend who retired from the circuit after winning world champion at Memphis in May four times in a row, stops in for a visit and a taste.

"In all honesty, Kenny, I'm not getting any bump at the end," he says. "I'm going to call it bland because I don't have a finish. I need something that makes me want another bite." Stage looks to

Callaghan. "A little more heat and sugar in the glaze?" Callaghan nods and tweaks it with chili sauce and honey. Mills takes a bite of the newly enhanced pork. "Yes, I've got something left in my mouth now." The ribs are ready for the judges.

RULE NUMBER 5

Don't sweat your critics.

Once the blind box is on its way, the mood inside the tent turns serious. Wanda Barzizza, the first of three judges, arrives at the 'Cue Crew tent. Callaghan delivers his well-practiced spiel: "We're here to win, not to party. We know it takes a 10 to win, and we're confident our ribs are a 10."

Build a Backyard Rig

Create a championship-worthy smoker with the following essential components.

THE GRILL Gas grills can't sustain the low temperatures needed for barbecue, so you'll need a charcoal grill. Models range from the basic (a kettle grill or an upright bullet smoker) to elaborate rigs with separate smoke boxes. A kettle grill is more versatile than a bullet smoker, since you can use it for both direct, high-heat grilling and indirect-heat cooking. Seek out a model with a wide cooking surface and a built-in thermometer, like the Weber One-Touch Gold 26.75" grill ($300, amazon.com).

THE COALS Even though briquettes are cheaper and easier to find, they have chemical binders that affect your food's taste, says Joe Carroll. Pick hardwood charcoal instead. "It produces a deep, smoky flavor that matches barbecue perfectly." We like Frontier Hard Lump Charcoal ($12 for a 20-pound bag, ace-hardware.com).

THE WOOD Real barbecue means smoky barbecue, and that's where wood comes in. Adding a fragrant wood creates smoke that infuses your food as it cooks. Match lighter proteins like chicken or turkey with fruitwoods like apple or cherry. Richer meats like beef or pork can stand up to stronger hickory wood. If you can't find any suppliers in your area, try firewood.com.

He goes into detail about the humanely raised pork, but the judge needs no convincing. The ribs speak for themselves: Barzizza devours them and gnaws the bones. As she leaves the tent, the entire team gives her a big round of applause. The next two judges seem to dig the pig just as much as the first one did. Then judging is over.

After a couple hours of drinking and waiting, the 'Cue Crew hears the verdicts: The team didn't make the top three. In fact, their ribs placed a respectable but unspectacular 57th out of 113, while the beef ranked 40th out of 92. The chicken tanked entirely, probably a victim of undercooking. There will be no fist-pumping on the awards stage today. But none of that seems to matter to the team. As the party begins to flow, more ribs land on the table, along with gifts from neighbors—a tray of steaming crawfish, a bag of frozen Jell-O shots.

"If those ribs weren't right, I'd be the first one to say so," Stage says, sucking down a purple lozenge of Jell-O and wincing. "But I was really proud of the ribs we turned in."

Through the haze of smoke and trash talk, mud and booze, bare-bones equipment and tight timelines, the 'Cue Crew have managed to hold their own against some of the best barbecue in the country. And as they toast their fortitude, Samuel puts the experience into perspective for men everywhere. "Real barbecue isn't about winning over anonymous judges anyway," he says. "It's about making your family and friends happy. And once you start doing that, you won't ever stop."

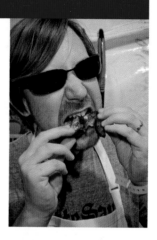

Joe Carroll

Pair this delicious chicken with
Central BBQ's Baked Beans.

Cumin and Espresso Chicken

- **1** cup dark-brown sugar
- **1** cup kosher salt
- **1** cup ground espresso-roast coffee
- **2** tbsp ground cinnamon
- **2** tbsp garlic powder
- **2** tsp ground cumin
- **1** tsp cayenne pepper
- **1** whole chicken (3 to 4 pounds)
  Butter or olive oil, for basting
- **1** to 2 fruitwood chunks or 1 cup of chips, soaked in water for 20 minutes and then drained

Pour 2 gallons of hot water into a large stockpot. Mix in the sugar, salt, coffee, cinnamon, garlic powder, cumin, and cayenne and stir until dissolved. Let the brine cool, then add the chicken and refrigerate it for 24 to 48 hours.

Fire up your barbecue and add the wood. (See "Go Low and Slow" on page 61.) Remove the chicken from the brine, wipe off the spices with a paper towel, and pat the chicken dry. Rub a generous amount of butter or oil under and over the skin.

Place the chicken on the grill, breast side up. Cook at 225° to 250°F, basting occasionally, until the juices run clear when you pierce the chicken at the hip joint, or the internal temperature reaches 165°F—about 2 hours. Let it rest for 10 minutes before carving.

Makes 4 servings

**Per serving: 519 calories, 41 g protein,
2 g carbohydrates, 37 g fat, 12.6 g saturated fat,
0 g fiber, 959 mg sodium**

Central BBQ Baked Beans

A few cans of baked beans isn't where this classic side dish ends—it's where it begins. At Central BBQ, in Memphis, fresh vegetables and spices amp up the flavor.

- **3** cans (28 oz each) baked beans (any brand)
- **½** red bell pepper, chopped
- **½** green bell pepper, chopped
- **¼** cup brown sugar
- **1** tbsp fresh garlic, minced
- **½** tbsp cayenne pepper
- **1** tbsp chili powder
- **1** onion, diced
- **¼** tsp white pepper
- **½** cup yellow mustard
- **½** cup BBQ sauce (any brand)

Preheat the oven to 275°F.

In a large bowl, combine all ingredients and pour into a 2-quart baking dish. Bake until the vegetables are tender and the flavors have blended, about 1½ hours.

Makes 12 servings

**Per serving: 260 calories, 11 g protein,
51 g carbohydrates, 4 g fat, 1 g saturated fat,
12 g fiber, 1,870 mg sodium**

John Stage and Kenny Callaghan

Pair these, and you'll never hit the (barbecue sauce) bottle again.

John Stage and Kenny Callaghan, part of the *Men's Health* 'Cue Crew.

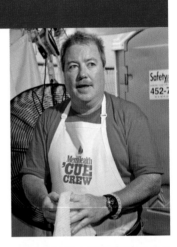

Backyard Baby Backs

Rib Rub
Real BBQ Sauce
2   slabs (2 pounds each)
    baby back or loin back ribs
¼   cup pineapple juice
    Plus 3 cups wood chips
    (apple or cherry), soaked
    20 minutes and drained

Fire up the grill and add the wood. (See "Go Low and Slow" on page 63.) Pour ⅛ inch of water into a large foil pan. Remove the grill grate, place the pan next to the coals, and replace the grate.

In a bowl, combine the Rib Rub ingredients. Coat the ribs on both sides with ¼ cup rub. Place the ribs opposite the fire, over the water pan. Cover and cook at 250°F.

Meanwhile, make the Real BBQ Sauce. After the ribs have cooked for 2 hours, remove them and place each rack on a large sheet of foil. Add 2 tablespoons of pineapple juice to each rack, wrap them tightly, and return them to the grill.

Cook the ribs until the meat begins to loosen from the bone, 45 to 60 minutes. Remove the ribs from the foil and return them to the grill, sprinkling them lightly with more rub.

Cook the ribs for 20 more minutes, then brush the glaze on both sides. Keep cooking the meat until it tears easily between the bones and the rack bends when you hold it in the middle with tongs, another 25 to 40 minutes.

Makes 8 servings

Per serving: 688 calories, 37 g protein, 11 g carbohydrates, 54 g fat, 20 g saturated fat, 0 g fiber, 388 mg sodium

Real BBQ Sauce

2   tbsp vegetable oil
½   cup minced onion
¼   cup minced green pepper
½   jalapeño pepper,
    seeded and minced
1   tbsp minced garlic
    Pinch kosher salt
1   can (15 oz) tomato sauce
1   cup ketchup
½   cup honey
½   cup water
6   tbsp dark brown sugar
6   tbsp Worcestershire sauce
¼   cup apple-cider vinegar
2   tbsp lemon juice
2   tbsp molasses
2   tbsp sambal chili sauce
2   tbsp cayenne-pepper sauce,
    such as Frank's Red Hot
2   tbsp spicy brown mustard
½   tbsp chili powder
1   tsp coarsely ground black
    pepper
¼   tsp ground allspice
½   tbsp liquid smoke (optional)

In a large saucepan, heat the oil and add the onion, green pepper, jalapeño, and garlic, cooking them until soft, about 10 minutes. Add the kosher salt, tomato sauce, ketchup, honey, water, sugar, Worcestershire sauce, vinegar, lemon juice, molasses, chili sauce, cayenne-pepper sauce, brown mustard, chili powder, black pepper, allspice, and liquid smoke, if using, and bring the mixture to a boil, stirring occasionally. Pour the sauce into a container and set aside.

Makes about 5 cups

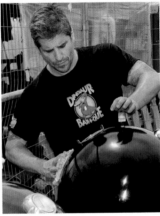

Rib Rub

¼   cup paprika
¼   cup kosher salt
¼   cup dark brown sugar
2½   tbsp granulated garlic
2   tbsp granulated onion
2   tbsp chili powder
1   tbsp coarsely ground black
     pepper
2   tsp ground cumin
½   tsp cayenne pepper

In a medium bowl, mix all ingredients together. Pour into a container and set aside.

Makes 1⅓ cups

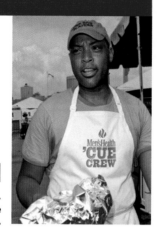

Craig Samuel

Try this fall-off-the-bone meat.

**Craig Samuel, part of the
Men's Health 'Cue Crew.**

Smoke Joint Prime

1½ cups dark brown sugar
½ cup kosher salt
½ cup butcher-grind black pepper ($4, spicebarn.com)
or coarsely ground black pepper
3 tbsp paprika
1 tbsp smoked paprika or chili powder
1 tsp cayenne pepper
1 tsp garlic powder
½ tsp onion powder
½ tsp mustard powder
1 boneless rib eye roast (10 to 14 pounds)
1 to 3 hickory chunks, or 2 cups chips soaked for 20 minutes and then drained

In a large bowl, combine ½ cup of the brown sugar with the salt, black pepper, paprika, smoked paprika or chili powder, cayenne pepper, garlic powder, onion powder, and mustard powder. Generously coat the roast with the mixture, but don't rub it in. Loosely cover the roast and refrigerate it for at least 4 hours or up to overnight.

An hour before cooking, remove the roast from the fridge and let it rest at room temperature. Pat the roast dry with a paper towel, taking care not to loosen the spices. Then press the remaining cup of brown sugar onto all sides of the roast.

Fire up the barbecue and add the wood. (See "Go Low and Slow" on page 63.) Fill a large foil pan with ⅛ inch of water. Remove the grill grates, place the pan in the center of the grill (away from the coals), and replace the grates.

Cook at 250°F until a meat thermometer in the thickest part of the meat registers 130°F for rare, around 3½ to 4 hours.

Let the roast rest for 30 minutes before carving, and serve it with the cooking juices from the foil pan.

Makes 10 to 15 servings

Per serving: 529 calories, 68 g protein, 8 g carbohydrates, 24 g fat, 10 g saturated fat, 0.5 g fiber, 1,095 mg sodium

Neely's

Nowadays, Pat and Gina Neely are famous for their Food Network show, but it all started with their first restaurant, Neely's Bar-B-Que, in Memphis. This recipe is a fixture on the menu.

Sweet and Spicy Coleslaw

2 pounds green cabbage
4 carrots
1 medium yellow onion
½ cup mayonnaise
¼ cup mustard
2 tsp apple-cider vinegar
1 cup sugar
1 tsp black pepper
½ tsp cayenne
Salt
Freshly ground black pepper

Quarter the cabbage and remove the core, and cut the carrots and onion into chunks.

In a food processor, grate the vegetables, using the large-holed grater attachment. In a large bowl, toss the vegetables together.

For the dressing, in a medium bowl, whisk together the mayonnaise, mustard, vinegar, sugar, black pepper, and cayenne. Toss the dressing with the vegetables, add salt and pepper to taste, and chill for at least 2 hours.

Makes 8 servings

Per serving: 256 calories, 2 g protein, 37g carbohydrates, 11 g fat, 1.5 g saturated fat, 4 g fiber, 230 mg sodium

BBQ, Rebooted

Want to try a different style of barbecue? Master the art of Korean barbecue and you'll unlock summer's quickest path to an incredible feast.

Talk about an overachiever. Korean barbecue would be plenty tasty even in its simplest state—soy-marinated meat, grilled until its edges become deeply caramelized. But when Korean BBQ hits the table, it comes with a posse: a greed-satisfying spread of cool vegetable salads, spicy kimchi, and crisp lettuce that transforms a dose of protein into an all-star feast. And it all comes together in record time.

"Korean-style barbecue is so simple and so flavorful it will change the way you cook," says Wuchung Kim, executive chef at Don's Bogam, in Manhattan's Koreatown.

Start by steaming rice and prepping the sides, then turn to the meat. Boneless beef short rib, a fatty, flavorful cut, is a classic choice. Kim slices it thin, massages it with an intense marinade, and grills it until it's as tender as a slow-cooked brisket, as full-flavored as a New York strip, and as satisfying as a quarter-pound patty.

At the table, the spectrum of sides and toppings pays off big time. Wrap a piece of meat in a lettuce leaf, and then experiment. Like it spicy? Add kimchi. Want crunch? Tuck in carrot slices. With Korean BBQ, you can customize every bite.

Marinated Beef Kalbi

This Korean standard combines tender, well-marbled beef short ribs with a potent marinade.

- **1** cup low-sodium soy sauce
- **¾** cup sugar
- **2** cups water
- **¼** cup grated onion (see note)
- **¼** cup grated pear, peeled and cored, with juices
- **3** garlic cloves, chopped
- **3** tbsp sake (see note)
- **1** tbsp toasted sesame oil
  Pinch of freshly ground pepper
- **2** pounds lean boneless beef short ribs (or 4-pound bone-in beef short ribs, deboned), sliced ¼" thick (see note)
  Korean hot pepper paste (optional)

In a medium saucepan, bring the soy sauce, sugar, and water to a boil. Remove the pan from the heat, and let cool to room temperature. Stir in the onion, pear, garlic, sake, sesame oil, and pepper, and pour most of the marinade into a large shallow dish, reserving 1½ cups of sauce for serving.

Using a sharp knife, gently score the beef on each side. Add it to the marinade and massage the liquid into the meat. Let stand for 5 minutes.

Heat a grill to medium high. Add the meat and grill until well seared, 3 to 4 minutes on each side. (Turn the meat when blood starts to seep through the surface.)

Cut the meat into bite-size pieces. (Try kitchen shears.) Serve with the reserved marinade and Korean hot-pepper paste for another dose of flavor.

Makes 4 servings

Per serving: 492 calories, 45 g protein, 19g carbohydrates, 25 g fat, 10 g saturated fat, 0.4 g fiber, 1,046 mg sodium

NOTES:

For a faster way to grate, toss the ingredients into a blender or food processor and whir until mostly smooth.

Chef Kim says cheap sake will ruin the taste of the marinade, but expensive sake is for drinking. For best results, use medium-grade sake. Try Gekkeikan brand.

If you can't find boneless short ribs, bone them yourself. Work the tip of a long, thin knife along the bones, peeling the meat away from the ribs. Trim away most of the fat, but leave some for flavor.

Korean-Style Spinach

Sesame oil heightens the earthy flavor of spinach in Chef Kim's easy side. You can also use baby spinach.

2 tbsp toasted sesame oil
1 tbsp minced garlic
1 pound leaf spinach, washed and stems removed, coarsely chopped
2 tbsp soy sauce
1 tbsp sugar
  Pinch of freshly ground pepper
  Toasted sesame seeds

In a large skillet, heat the oil over medium heat until it shimmers. Add the garlic and cook, stirring constantly, for 1 minute, and immediately add the spinach. Cook until the spinach is wilted, about 3 minutes, and reduce the heat to low.

In a small bowl, stir together the soy sauce, sugar, and pepper. Add to the spinach, mix, and remove from the heat. Top with the sesame seeds.

Makes 4 servings

Per serving: 131 calories, 5 g protein, 9 g carbohydrates, 9 g fat, 1 g saturated fat, 3 g fiber, 750 mg sodium

Scallion Salad

The heat of the grilled beef brings out the flavor of this unabashedly oniony salad. Thinly sliced red onion also would work well here instead of the scallions.

4 scallions, trimmed
1 head curly-leaf lettuce, shredded
3 tbsp toasted sesame oil
2 tbsp rice vinegar
1 tsp Korean chili powder (available at Asian markets) or ½ tsp red-pepper flakes
  Salt

Cut the scallions into 2-inch lengths, then cut those pieces lengthwise into thin strips.

In a large bowl, toss together the scallions and lettuce. Add the oil, vinegar, chili powder, and salt to taste. Toss.

Makes 4 servings

Per serving: 122 calories, 2 g protein, 6 g carbohydrates, 11 g fat, 1.5 g saturated fat, 4 g fiber, 15 mg sodium

Sesame Bean Sprouts

This simple Korean BBQ sidekick lends a fresh, crisp contrast to the savory marinated meat.

½ cup water
½ pound mung bean sprouts, rinsed
1 scallion, chopped
½ clove garlic, minced
1½ tsp toasted sesame seeds
1½ tsp Asian sesame oil
¾ tsp salt

In a large pot, bring the water to a boil. Add the sprouts, cover, and boil until just tender, 2 to 3 minutes. Immediately transfer to a colander and rinse with cold water. Drain and squeeze out any excess liquid.

Place the sprouts in a medium bowl. Add the scallion, garlic, sesame seeds, oil, and salt, and stir to combine. Serve warm or chilled.

Makes 4 servings

Per serving: 42 calories, 2 g protein, 4 g carbohydrates, 2 g fat, 0.2 g saturated fat, 1.2 g fiber, 443 mg sodium

The Sides

Serve your Korean barbecue family-style, with a stack of washed, well-dried lettuce leaves (red leaf or Boston varieties work best), thinly sliced carrots, kimchi (spicy Korean pickled cabbage found in Asian markets), and thinly sliced jalapeño. Steamed rice and your pick of these classic Korean side dishes (called banchan) will round out the meal.

Scallion Salad and Sesame Bean Sprouts recipes courtesy of Cecilia Hae-Jin Lee, adapted from Quick & Easy Korean Cooking (Chronicle Books)

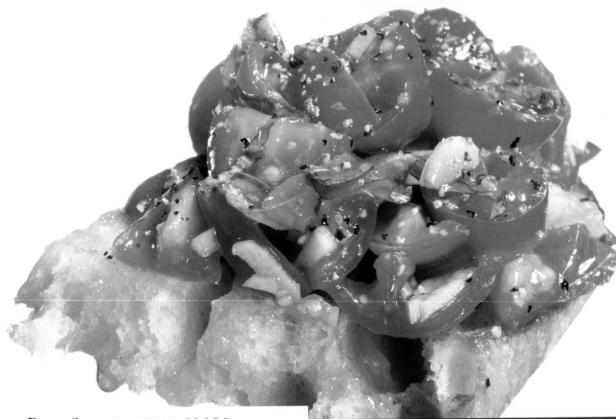

46 Best Snacks for Men

A snack between meals isn't bad for you. But hold off on that chip bag!

You might be surprised to hear that two snacks a day may help charge your metabolism for all-day fat loss. "A good snack has protein or fiber and healthy fats to fill you up so you won't be hungry again in an hour," says Valerie Berkowitz, RD, a nutrition expert at the Center for Balanced Health. Power your diet with these snacks and never go hungry again.

1 This is a simple, elegant snack.

Bruschetta

1 baguette, cut on the diagonal into ½" slices
2 large tomatoes, seeded and chopped
2 cloves garlic, minced
½ cup chopped fresh basil
1 tbsp olive oil
 Salt
 Freshly ground black pepper

Preheat the oven to 450°F.

Place the baguette slices on a baking sheet and bake until they're lightly browned but still soft in the middle.

While the bread bakes, in a medium bowl, mix the tomatoes, garlic, basil, and oil. Season with salt and pepper.

Remove the bread from the oven and arrange on a large serving plate. Top with the tomato mixture.

Makes 4 servings

Per 2 slices: 200 calories, 6 g protein, 35 g carbohydrates, 4 g fat, 0.5 g saturated fat, 1 g fiber, 411 mg sodium

2 Pop a 1.6-ounce bag of plain popcorn. Pour the popcorn into a bowl and toss it with chopped rosemary, olive oil, and finely grated Parmesan. Share with her for an inexpensive gourmet alternative on date night.

Per batch: 313 calories, 7 g protein, 34 g carbohydrates, 17 g fat, 3 g saturated fat, 6 g fiber, 80 mg sodium

3 Spread a dollop of gua-camole on a slice of smoked turkey, then roll the turkey up in a slice of Swiss cheese. Secure with a toothpick. Make a batch and serve them on game day.

Per roll-up: 173 calories, 14 g protein, 5 g carbohydrates, 11 g fat, 6.4 g saturated fat, 7 g fiber, 536 mg sodium

4 Remove the pits from a few dates. Stuff each date with an almond and some blue cheese and wrap it tightly with half a strip of bacon. Secure with toothpicks and bake at 400ºF until the bacon is crisp, about 25 minutes. These make amazing party appetizers, too.

Per date: 91 calories, 2 g protein, 6 g carbohydrates, 6.5 g fat, 2.3 g saturated fat, 0.7 g fiber, 134 mg sodium

5 This bagel sandwich really satisfies.

Vegetable Bagel Grinder

1 bagel, split
1 tbsp fat-free cream cheese
⅓ cucumber, thinly sliced
⅓ tomato, finely chopped
1 portobello mushroom, thinly sliced
2 slices reduced-fat or fat-free Swiss cheese

Preheat the broiler.

In a toaster oven, lightly toast the bagel halves. Top them with the cream cheese, cucumber, tomato, mushroom, and cheese. Place them on a broiler rack and broil for 4 minutes, or until the cheese is melted.

Per bagel half: 268 calories, 16 g protein, 41 g carbohydrates, 5 g fat, 2 g saturated fat, 3 g fiber, 436 mg sodium

6 Sandwich a hunk of mozzarella or Swiss between two olives on a toothpick. (Pesto drizzle optional.)

Per 2-hunk serving: 201 calories, 12 g protein, 2.5 g carbohydrates, 16 g fat, 9.1 g saturated fat, 0.5 g fiber, 389 mg sodium

7 One wouldn't think a snack called "towers" could be healthy, but this one is.

Caprese Tomato Towers

- **4** medium tomatoes (preferably heirloom tomatoes of various colors)
- **6** ounces fresh mozzarella
- **16** large fresh basil leaves
- **1** tbsp olive oil
- **½** tsp balsamic vinegar
  Salt
  Freshly ground black pepper

Cut the tomatoes into thick slices. (One should yield four or five slices.) Slice the cheese into slightly thinner discs. (You should have an equal number of tomato and cheese slices.)

Place a tomato in the center of a small plate. Top with a mozzarella slice and a single basil leaf. Repeat until you've used up one-fourth of the tomatoes, cheese, and basil. (If you really want to nail this, salt and pepper each individual layer.) If you're using tomatoes of different colors, alternate the slices. Repeat with the rest of the tomatoes, cheese, and basil, making four towers in all.

Drizzle each tower with a bit of olive oil and balsamic vinegar, and season again with salt and pepper.

Makes 4 servings

Per serving: 189 calories, 10 g protein, 6 g carbohydrates, 14 g fat, 7.2 g saturated fat, 1.5 g fiber, 219 mg sodium

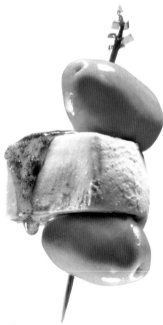

8 Lay out slices of prosciutto or another type of thinly sliced ham. Mix chopped olives and sun-dried tomatoes with fresh ricotta, then place a spoonful on the center of each prosciutto slice. Wrap and eat like a soft taco—a guilt-free soft taco, that is.

Per 2 wraps: 144 calories, 12 g protein, 5 g carbohydrates, 9 g fat, 3.8 g saturated fat, 1 g fiber, 1,013 mg sodium

9 Teriyaki Scallops: Toss 8 large sea scallops with ¼ cup teriyaki marinade and marinate them for 30 minutes in the refrigerator. Preheat the broiler. Wrap each scallop with ½ to 1 strip bacon to encircle it fully without overlapping. (Stretch the bacon fairly thin—it crisps up better that way.) Thread a toothpick through each wrapped scallop to secure the bacon. Brush with a bit more teriyaki marinade, then place the scallops in the oven 6 inches beneath the broiler. Cook for 10 to 12 minutes, until the scallops are firm and the bacon is fully cooked.

Per 2 scallops: 135 calories, 8 g protein, 2 g carbohydrates, 10 g fat, 3.4 g saturated fat, 0 g fiber, 444 mg sodium

10 These mini pizzas are sure to satisfy.

Pesto–Goat Cheese Mini Pizzas

- **2** tbsp basil pesto
- **2** English muffins, split
- **4** tbsp goat cheese
- **2** tbsp chopped green or kalamata olives
- **4** jarred or canned artichoke hearts, quartered

Preheat the oven to 425°F.

Divide the pesto among the four muffin halves, then add the cheese, olives, and artichokes. Place the muffins on a baking sheet and bake for about 5 minutes, until the cheese is melted and the bottoms are slightly crisp.

Makes 4 servings

Per muffin half: 161 calories, 6 g protein, 16 g carbohydrates, 8 g fat, 3.1 g saturated fat, 1.5 g fiber, 382 mg sodium

11 Arrange marinated artichoke hearts, roasted red peppers, and good olives on a platter with a chunk of real Parmesan (or manchego or Gruyére) and a thin slice of nice ham.

Per two pieces each of artichoke, pepper, and cheese, plus four olives and one slice of ham: 216 calories, 16 g protein, 13 g carbohydrates, 12 g fat, 5.6 g saturated fat, 4 g fiber, 1,073 mg sodium

12 Thread chunks of watermelon, cherry tomatoes, small balls of fresh mozzarella, and a few basil leaves on wooden skewers. It's summer on a stick.

Per two tomatoes, two chunks of melon, and one cheese ball: 142 calories, 8 g protein, 6 g carbohydrates, 10 g fat, 6 g saturated fat, 0.6 g fiber, 27 mg sodium

13 Not all healthy snacks require chewing. Try this mocktail: Pour ¾ cup of vegetable juice and stir in 1 teaspoon each of horse-radish and hot sauce. (Recipe by Valerie Berkowitz, RD.)

Per ¾-cup serving: 43 calories, 1 g protein, 9 g carbohydrates, 0 g fat, 0 g saturated fat, 12 g fiber, 267 mg sodium

14 Skip the frozen concoctions and make these handmade crab cakes instead.

Crab Cakes

1 can (16 ounces) jumbo lump crab meat
2 tbsp minced jalapeño
2 scallions, chopped
½ cup minced red bell pepper
1 egg, lightly beaten
2 tsp Dijon mustard
Juice of 1 lemon
¼ tsp Old Bay seasoning
½ tsp salt
¾ cup bread crumbs

Preheat the oven to 425°F.

In a medium bowl, gently mix together the crab meat, jalapeño, scallions, pepper, egg, mustard, lemon juice, Old Bay seasoning, salt, and ¼ cup of the bread crumbs. Using your hands, loosely form the crab mixture into eight patties.

Spread the remaining bread crumbs on a plate and roll each patty over the crumbs to lightly and evenly coat it. Shape the crab cakes, using the palm of your hand to press each one into an evenly shaped disk the size of a small hockey puck. Place them on a nonstick baking sheet or in a baking dish that you've coated with nonstick cooking spray.

Bake for 12 to 15 minutes, until golden brown on the outside.

Makes 4 servings

Per 2 crab cakes: 212 calories, 25 g protein, 19 g carbohydrates, 3.6 g fat, 1 g saturated fat, 1 g fiber, 910 mg sodium

15 Wrap a strip of prosciutto or good Spanish ham around a slice of honeydew melon or cantaloupe. The salty-sweet combo blows away chocolate–covered pretzels.

Per wrapped slice: 88 calories, 5 g protein, 15 g carbohydrates, 2 g fat, 0.6 g saturated fat, 1 g fiber, 404 mg sodium

16 Halve an avocado, remove the pit, and drape each piece with two anchovy fillets. Drizzle with olive oil. Eat the avocado directly out of the skin with a spoon for easy cleanup.

Per avocado half: 188 calories, 4 g protein, 9 g carbohydrates, 17 g fat, 2.4 g saturated fat, 7 g fiber, 300 mg sodium

17 Place a hunk of halloumi cheese (buy it at Whole Foods or in Greek markets) directly on the grill. Cook until lightly charred on the outside, about 2 minutes a side. Top with olive oil and fresh herbs. Serve on a salad, atop thin crackers or toast, or eat as is.

Per 1.5-ounce slice: 145 calories, 8 g protein, 1.5 g carbohydrates, 18 g fat, 9.2 g saturated fat, 0 g fiber, 660 mg sodium

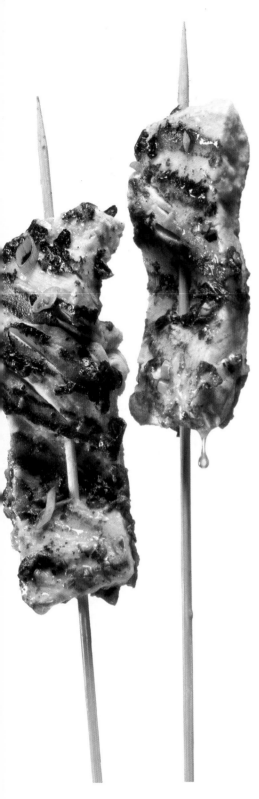

18 Peel a mango and cut it into spears. Top with fresh lime juice and a couple of shakes of chili powder. It'll satisfy both sweet and spicy cravings.

Per mango: 139 calories, 1 g protein, 37 g carbohydrates, 0.6 g fat, 0.1 g saturated fat, 4 g fiber, 6 mg sodium

19 Top whole–wheat crackers with a schmear of low–fat cream cheese, smoked salmon, thinly sliced red onion, a few capers, and a squirt of lemon juice.

Per 2 crackers: 259calories, 36 g protein, 8 g carbohydrates, 9 g fat, 2.5 g saturated fat, 1 g fiber, 237 mg sodium

20 At first, tuna and peanut butter might seem like an odd combo, but it works!

Tuna Skewers

½ tablespoon peanut or vegetable oil
1 tbsp minced fresh ginger
1 clove garlic, minced
2 tbsp peanut butter
1 cup light coconut milk
½ tbsp low-sodium soy sauce
   Juice of 1 lime
1 tsp sriracha or other hot sauce
1 pound ahi tuna, cut into 8 long pieces
8 wooden skewers, soaked in cold water for at least 20 minutes

In a medium saucepan, heat the oil over medium heat. Cook the ginger and garlic until lightly toasted, about 1 minute. Add the peanut butter, coconut milk, and soy sauce. Simmer on low heat for 10 minutes. Add the lime juice and sriracha and remove from the heat.

Heat a grill or stovetop grill pan. Thread each piece of tuna onto a skewer and brush it all over with the sauce. Cook for about 2 minutes on each side, until charred on the outside but still pink in the center. Serve the skewers with the remaining sauce.

Makes 4 servings

Per 2 skewers: 230 calories, 29 g protein, 4 g carbohydrates, 10 g fat, 4.4 g saturated fat, 1 g fiber, 181 mg sodium

21 Toss pumpkin seeds with olive oil and salt, and toast the seeds in a 375°F oven until puffed and golden, about 30 minutes. Finish with lemon juice and a dusting of Spanish paprika. (Recipe by Seamus Mullen, chef at Boqueria in New York.)

Per 2 tablespoons: 149 calories, 5 g protein, 3 g carbohydrates, 13 g fat, 2 g saturated fat, 0.7 g fiber, 585 mg sodium

22 Chop two hard–boiled eggs and mix with diced pickles, a spoon of olive–oil mayonnaise, spicy mustard, and a pinch of cayenne. Spoon the egg salad onto romaine or Bibb lettuce and eat like a burrito.

Per 2 eggs: 194 calories, 13 g protein, 2 g carbohydrates, 14 g fat, 4 g saturated fat, 0.5 g fiber, 298 mg sodium

23 Yes, you can have chips—these chips, anyway.

Spiced Sweet-Potato Chips

- **1** sweet potato, peeled (12 ounce)
- **½** tsp ground cumin
- **¼** tsp sugar
- **¼** tsp chili powder
- **¼** teaspoon salt

Preheat the oven to 375°F. Coat two baking sheets with cooking spray.

Cut the potato into very thin slices. Arrange the slices on the sheets in a single layer and lightly coat the slices with cooking spray. Bake for 7 minutes, until they've barely started to brown. Remove, turn them over, return to the oven, and bake 7 to 10 more minutes, until lightly browned. Transfer to a bowl, and repeat with the remaining potato slices.

Meanwhile, in a small bowl, combine the cumin, sugar, chili powder, and salt. Pour over the chips, toss well, and serve immediately.

Makes 2 servings

Per serving: 151 calories, 3 g protein, 35 g carbohydrates, 0 g fat, 0 g saturated fat, 5 g fiber, 385 mg sodium

24 Slice half of a small apple into 4 ounces of cottage cheese. Stir in a little cinnamon and honey.

Per 4 ounces: 156calories, 13g protein, 1.5 g carbohydrates, 5 g fat, 2 g saturated fat, 2 g fiber, 413 mg sodium

25 Combine a sliced Fuji apple with ½ fennel bulb, shaved; 2 tablespoons

red-wine vinegar; and 1 tablespoon Parmesan cheese. (Recipe by Mike Price, chef at Market Table in New York.)

Per apple: 144 calories, 5 g protein, 29 g carbohydrates, 1 g fat, 7 g saturated fat, 7 g fiber, 187 mg sodium

26 Slice an Asian pear in half and eat with a little blue cheese for a tasty protein kick.

Per pear half: 158 calories, 7 g protein, 15 g carbohydrates, 8 g fat, 5.3 g saturated fat, 5 g fiber, 395 mg sodium

27 Munching on potato skins like these is a better choice than tearing open a bag of chips.

Spicy Potato Skins

- **4** small russet potatoes
   Olive oil
   Salt
   Freshly ground black pepper
- **1** cup 2% milk
- **2** tbsp butter
- **½** cup shredded sharp Cheddar cheese, plus more for garnish
- **4** scallions, chopped, plus more for garnish
- **½** tbsp minced chipotle pepper
- **¼** cup sour cream
- **6** strips bacon, cooked and crumbled
   Pickled jalapeños

Preheat the oven to 400°F. Rub the potatoes with a bit of olive oil and lightly salt the skins. Bake for 35 to 40 minutes, until tender.

Halve the potatoes lengthwise and, when they're cool enough to

handle, carefully scoop out the warm flesh into a bowl. (Leave a thin layer of potato intact around the skin to help prevent it from tearing.) Add the milk, butter, cheese, and scallions, and stir with a wooden spoon until smooth. Season with salt and pepper.

Preheat the broiler. Carefully scoop the mashed potatoes into the hollowed-out potato halves. Top with a bit of extra cheese and place under the broiler until the tops are brown and crispy, 3 to 5 minutes.

In a small bowl, mix the chipotle pepper with the sour cream and place a dollop on top of each potato half. Finish each with a bit of crumbled bacon and jalapeños.

Makes 4 servings

Per potato half: 243 calories, 8 g protein, 20 g carbohydrates, 15 g fat, 6.7 g saturated fat, 1 g fiber, 307 mg sodium

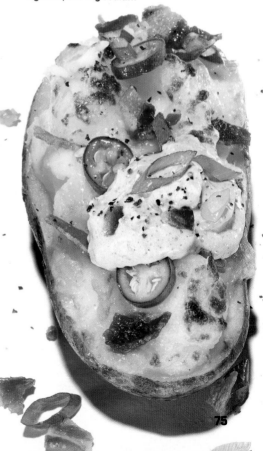

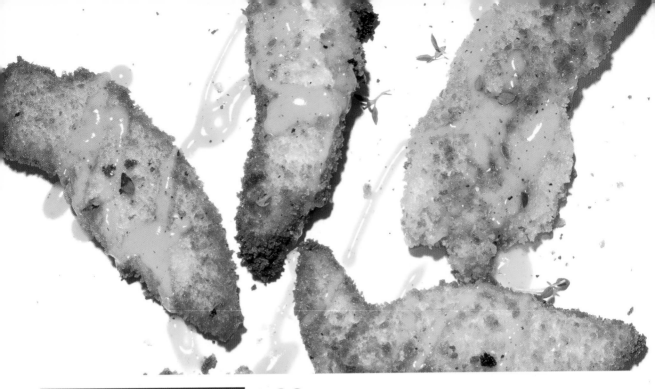

Nine More Fast, Easy Snacks

BEST SNACK FOR A DESK DRAWER:
2 tablespoons peanuts, 4 tablespoons dried cranberries

BEST SNACK FOR THE OFFICE MINI-FRIDGE: 2 cups baby carrots plus 4 tablespoons hummus

BEST CHEESE SNACK: Laughing Cow Mini Babybel (3 pieces)

BEST LATE-NIGHT AFTER-THE-BAR SNACK: 2 eggs with one slice wholewheat toast

BEST SNACK FOR YOUR GLOVE COMPARTMENT: Golden Valley Natural Beef Jerky (1 ounce)

BEST SNACK FOR POTATO-CHIP CRAVINGS: Popchips (1 ounce)

BEST ANYTIME SNACK: 1 tablespoon peanut butter

BEST CHOCOLATE CRAVING CRUSHER: Emerald Cocoa Roast Almonds, Dark Chocolate (1 ounce)

BEST ON-THE-GO BAR: Larabar Pecan Pie

28 Don't drive-thru; make these chicken fingers at home.

Chicken Fingers

1	pound boneless, skinless chicken tenders
	Salt
	Freshly ground black pepper
3	egg whites, lightly beaten
2	cups panko bread crumbs
2	tbsp Dijon mustard
1	tsp chipotle pepper puree
1	tbsp honey

Preheat the oven to 450°F. Coat a baking sheet with cooking spray.

Season the chicken with salt and pepper.

In a shallow bowl, place the egg whites. On a plate, place the crumbs (season them too). Dip the chicken into the egg and toss them in the crumbs.

Place the breaded chicken pieces on the prepared baking sheet. Bake for 10 to 12 minutes, until the crumbs have browned and the chicken is firm.

In a large bowl, combine the mustard, chipotle, and honey. Toss the cooked chicken tenders in the mixture so they are all evenly coated.

Makes 4 servings

Per serving: 276 calories, 31 g protein, 26 g carbohydrates, 4 g fat, 0.6 g saturated fat, 1 g fiber, 474 mg sodium

29 Skip sweetened yogurts. Instead, try FoodShouldTasteGood chocolate tortilla chips. Crush a few into a cup of fat-free vanilla yogurt.

Per cup: 293 calories, 14 g protein, 51 g carbohydrates, 4 g fat, 0.7 g saturated fat, 1.5 g fiber, 208 mg sodium

30 Mix a variety of cooked beans, red-wine vinegar, extra-virgin olive oil, finely chopped red onions, thyme, and rosemary. Add salt and pepper. (Recipe by Cesare Casella, chef at Salumeria Rosi Parmacotto, New York.)

Per half cup: 246 calories, 8 g protein, 22 g carbohydrates, 14 g fat, 2 g saturated fat, 7 g fiber, 506 mg sodium

31 Use snacks to complete your nutrition plan, not wreck it.

Pot Stickers

- 24 frozen pot stickers (chicken, pork, or vegetable)
- 1 tbsp sesame or peanut oil
- 4 ounces mushrooms (preferably shiitake), stems removed, sliced
- 2 cups sugar snap or snow peas, tough ends removed
- 1 tbsp soy sauce
- 1 tbsp rice vinegar
  Sriracha hot sauce
  Sesame seeds (optional)
  Sliced scallions (optional)

Bring a large pot of water to a boil. Drop in the pot stickers and cook for a few minutes, until they're tender but not gummy. Drain.

In a large nonstick skillet or sauté pan, heat the oil over medium heat. Add the mushrooms and cook for 2 to 3 minutes, until lightly browned. Add the cooked pot stickers to the pan and cook, undisturbed, until they're crispy and browned on the bottom, 2 to 3 minutes on each side. In the last minute of cooking, toss in the peas and warm through.

Remove the pan from the heat. Stir in the soy sauce, vinegar, and sriracha to taste. Divide among four bowls and, if you choose, garnish with sesame seeds and scallions.

Makes 4 servings

Per serving: 513 calories, 22 g protein, 57 g carbohydrates, 22 g fat, 6 g saturated fat, 5 g fiber, 2,272 mg sodium

32 Peanuts are very rich in nutrients. Here's an unusual way to enjoy them.

Curried Peanuts

- 2 tsp canola oil
- 1 cup dry-roasted unsalted peanuts
- 1 tsp curry powder
- ¼ onion, chopped
- 2 tbsp chopped cilantro
- ⅛ tsp salt
  Pinch of red pepper

In a skillet, heat the oil for 1 minute on medium. Add the peanuts and curry powder. Cook, stirring constantly, for about 2 minutes, or until golden. Add the onion, cilantro, salt, and ground red pepper. Cook for 2 minutes. Serve warm or at room temperature.

Makes 8 servings

Per serving: 119 calories, 4 g protein, 4 g carbohydrates, 10 g fat, 1.3 g saturated fat, 2 g fiber, 37 mg sodium

33 Hit the sushi section for seaweed salad, which packs plenty of vitamins and minerals.

Per 4 ounces: 91 calories, 3 g protein, 10 g carbohydrates, 5 g fat, 0.8g saturated fat, 0.5 g fiber, 989 mg sodium

34 Pour 1 tablespoon of olive oil onto a plate and add a dash each of salt, pepper, dried rosemary, and dried thyme. Dip a hunk of whole-wheat bread.

Per slice: 196 calories, 4 g protein, 12g carbohydrates, 15 g fat, 2.2 g saturated fat, 2 g fiber, 278 mg sodium

35 Place halved, pitted peaches on a foil-lined baking sheet. Top with a dab of butter and a sprinkle of sugar. Cook at 400ºF for a half hour. Finish with cinnamon.

Per 2 peach halves: 112 calories, 1 g protein, 20 g carbohydrates, 4 g fat, 2.5 g saturated fat, 3 g fiber, 1 mg sodium

36 Baba ghanoush is made from eggplant, which gives it a creamy texture. Scoop it with a handful of pita chips.

Per cup: 293 calories, 14 g protein, 51 g carbohydrates, 4 g fat, 0.7 g saturated fat, 1.5 g fiber, 208 mg sodium

37 Fried calamari clobbers your gut. Try it sautéed.

Sautéed Calamari

- 2 tsp olive oil
- 2 cups calamari
  Salt
  Freshly ground black pepper
  Spanish paprika
  Lemon juice

In a sauté pan, heat the oil on medium high. Season the calamari with salt and pepper and cook it for 2 to 4 minutes, stirring frequently, until the flesh turns white. Serve sprinkled with paprika and drizzled with lemon juice.

Makes 4 servings

Per serving: 125 calories, 18 g protein, 4 g carbohydrates, 4 g fat, 0.7 g saturated fat, 0 g fiber, 86 mg sodium

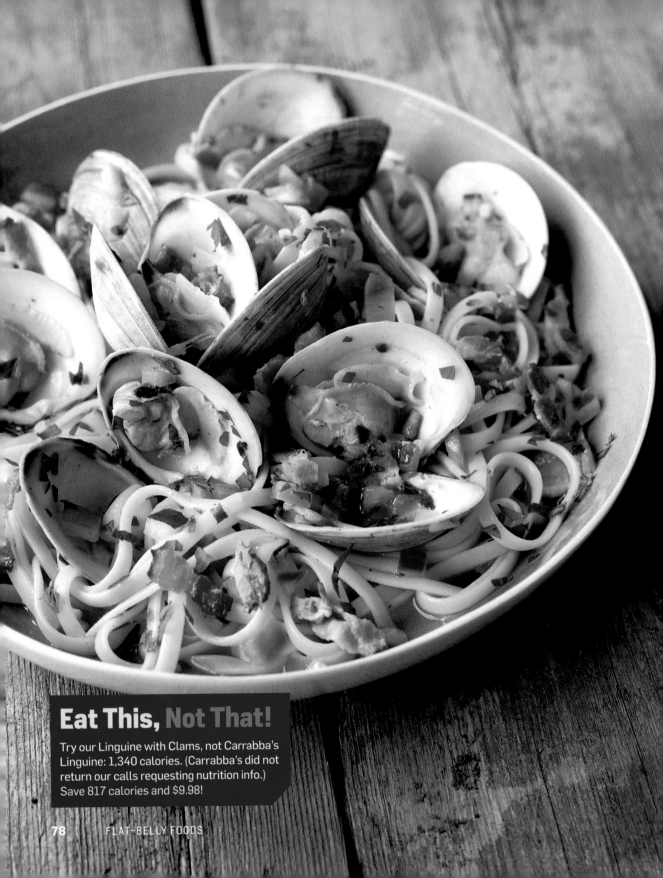

Eat This, Not That!

Try our Linguine with Clams, not Carrabba's Linguine: 1,340 calories. (Carrabba's did not return our calls requesting nutrition info.) Save 817 calories and $9.98!

Your Favorite Restaurant Dishes— At Home

Cook this, not that—cheaper, healthier, and tastier

Your most important food decision isn't what to order from a menu. It's whether to hop into the car, drive to a restaurant, wait for a table, and pick up that menu in the first place.

By the time you've made the trip and scored a table, you could be sitting down at home to a meal that tastes better, costs less, and is much healthier than the caloric bombs you'd tip a waitress to bring you.

The restaurant world is hazardous for any man hoping to control his weight. If you're looking for a burger, a plate of pasta—or even just a salad—it's difficult to find an entree that comes in under 1,000 calories. What's worse, you could end up ingesting a few days' worth of sodium, bad fats, and refined carbs.

There's a better way. In this excerpt from our new book, *Cook This, Not That!* we'll show you how to whip up the kind of food men typically go out for. But you'll make it better. Best of all, these meals are easy (dare we say fun?), especially with a helper and a glass of wine. Let's get started.

Linguine with Clams

Traditionalists cringe, but using lots of sauce and not much pasta saves calories and boosts taste.

Much has been said about the fact that in Italy, sauce comes second; for true paisanos, it's all about the noodle. Call it sacrilege, but we love sauce, and we love to be able to eat a bowl of pasta without ingesting the caloric equivalent of nearly seven glazed doughnuts. We favor a high sauce-to-noodle ratio to maximize flavor and nutrition and minimize waistline expansion.

- **4** bacon slices, cut into thin strips
- **1** red onion, diced
- **2** cloves garlic, minced
  Red pepper flakes (generous pinch)
- **32** littleneck clams
- **1** cup dry white wine
- **12** ounces whole-wheat linguine
- **¼** cup fresh chopped parsley leaves

Heat a large sauté pan on medium and add the bacon. Cook for about 5 minutes, until the fat is rendered and the bacon is browned. Take the pan off the heat. Remove the bacon and set it aside, and pour out all but a film of the fat.

Return the pan to the stove and add the onion, garlic, and pepper flakes. Cook, stirring occasionally, until the onion is translucent, about 3 minutes. Add the clams and white wine and continue to cook over medium heat for about 10 minutes, until most of the wine has evaporated and the clams have opened. (If the clams aren't opening, top the pan with a lid until they do. Discard any clams that never open.)

Bring a large pot of water to boil and cook the linguine according to the package instructions. When the pasta is al dente, drain it, reserving a bit of the cooking water. Add the cooked linguine directly to the sauté pan with the clams. Stir in the parsley and cook for 30 seconds, adding a bit of pasta water if the noodles look dry. Divide the clams and pasta among four warm bowls and serve immediately.

Makes 4 servings

Per serving: 523 calories, 26 g protein, 66 g carbohydrates, 16 g fat, 4.2 g saturated fat, 13 g fiber, 595 mg sodium

Cost per serving: $5.27

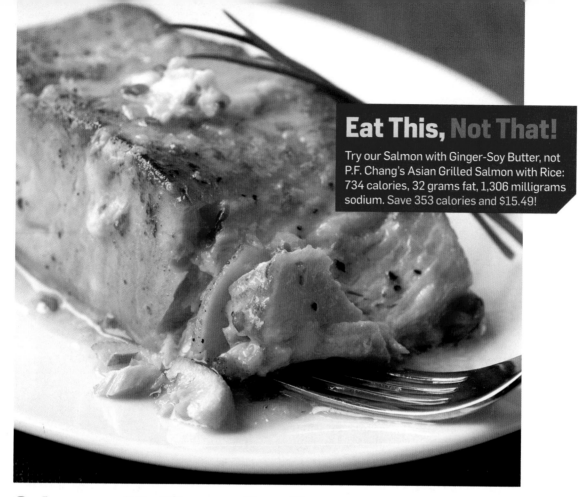

Salmon with Ginger-Soy Butter

Not only can you outcook P.F. Chang's with this salmon dish, but you'll save more than 15 bucks.

Yes, even salmon can suffer at the hands of a restaurant chef who uses oil as a condiment and salt as a main ingredient. A third of salmon's fat is of the heart-healthy monounsaturated variety, but P.F. Chang's has found a way to cram roughly three-quarters of a day's worth of saturated fat into this otherwise super food. Cook it this way instead.

2	tbsp unsalted butter, softened at room temperature for an hour or two
½	tbsp minced chives
½	tbsp fresh ginger, peeled and grated (or minced)
	Juice of 1 lemon
½	tbsp low-sodium soy sauce
1	tbsp olive oil or canola oil
4	salmon fillets, 4 to 6 ounces each
1	tsp salt
	Freshly ground black pepper

In a bowl, combine the butter, chives, ginger, lemon juice, and soy sauce and stir vigorously with a wooden spoon until the ingredients are incorporated. Set aside.

In a large stainless-steel sauté pan, heat the oil over medium-high heat. Season the salmon with salt and pepper; when the oil is lightly smoking, add the fish to the pan, flesh side down. Cook for 4 to 5 minutes, until the skin is lightly charred and crisp. Flip the fish and cook for 2 to 3 minutes more, until the flesh flakes with gentle pressure from your finger but is still slightly translucent in the middle. (Salmon is best served medium, but if you want yours completely cooked, sauté for another 2 to 3 minutes.)

Serve the salmon with a generous spoonful of the flavored butter, which should begin to melt on contact.

Makes 4 servings

Per serving: 381 calories, 29 g protein, 1 g carbohydrates, 28 g fat, 8.4 g saturated fat, 0 g fiber, 733 mg sodium

Cost per serving: $2.46

Sliders Two Ways

Frying up your own sliders produces a tastier, healthier appetizer—or main course.

Never order a menu item described as "mini." Most so-called mini bites come with max fat saturation. Instead, cook up these tasty little burgers at home.

Sliders

½ pound lean ground sirloin
4 small rolls, about 2" round
   Salt
   Freshly ground black pepper

Chipotle-Bacon Topping

2 tbsp mayonnaise
1 tbsp chipotle pepper, chopped
½ ounce shredded sharp Cheddar cheese
4 strips cooked bacon
½ cup caramelized onions

To make Chipotle-Bacon Sliders

In a small bowl, mix the mayo and chipotle together.

Heat a grill pan or cast-iron skillet over medium heat. Season the sirloin with salt and pepper, and lightly form into 4 patties. Add the burgers and cook for 3 minutes on the first side, then flip. Top each patty with Cheddar and continue cooking until the patties are firm and the cheese starts to melt.

Toast the rolls in the pan and spread each with some of the mayo mixture. Top with burgers, bacon, and caramelized onions.

Makes 4 sliders

Per serving: 266 calories, 18 g protein, 14 g carbohydrates, 15 g fat, 4 g saturated fat, 1 g fiber, 455 mg sodium

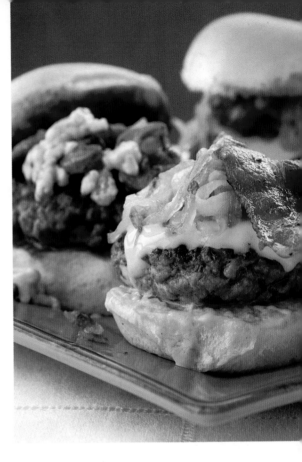

Mushroom–Blue Cheese Topping

2 teaspoons olive oil
1 clove garlic, minced
1¼ cups sliced mushrooms
   Salt
   Freshly ground black pepper
2 tbsp steak sauce
¼ cup crumbled blue cheese

To make Mushroom–Blue Cheese Sliders

Heat a grill pan or cast-iron skillet over medium heat. Add the oil and garlic and sauté for 60 seconds, until fragrant but not brown. Add the mushrooms; sauté for 2 to 3 minutes, until the mushrooms are caramelized. Season with salt and pepper.

Cook the burgers as above, brushing them with steak sauce before and after and topping with blue cheese crumbles after flipping.

Place the burgers on toasted buns brushed with steak sauce, and top with mushrooms.

Makes 4 sliders

Per serving: 204 calories, 17 g protein, 16 g carbohydrates, 9 g fat, 3.3 g saturated fat, 1 g fiber, 472 mg sodium

Cost per serving: $2.09

Dr Pepper Ribs

We tap into the surprisingly complex flavor of Dr Pepper to create a perfectly balanced sauce.

Order ribs at a restaurant and you could gain a full pound by the time the bill comes. Think we're kidding? Outback's ribs have more calories than 15 Krispy Kreme Original doughnuts and more saturated fat than you should consume in 4 days. With our at-home option, we suggest half a rack.

2 racks baby back ribs
1 large (2-liter) bottle of Dr Pepper
¼ cup salt
1 tbsp chili powder
1 cup water
½ tbsp canola oil or vegetable oil
½ onion, minced
1 clove garlic, minced
½ cup ketchup
2 tbsp Worcestershire sauce
2 tbsp cider vinegar
⅛ teaspoon cayenne pepper

In a large baking dish, place the ribs. Pour in Dr Pepper to cover them, reserving at least ½ cup for the sauce. Add the salt and soak the ribs in the fridge overnight (or at least 2 hours).

Preheat the oven to 350°F.

Remove the ribs from the liquid, dry them, and rub with the chili powder. Place them on a baking dish, add the water, and cover tightly with foil. Cook for 2 hours, until the meat nearly falls off the bone.

For the barbecue sauce, in a saucepan, heat the oil over medium heat. Sauté the onion and garlic until they're soft and fragrant, and add the ketchup, Worcestershire, vinegar, cayenne, and ½ cup of Dr Pepper. Simmer for 15 to 20 minutes, or until the sauce thickens.

Fire up the grill, and brush the ribs with sauce. When the grill is hot, cook them bone side down on a cooler part for 10 to 15 minutes. Flip them and cook until lightly charred and smoky. Remove, and brush on more sauce.

Makes 4 servings
Per serving: 921 calories, 47 g protein, 27 g carbohydrates, 69 g fat, 25 g saturated fat, 1g fiber, 4,160 mg sodium
Cost per serving: $5.17

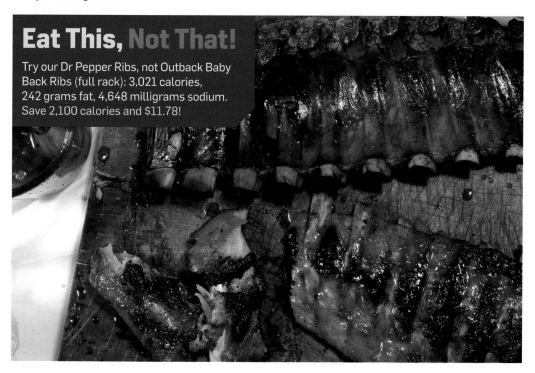

Eat This, Not That!

Try our Dr Pepper Ribs, not Outback Baby Back Ribs (full rack): 3,021 calories, 242 grams fat, 4,648 milligrams sodium. Save 2,100 calories and $11.78!

Beer-Can Chicken

The beer you left in the can (you left some, right?) keeps the chicken moist and tender.

Whole chickens mounted on beer cans have become familiar sights in backyard barbecues. And for good reason: The liquid creates steam that helps cook the chicken from the inside and keep it moist. Also, standing the bird vertically means the legs, which take the most time to cook, are exposed to the most intense heat. That way it cooks evenly without drying out the breast. The result: one of the tastiest chickens imaginable. Serve with baked beans and coleslaw.

1	whole chicken (3 to 4 pounds)
24	ounces Coca-Cola
¾	tsp salt
	Freshly cracked pepper
1	can (12 ounces) beer

Place the chicken in a covered dish or zip-lock bag. Pour in the Coke and soak in the fridge overnight (or for at least 2 hours).

Preheat a grill. If you're using charcoal, bank the hot coals to one side to create a cooler section for indirect cooking. If you're using a gas grill, leave one section of burners off and the others set on medium. Remove the chicken from the liquid, dry it, and rub it with salt and pepper.

Open the beer and drink half of it. Then mount the chicken on top of the can, firmly lodging the can in the chicken's cavity until the bird stays upright on its own. Place it on the cool side of the grill, close the lid, and cook until it reaches an internal temp of 165°F, about 1 to 1½ hours. (You can baste the chicken with your favorite barbecue sauce in the last 20 minutes or so, but it will be so moist you won't really need it.)

Remove the chicken and let it rest for 15 minutes before carving.

Makes 4 servings
Per serving: 538 calories, 42 g protein, 11 g carbohydrates, 34 g fat, 9.7 g saturated fat, 0 g fiber, 596 mg sodium
Cost per serving: $3.09

Fast-Food Fixes

Many restaurants have hidden menus—stuff they'll make if you know to ask. We dug deep to find options that are healthier than some actual menu fare.

1 STARBUCKS

A "short" drink: Upon request, your barista will serve you a "short" 8-ounce cup. A grande White Chocolate Mocha, for example, has 400 calories—the equivalent of about three Starbucks double fudge mini doughnuts. The short has half that amount.

2 RED ROBIN

The "petite" burger: This small burger was removed from the menu, but the kitchen still makes it, and it has about half the calories of the standard 931-calorie cheeseburger. If you're embarrassed asking for a petite, just ask for the "smaller" size.

3 CHIPOTLE

Customized tacos: Ask for three crispy tacos with black beans, fajita vegetables, tomato salsa, and lettuce. That saves you 615 calories and 28 grams of fat over a chicken burrito with black beans, rice, green salsa, cheese, and sour cream.

4 SUBWAY

6-inch chicken marinara sub: The meatball marinara sub tastes great, but it costs you 580 calories and 23 grams of fat. If they use oven-roasted chicken instead, you save 260 calories and 19 grams of fat. Top with oregano and a few black olives.

5 IHOP

Real fruit on top: Many of the menu's pancakes and waffles come with fruit "toppings," which are often preserved fruit swimming in a sauce of extra calories. Order a short stack of buttermilk pancakes, and ask them to top it with whatever fruit is available.

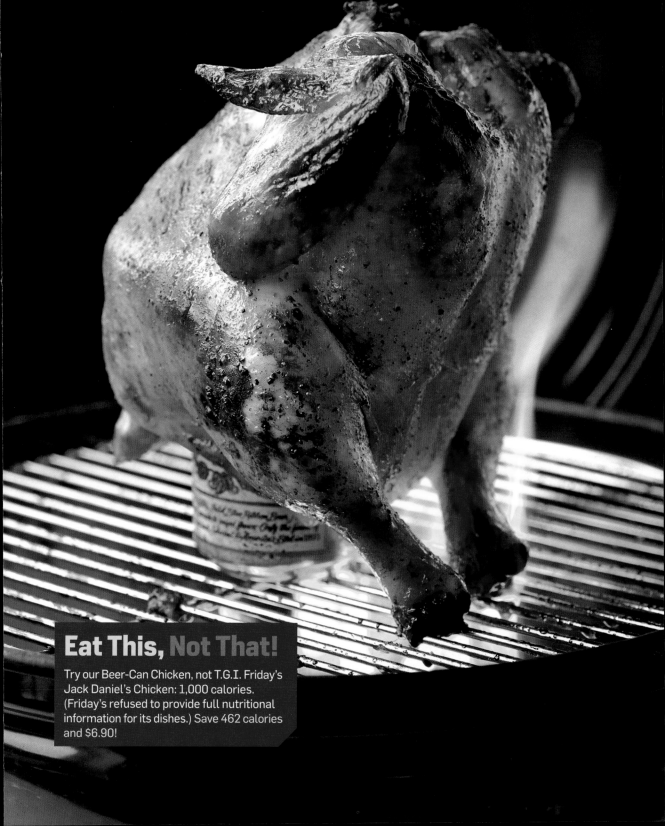

Eat This, Not That!
Try our Beer-Can Chicken, not T.G.I. Friday's Jack Daniel's Chicken: 1,000 calories. (Friday's refused to provide full nutritional information for its dishes.) Save 462 calories and $6.90!

Street Food Revolution

Modern chain restaurants nearly ruined fast food, but now the truck is here to save it. Join writer Matt Goulding on the trail of some of the most delicious (and creative) guy foods on the planet.

The group of tourists walking by me can't help but stare in horror. But beneath it all, what's really at work is simple jealousy. Before me are a half dozen dishes worthy of feverish envy, from spring-onion pizza and meat-covered fries to an embarrassment of tacos and grass-fed burgers. I'm no depraved glutton, though; this feast constitutes vital street-food research.

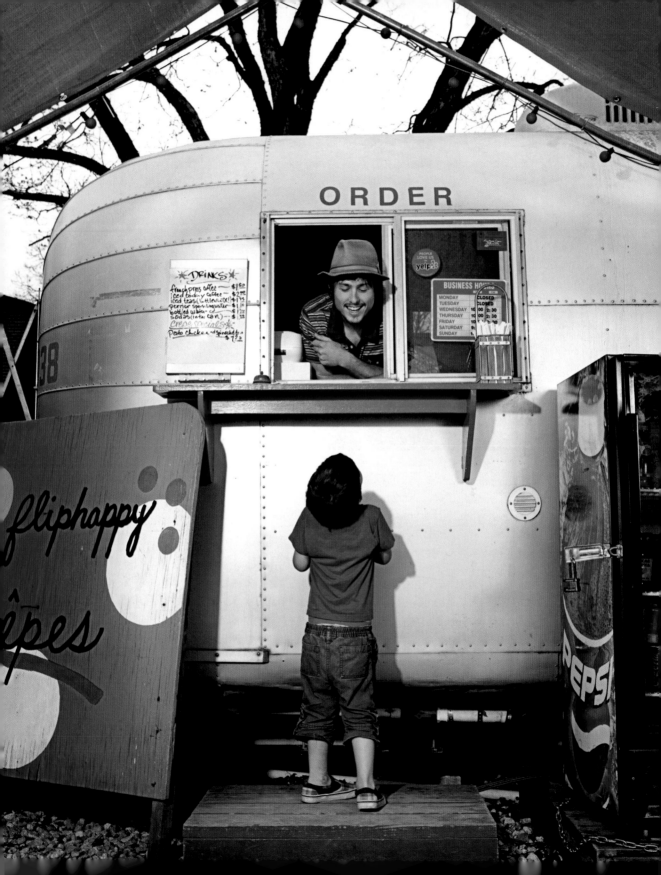

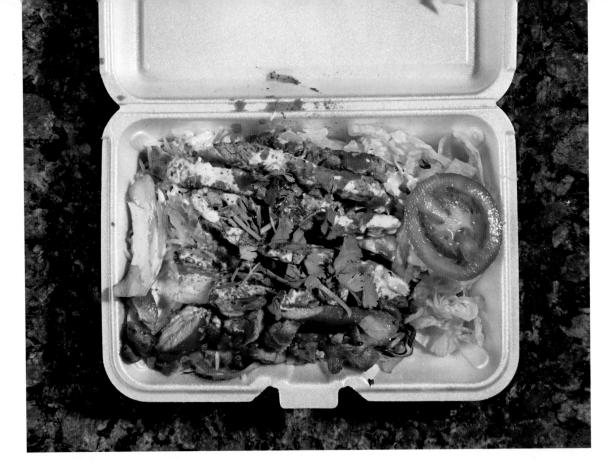

Over the past 3 years, mobile eats have transcended tube steak and mystery meat. Armed with tricked-out trucks, Twitter feeds, and plenty of culinary swagger, chefs and entrepreneurs have taken to the streets in record numbers. And time has taught us that it isn't a mere fad. These itinerant eateries are fast becoming permanent fixtures on America's culinary landscape, places that will feed us better and help teach us how to feed ourselves. With this in mind, I've set out to consume as much of this movement as possible, traveling to seven cities in 7 days to sample 178 dishes from 69 establishments, for a grand total of 63,000 calories. Does street grub really deserve your hard-earned dollars (and even harder-earned stomach real estate)? Can

a man live off this stuff without seriously jeopardizing his well-being? Let's hit the road to find out.

DAY 1
New York

The New York street-food scene has two archetypes: the Middle Eastern stands, home to foam containers of chicken and rice, and the dirty-water dog guys, who fill Manhattan with a thick funk of processed pig. But does the stereotype of street food—that it's dominated by grease and empty calories—hold true in this new era? My copilot today, Keith Berkowitz, MD, a nutrition authority and medical director of Manhattan's Center for Balanced Health, will weigh in.

Biryani Cart is a midtown favorite, winner of a 2008 Vendy (New York City's official street-food award). That's in no small part due to its kati roll, a thin flatbread stuffed with juicy chunks of marinated chicken and drizzled with spicy sauce. Dr. Berkowitz inhales his roll.

"Unprocessed protein with nonstarchy vegetables," he says. "Lots of turmeric, a cancer fighter. Nicely spiced, not overly sauced, and the bread doesn't dominate. Most important, it's natural."

Two blocks away, we find people lined up 25 deep at Frites 'N' Meats, a brand-new truck with glossy menus, an active Twitter feed, and a snappy (if inane) tagline, "Saving the world one burger at a time." Here there's another trademark of the 21st-century food truck: ingredient fetish. After a 30-minute wait, I take a bite of the grass-fed burger. It's topped with nutty Gruyère and served on a potato-onion roll from Balthazar, one of the best bakeries in the city. The patty is juicy and perfectly pink, while the cara-melized onions add a sweet counterpoint.

I ask Dr. Berkowitz if it would concern him if a patient of his had a proclivity for street food. "You can still go wrong, of course, but on the whole, some of it's a lot more balanced than food you'd find at restaurants in the neighborhood."

With his blessing, I eat my way through the city—duck dumplings at Rickshaw Dumpling Truck, near Central Park; pork schnitzel and potato salad at Schnitzel & Things, near Wall Street; and finally, a Salty Pimp—soft serve with dulce de leche, sea salt, and chocolate—from Big Gay Ice Cream Truck. The journey has begun.

STREET LESSON #1

Bulk Up Your Breakfast

In cities like Philadelphia and New York, trucks and street carts dish out substantial handheld breakfasts for the briefcase and blue-collar sets alike. Capable cooks shorten the wait by cooking vegetables, meat, and eggs in one batch over a vigorous heat. This ingenious twist to the standard breakfast sandwich is never more than 5 minutes away. It's serious (and seriously fast) fuel for a weekday morning. The following recipe was inspired by Mikey D's, in Philadelphia.

Broccoli Rabe and Egg Sandwich

½	tablespoon olive oil
¼	bunch broccoli rabe or spinach, washed
1	clove garlic, minced
1	tsp red-pepper flakes
2	eggs
	Salt
	Freshly ground black pepper
1	slice sharp provolone
1	soft hoagie roll, split

In a medium sauté pan, heat the oil over medium-high heat. Add the greens, garlic, and red-pepper flakes and sauté for about 5 minutes, until the greens are soft and cooked through.

In a bowl, crack the eggs, add a pinch of salt and pepper, and add them to the pan. Scramble, stirring constantly, until the eggs are set. Lay the provolone inside the roll and top it with the egg-and-greens scramble.

Makes 1 sandwich

Per sandwich: 549 calories, 30 g protein, 40 g carbohydrates, 31 g fat, 11 g saturated fat, 3 g fiber, 951 mg sodium

DAY 2
Philadelphia

Today I ended up eating 18 sandwiches. I strike out early, venturing straight from 30th Street Station to a nearby cluster of food trucks. Richky Cafe serves a Philly classic: an egg-cheese-and-scrapple hoagie. Scrapple, a pork loaf thickened with cornmeal, is crisped up on the

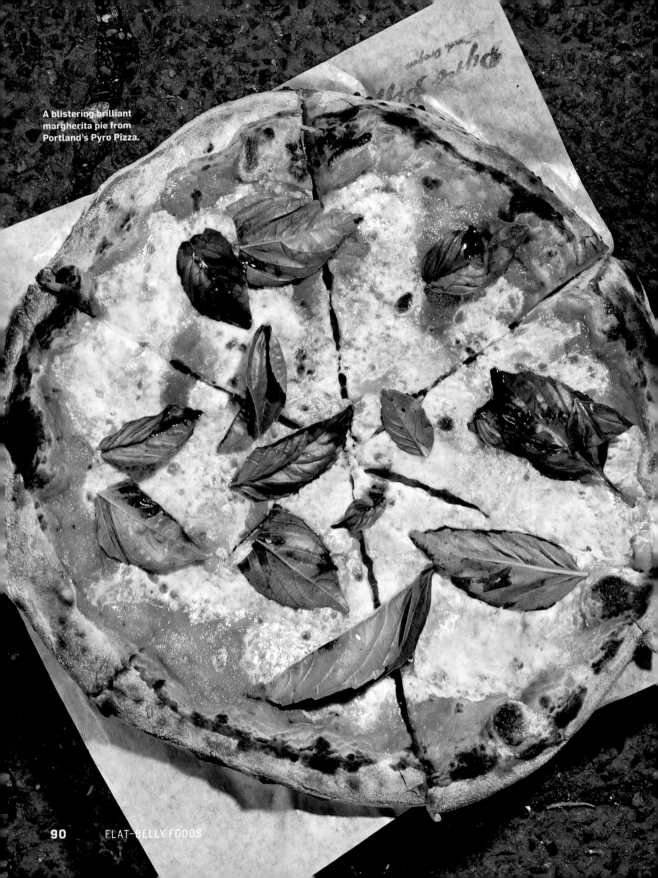

A blistering brilliant margherita pie from Portland's Pyro Pizza.

griddle. It's a rich, resoundingly delicious stand-in for bacon or sausage. A triumph of a breakfast sandwich.

Philly, more than any other city in the United States, is a sandwich town. Credit the bread, says Rick Nichols, a food columnist for the *Philadelphia Inquirer* and a sandwich savant of the highest order.

"The South Philly bakeries set the pace decades ago with a light, crispy Italian roll with a stretchy interior, he says. "And now a new breed of Philly-style sandwich guys have stepped up in the face of hoagie interlopers like Subway."

If any street sandwich is worthy of beatification, it's the Italian pulled pork, a heroic ensemble that has lived far too long in the cheesesteak's greasy, 12-inch shadow. For lunch, we head straight for Nichols's favorite version at DiNic's, inside the Reading Terminal Market. There they combine slow-cooked pork with classic Philly supporting players: sharp provolone, sautéed broccoli rabe, and a hit of pickled hot peppers on a long Italian roll.

Not far behind is another Philadelphia classic, the hot-sausage sandwich topped with pepper hash and a crispy fish cake at Johnny's Hots. The spice of the sausage is mitigated by the creamy, potato-rich cake, and the tangy relish provides the bridge between them.

Paesano's is owned by Peter McAndrews, a thick, cheery Irishman who also runs Modo Mio, one of Philly's best Italian restaurants. His menu reflects a man with an appetite: a hot dog wrapped in soppressata and covered in cheese and Bolognese sauce; a braised brisket sandwich slathered in horseradish mayo, sharp

provolone, roasted tomatoes, and pepperoncini, and crowned with a fried egg; and best of all, the Daddy Wad. That's prosciutto and mortadella, along with arugula, peppers, and—for just the right bite—razor-thin slices of raw onion.

And yes, there is a single Philly cheesesteak, from Jim's Steaks on South Street, that I eat at one in the morning with the buzz of a few cocktails rekindling my appetite. Covered in Cheez Whiz (the industrial gloop is traditional) and half-cooked onions, it's the worst sandwich I've had all day, which, in a town like Philadelphia, is still pretty damn good.

DAY 3
Chicago

You might expect Chicago, home to world-famous hot dogs, succulent Italian

STREET LESSON #2

Reinvent the Wheel

Anyone can slap a Kraft Single between two slices of Wonder bread, but Portland's Grilled Cheese Grill cart attracts throngs by reimagining what this simple sandwich can really be. According to co-owner Bill Bunkley, there are three tricks to crispy, melty, grilled-cheese perfection: Butter the bread (not the pan), cook over medium-high heat, and use a lid to cover the sandwich while it cooks. "The ambient heat melts the cheese perfectly." Try this technique with one of these five flavor combinations for spectacular results.

· **Sautéed mushrooms and Swiss on rye**
· **Tomato, havarti, honey mustard, and ham on wheat**
· **Bacon, apples, blue cheese, and Swiss on sourdough**
· **Roasted jalapeños, Colby Jack, cream cheese, and crushed tortilla chips on sourdough**
· **Mascarpone, Nutella, and banana on cinnamon-raisin bread**

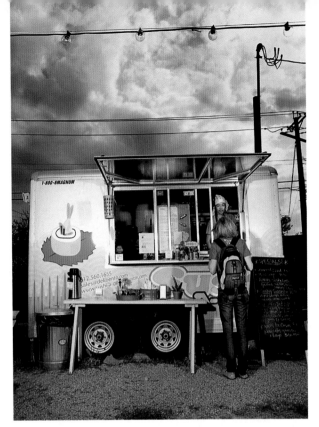

Raw fish on the road at Austin's Sushi-A-Go-Go.

beef sandwiches, and a staggering array of regional Mexican cuisine, to be the white-hot center of the street-food universe. You would be wrong. Chicago city ordinances have long banned the preparation of food in mobile kitchens. It's like banning prayer in St. Peter's Square, for... Pete's sake.

In search of answers, I head straight to Xoco, the newest restaurant from the city's most famous chef, Rick Bayless, who's one of the original proponents of street food. One thing is clear: Bayless is not happy about the ban.

"The health department is trying to destroy American cuisine," Bayless says. "The truck people want to prepare fresh food on the spot, but the health department would prefer if we bought all our food frozen and cooked it in a microwave."

Dedicated to the food of the markets and sidewalks of Mexico, Xoco is Bayless's reminder to the citizens and officials of Chicago just what street-food culture would taste like in their city: tortas, sandwiches stuffed with smoky roasted goat and suckling pig; and hot, cinnamon-dusted churros so perfectly fried you're willing to scorch the roof of your mouth just to feel their warm, crunchy embrace.

"America is about to fully recover from the bland-food movement of the '50s and '60s, and it's the street vendors who will take us there," says Bayless. "But first we have to let them. Don't they see Chicago wants this?" As if to prove his point, he glances over his shoulder to the line of people spilling out onto the sidewalk.

Chicagoans do not suffer alone; cities like Atlanta and Boston have similar restrictions. But a street-food movement is forming in Chicago, led by Matt Maroni and Phillip Foss, two local chefs who founded Chicago Food Trucks in 2010. They've even drafted legislation that would effectively lift the ban.

"It's a win-win-win situation. You're creating jobs, you're creating business growth, and you're giving people what they want," says Foss. "This is not the first time this movement has been initiated, but God willing, it will be the last," says Foss. "Enough is enough already."

DAY 4
Austin

Easter Sunday. As priests in silken robes announce the resurrection of Christ to the spiritually hungry, I'm seeking out nondenominational sustenance in a gravel parking lot, knocking back bottles of Lone Star, mopping up barbecue sauce with squishy pieces of white bread. Swill for the soul; food for the gods. Hallelujah: Austin.

Austin takes pride in being atypical in nearly every regard, and its sprawling, funky, disparate street-food scene is not only one of the most unconventional you'll stumble across, but also one of the finest in America.

"There are something like 5,000 food-service permits issued in Austin, and 900 of them are for mobile food vendors," says Mike Sutter, food critic for the *Austin American-Statesman*.

John Anthony Galindo III, owner of Izzoz Tacos, bought one. He tells a tale that's familiar among emerging street-food

STREET LESSON #3:

Be a Condiment King

If street food has taught us anything, it's that a good condiment can turn decent cooks into culinary geniuses. Here are three of the best flavor boosters used on the street today.

$$$ Sauce

Use this sauce on hot dogs, grilled sausages, grilled chicken sandwiches, or burgers.

- **3** tbsp yellow mustard
- **3** tbsp sambal (or other Asian chili relish)
- **4** tbsp low sodium soy sauce
- **3** tbsp water
- **3** tbsp honey

Combine all ingredients in a bowl and mix well.

Makes 3¹/₂ cups

Per 2oz serving: 28 calories, 1 g protein, 7 g carbohydrates, 0 g fat, 0 g saturated fat, 1 g fiber, 278 mg sodium

Note: *This recipe was adapted from 4505 Meats in San Francisco.*

Kimchi

If there's one thing home cooks can learn from the mobile movement, it's that a few spicy strands of kimchi—Korean-style fermented cabbage—on a hot dog or a burger turns you into a gourmet. Pick up a jar of the stuff at an Asian market, or grab one from grannychoe.com. Use it on quesadillas, hot dogs, or burgers, or serve pureed on thick slices of grilled steak or pork.

Pepper Hash

This keeps in the fridge for up to 2 weeks. Use on hot dogs, sausage, or pulled pork, or as a sidekick to anything off the grill.

- ½ medium head cabbage, chunked
- ¾ green bell pepper
- ½ medium carrot
- **2** cloves garlic, grated on a zester
- ¼ cup cider vinegar
- ¼ cup water
- ¼ cup sugar
- ½ tbsp salt
  Pinch of red-pepper flakes

In a food processor, pulse the cabbage, pepper, carrot, and garlic until finely chopped.

In a bowl, mix the vinegar, water, sugar, salt, and red pepper, then add the vegetables and mix well.

Makes 1 cup

Per serving: 255 calories, 5 g protein, 69 g carbohydrates, 2 g fat, 0.1 g saturated fat, 2 g fiber, 3,818 mg sodium

Note: *This recipe is from Johnny's Hots in Philadelphia.*

Is Street Food Safe?

We took samples from 15 New York City food carts and had them tested for the three most common (and dangerous) food-borne bacteria: *E. coli* O157:H7, *Salmonella,* and Campylobacter. Two were positive for "generic" strains of *E. coli.* While these varieties are harmless, says Catherine Cutter, PhD, food safety extension specialist at Penn State University, they still indicate that the food was probably undercooked, cross-contaminated, or touched by dirty hands. Whittle your risk of a health threat by always checking street carts for four common types of poor handling.

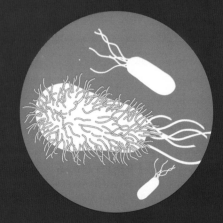

BARE HANDS ON FOOD

There should be a barrier between your food and the cook's digits. Tongs, wooden skewers, paper napkins, and clean gloves all do the trick.

CROSS-CONTAMINATION

If the cook handles raw meat and then grabs a roll with the same glove, then he or she could transfer bacteria to your food. To a lesser extent, the same thing can happen when a cook handles money while preparing food.

WARM (NOT HOT) FOOD

Meat should be stored at either very hot or very cold temperatures; if food stays at warm temperatures for an extended time, it's an ideal environment for bacterial growth. If you see meat sitting off to the side of the grill, especially when business is slow, don't eat it.

UNDERCOOKED MEAT

Even meat that's been cooked past the pink stage can be underdone. So focus on temperature. Hold your hand near the food. Heat should be radiating from it, and the food should be too hot to bite into right away.

vendors: Once an executive chef at an upscale restaurant, Galindo sold his place just before the market tanked. Rather than invest a few million in another restaurant, he spent about $25,000 on a trailer that had been converted into a kitchen, and to pay the fees to open a food stand. Galindo runs his joint like a full-scale professional kitchen, and the proof is in the taco: His seared ahi tuna version with pickled red onions is outdone only by his spicy ground beef taco, the flavor of a dozen standard Tex-Mex tacos concentrated into one shatteringly crisp shell.

What else are you willing to eat in the street? Hot dogs? Maybe a bit of mystery meat? How about raw fish from a trailer parked at a gas station? Sushi-A-Go-Go is helmed by husband and wife Take and Asazu Kayo. "Sushi started out as street food in Japan 200 years ago," says Asazu, "so why not now?" Take quickly makes a believer out of me with their best-selling roll, a combo of salmon, avocado, and fresh mango that hits all the right notes: sweet, creamy, fatty. Gorgeous.

Dessert means doughnuts, or at least it should in Austin, where Gourdough's is doing some of the funkiest fried-dough concoctions in the country. Think bacon and maple syrup, fried chicken with honey butter, and the Porkey's, complete with whipped cream cheese, jalapeño jelly, and Canadian bacon. If dinner was trailer sushi, you can afford to splurge on trailer doughnuts.

I've dined like a roving king in Austin's balmy embrace, but as I head toward the airport, something's amiss. The barbecue just wasn't as bliss-inducing as you'd

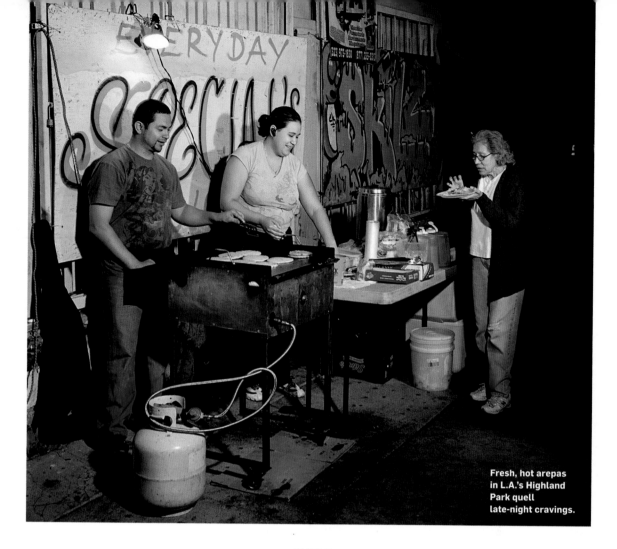

Fresh, hot arepas in L.A.'s Highland Park quell late-night cravings.

expect from the Lone Star State. Then suddenly there's a vision on the horizon: a school bus in a lumberyard, its retrofitted exhaust vent billowing meat smoke from the roof. Inside Old School BBQ and Grill, sweaty men in bandannas serve meat with the deep, caramelized exterior that bespeaks hours—even days—of slow, steady smoking.

I dive into the to-go container mere feet from the airport security line, devouring shards of charred, tender brisket, soft white bread, and pickle slices. A religious experience.

DAY 5
Portland

It's the world's most diverse and fulfilling food court, an Epcot of grub contained within two blocks of downtown concrete. On Alder Street, you can order Japanese bento boxes or Hungarian chicken paprikash; slurp rice noodles from Vietnam or a fiery chili-laced broth from Korea; gnaw on pork ribs from the Deep South or overstuffed fried-fish burritos from the Even Deeper South; and wash it all down with a mango lassi or a world-class shot of espresso. This is Portlandia, kingdom of the street carts.

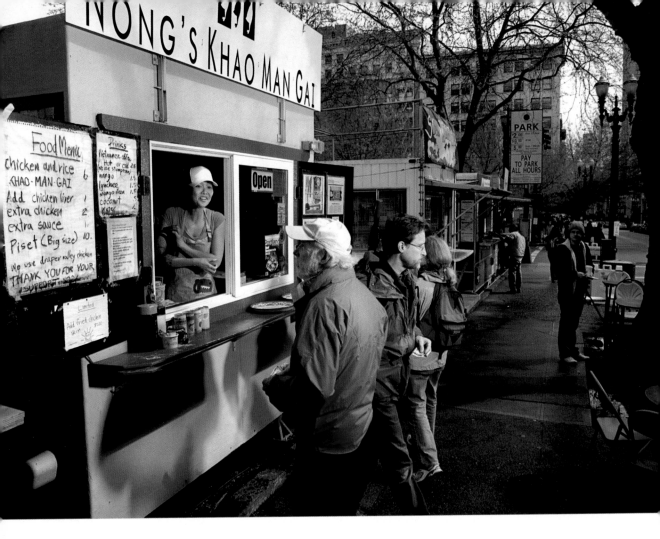

"Sometimes it feels as if people are spinning a giant wheel here. Whatever food it lands on, they decide to do a cart," is how one hungry denizen explains it to me. "We don't have a Himalayan cart, but soon enough . . ."

Give me the choice of just one cart, though, and I'll take Nong's Khao Man Gai. Nong Poonsukwattana dishes up the comfort food of her native Thailand: chicken and rice. The tender poached chicken breast, served over rice that's been cooked in chicken juices, exemplifies why street food can be better than restaurant food. While restaurant menus can be bogged down by entrees, many of them mediocre, Nong—like so many of her cart-confined cohorts—specializes in just one thing.

When night falls, I follow the burning glow from across the river to Portland's East Side. That's where obsessive pizza practitioners like John Eads are giving a mobile identity to the ongoing artisanal pizza revolution. The wood-fired oven he built inside his tiny trailer could rival the best in Naples. "I'm burning at 750°F to 800°F on the floor, with the ceiling at 1,000° or so. It takes 2 minutes to cook a pizza."

But it takes more than a hellfire oven to

The 10 Best Street Eats in America

1 Porchetta Sandwich, ROLIROTI, SAN FRANCISCO

Lean pork loin is wrapped in heritage pork belly and spit-roasted so the rendered fat from the belly bastes the loin and turns it crispy. Thick slices are served on rolls rubbed in a puddle of pork juices, then topped with shingles of crispy skin. It will forever change the way you look at pork.

2 Khao Man Gai, NONG'S KHAO MAN GAI, PORTLAND

This is Asian comfort food of the noblest order. Nong poaches organic chicken in a broth rich with Asian herbs and spices, and uses the same broth to cook her long-grain rice. The ginger sauce on the side should come with a straw.

3 Italian Pulled-Pork Sandwich, DINIC'S, PHILADELPHIA

Pork shoulders are braised with pork stock, caramelized onions, and wine, then shredded and stuffed into an Italian roll with that oh-so-Philly combo of provolone, sautéed broccoli rabe, and pickled peppers. The cooking juices spooned on at the end blast this sandwich into the stratosphere.

4 Margherita Pizza, PYRO PIZZA, PORTLAND

Their margherita, a perfect balance of creamy, handmade mozzarella, tangy tomato sauce, and sharp, fragrant basil, is a simple reminder of why pizza is one of the world's most popular foods.

5 Double Cheeseburger, 4505 MEATS, SAN FRANCISCO

A dry-aged mix of short rib and brisket is covered in Sonoma dry Jack cheese and special sauce, and tucked into a soft Parmesan-scallion sesame seed bun. It's one of the best burgers in America, indoors or out.

6 Brisket, OLD SCHOOL BBQ & GRILL, AUSTIN

The alchemy of true barbecue: meat, salt, smoke. The small plastic cup of sauce on the side went untouched. This is caveman food at its finest.

7 Crispy Taco, IZZOZ TACOS, AUSTIN

The beef is crumbly and deftly spiced, the baby spinach and tomato cool and bracing, and the shell, a freshly fried corn tortilla, shatters with the gentlest pressure from your teeth.

8 Peanut Butter–Banana Dream Oatmeal, BLOOP, PORTLAND

Who would have guessed a vegan oatmeal shack could put out something so memorable? Bob's Red Mill oats are cooked with almond milk, peanut butter, cinnamon, and agave until it's thick and creamy, then enhanced with bananas, almonds, and a drizzle of agave syrup. Steal this recipe now!

9 Peruvian Ceviche, BORDER GRILL TRUCK, LOS ANGELES

These guys do ceviche better than anyone, combining fresh chunks of mahi with plenty of lime juice, cilantro, and spicy aji amarillo. Break off pieces of the tortilla cone that it's served in and start scooping.

10 Salty Pimp, BIG GAY ICE CREAM TRUCK, NEW YORK CITY

Score another one for simplicity: vanilla soft serve and sea salt, drizzled with dulce de leche and enrobed in a chocolate shell. Try it at home: Drizzle a scoop of vanilla ice cream with caramel and a few pinches of coarse sea salt.

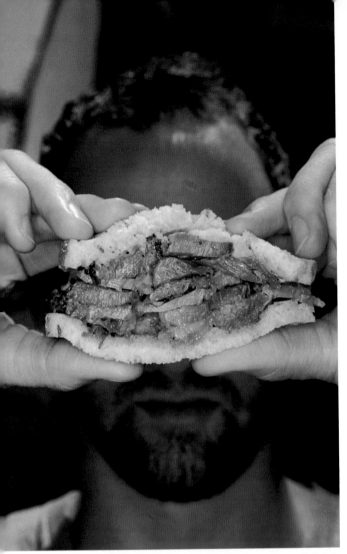

Juicy pastrami on seeded rye commands attention at Fresser's in L.A.

make a good pie. Eads constantly tweaks his dough recipe ("nothing is sacred"), sources local oils and cured meats, and, most important, pulls his own mozzarella by hand every night—a step that not even the finest pizzerias in New York bother with. Not surprisingly, the pies are exceptional: a luscious margherita with that homemade mozz; an all-white pizza goosed with a drizzle of locally produced white truffle oil; and a pizza with caramelized onions, blue cheese, and pistachios, a

symphonic experience of sweet, creamy, crunchy, and chewy. Why aren't you booking a flight to Portland right now?

DAY 6
San Francisco

The first thing the guy in cargo shorts passes through the truck window is a hockey puck of foie gras, topped with a toasted baguette slice and delicate micro-herbs. The foie gras has been as lovingly prepared as most renditions in white-linen restaurants around town . . . and at $12 a serving, it's just as expensive.

It was only a matter of time before street food went from hot dogs to foie gras, and no city ups the gastronomic ante more than San Francisco, a place where growing asparagus or churning butter can make you a celebrity.

Truth be told, carts like Spencer on the Go!—where I have my first street foie, not to mention my first street truffles and street snails—sometimes just feel silly. If I'm going to splurge on duck liver, I'd rather not eat it on a sidewalk. And in many cases, these high-end iterations aren't being cooked on the street at all. They're prepped in restaurant kitchens and brought to the cart to be reheated, hit with a few fancy garnishes, and served to people who enjoy a forkful of irony.

But when you combine serious kitchen skills with foods that are still street in spirit and shape, the results can be astounding. Don't believe me? Stop by the Ferry Building Marketplace and behold the splendor that is America's most amazing makeshift-food mecca.

Ryan Farr of 4505 Meats gave up gigs at some of San Francisco's finest restaurants (Fifth Floor, Orson) to make burgers and dogs instead.

"We buy whole grass-fed steers and dry-age them ourselves for up to 28 days," he says. Farr then butchers and grinds the meat fresh before each market day. He also grills up a variety of house-made sausages, including the formidable Dogzilla: a snappy bacon-infused hot dog tagged with special sauce, spicy cabbage, and a handful of chicharrones (deep-fried pork skins, a nice bonus dose of protein).

Other musts: the insanely addictive "gamja" fries from the Namu stand, topped with braised short ribs, scallions, kimchi relish, teriyaki sauce, and Kewpie mayo; iced chicory coffee from the Blue Bottle Coffee stand, where every cup is made to order; and, from the RoliRoti truck, spit-roasted meat that's bronzed and moist, like a bodybuilder lubed up for competition. If the Swiss-born chef, Thomas Odermatt, had a roof over his head and white linens beneath his plates, he could charge $20 for a portion of his porchetta. And I'd be the first guy on the phone, angling for a reservation.

DAY 7
Los Angeles

No city better encompasses the full spectrum of street eats than Los Angeles. On one end, you have illegal, unregistered carts; on the other, the masterfully marketed, Twitter-powered restaurants on wheels. I start with the urban underbelly, enlisting the help of Jonathan Gold,

STREET LESSON #4
Embrace the Neglected Cuts

How do carts keep prices so low? Low overhead, sure. But they also use cheaper cuts of beef, chicken, and pork, combined with vibrant seasonings. Here are three of our favorite cuts, plus street-inspired ways to cook them.

CHICKEN THIGHS

Why they're great: Dark-meat chicken generally costs about half as much as breasts, and it packs twice as much flavor.

Cook them street-style: Rub the thighs with curry powder or curry paste and grill. Serve over a bed of lettuce, sliced onions, tomatoes, and cucumbers with a dressing of yogurt, olive oil, minced garlic, and fresh lemon juice.

SKIRT STEAK

Why it's great: This robust-tasting cut is a favorite of Mexican streetfood vendors, and it stays tender when grilled medium rare.

Cook it street-style: Marinate 1 pound overnight in 1 cup orange juice, 2 tablespoons canned chipotle pepper, 1 teaspoon ground cumin, and a fistful of cilantro. Grill on high until charred. Serve with warm tortillas and guacamole.

PORK SHOULDER

Why it's great: After long, slow cooking, this cut turns soft and maddeningly delicious.

Cook it street-style: Rub a 5- to 6-pound shoulder with salt and pepper; roast in a 250°F oven until it can be shredded with a fork, about 3 hours. Toss with 1/2 cup cider vinegar mixed with a few drops of liquid smoke and a dash of cayenne. Serve on soft buns with coleslaw.

longtime omnivorous critic for *L.A. Weekly* and the only food writer to ever bring home a Pulitzer.

We hit El Pique Taco Truck on York in Highland Park, where tattooed skateboarders and moms driving Mercedes line up for first-rate carne asada tacos, then we chase those with brain and goat tacos from the Birria de Chivo Taco Truck down the street. I ask Gold how he chooses between the hundreds of taco trucks in his city: "The quality of the painting on the side of the truck helps. If there's a picture of a naked girl or a mermaid, there's a damn good chance some of the food will rock," he says.

Around midnight, we end up downtown in search of the city's most notorious carts: the danger dog dispensers. The "danger" refers to the makeshift griddles that the bacon-wrapped, mayo-slathered dogs are cooked on—made by heating sheet pans with small propane tanks. "When the city finds these carts, they literally tear them to pieces," says Gold. Right on cue, a bike cop rolls up, customers scatter, and the makeshift griddle is disassembled. When I ask the cop why so harsh, he's unequivocal: "A lot of people get sick eating from the dog guys. We can't be having that." When I ask the young cook for his side of the story, he shrugs. "I'd probably bust me, too."

Across town, though, there's street food of an entirely different stripe. Coolhaus, an old ice-cream sandwich trafficker in a converted mail truck, serves scoops of flavors, like pistachio with black truffle, between squishy brioche cookies. And the Border Grill Truck—the mobile unit for Mary Sue Milliken and Susan Feninger's popular Border Grill restaurants—have the masses clamoring for fiery, lime-lacquered mahi ceviche served in a corn tortilla cone. Despite the traffic, truck-hopping is a happy way to eat in Los Angeles.

I end my journey where this countrywide craze began—at the Kogi BBQ truck. Kogi was the first cart to take full advantage of Twitter to build a community of rabid followers. But tasting the revolution at its source isn't as easy as I'd hoped. The line stretches around the block, and when our photographer begins to shoot the truck, a nervous employee asks if I have permission from the Kogi corporate office. I make the phone call and try to set up an interview with owner Roy Choi.

"I'm sorry," says an office functionary. "You'll need to speak with his PR agent." (Sign #117 of the Apocalypse: A taco truck has a PR team.)

Is the food any good? The hot dog and the quesadilla are the kind of food you want when you stumble out of a bar at 2 a.m., but palate fatigue sets in almost immediately, and nothing's that groundbreaking. Fact is, in the 2 years since Kogi opened the floodgates, the rest of the country has caught up. New York added high-concept trucks to its plethora of ethnic carts. Philly reinforced its claim to sandwich supremacy. Austin pushed the boundaries of doughnuts and sushi. Portland established itself as the country's undisputed street-food king. San Francisco found porchetta. This is all excellent news for hungry Americans the country over. If trucks haven't started rolling through your town yet, don't worry. They're on their way.

The Unhealthiest Mobile Meals in America

There are plenty of lean, nutrient-dense meals to be found on carts and trucks across the country. There are also more than a few weapons of mass consumption. We ate them so you wouldn't have to.

Danger Dog, DOWNTOWN L.A.

Estimated calories:

500

Estimated chance of contracting food-borne illness: obscenely high. The cooking contraption is a shopping cart loaded with propane and topped with a sheet pan that could barely toast bread, let alone cook meat. The dogs, wrapped in raw bacon, roll around in a black hole of bacteria, only to be plucked from the pan, smothered in mayo, and distributed to unsuspecting downtown revelers.

Cheesus Burger, THE GRILLED CHEESE GRILL, PORTLAND

Estimated calories:

1,400

It's a ⅓-pound burger, and the cook eschews the bun in favor of a pair of grilled-cheese sandwiches. The tagline: "You won't need to eat again for 2 days."

Double Poutine, POTATO CHAMPION!, PORTLAND

Estimated calories:

1,200

This is the most egregious version of a troubling Canadian staple we've seen. A wheelbarrow of twice-fried potatoes strewn everywhere with squishy cheese curds and smothered in a salty sea of viscous gravy. Prepare to give up 2 days of sodium on top of the calories.

Tuscan Tony, PAESANO'S, PHILADELPHIA

Estimated calories:

850

If the huge spicy sausage doesn't get you, then the melted provolone might. If the provolone doesn't get you, then watch out for the salami slices and hot peppers. Survive that, and you still have a huge ladle of rich ragu Bolognese to contend with. Proceed with caution.

The Puddin' with Ice Cream, GOURDOUGH'S, AUSTIN

Estimated calories:

700

This sugar-spiked catastrophe takes the . . . cake. It's deep-fried until crisp and golden, filled with vanilla pudding, and topped with cream-cheese icing. Then it's gilded with bananas and crushed vanilla wafers, more pudding, and a scoop of ice cream. This is not a doughnut; it's a spare tire.

PROVE IT

START A FIRE

Behold the power of peppers. A recent Korean lab study found that the compound that makes chili spicy, capsaicin, can help kill colon-cancer cells. Previously, a Dutch study review had concluded that capsaicin encourages thermogenesis, the body's heat-generating response to food intake, which can help burn calories.

"For the thermogenic effect, it's best to eat chili-based foods on a daily basis," says Jeya Henry, PhD, who researches energy metabolism at Oxford Brookes University. The Scoville scale measures capsaicin content; the more capsaicin in the peppers you eat, the greater the benefit (and hotter the burn).

Type	Scoville Heat Units
Pure capsaicin	15,000,000
Capsicum oleoresin (used to make pepper spray)	1,500,000
Bhut Jolokia (hottest known chili variety)	1,000,000
Orange habanero	210,000
Tabasco (chili)	120,000
Thai hot	60,000
Ground cayenne	40,000
Serrano	25,000
Chipotle	5,000-10,000
Jalapeño	5,500
Pasilla	4,000
Tabasco sauce	3,750
Poblano	1,500
Mulato	1,000
Bell pepper	0

FUEL YOUR BRAIN

Eating vegetables can keep you smart into old age, say researchers in Germany. In their study, people who ate four or more daily servings (about 350 grams) of fruits and vegetables scored higher on cognitive tests than did those who took in less than a serving. They also had high blood levels of vitamin E, which can prevent degradation of nerve tissues.

GET THE ORGANIC EDGE

Pesticide-free foods might have another plus: more nutrients. Studies have already shown that organic kiwis and potatoes are more nutritious than conventionally grown ones. Now Spanish scientists say

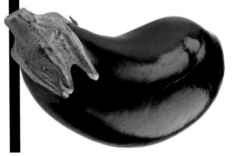

organically grown eggplants have 30 percent more phenolic compounds (disease-fighting antioxidants) than those treated with pesticides.

Toss cubes of organic eggplant with olive oil, salt, and pepper. Then skewer and grill them with your next round of kebabs.

EASE THE SQUEEZE

Rumbling bowels? The type of fiber you eat may reduce symptoms of irritable bowel syndrome (IBS), according to a study in the *British Medical Journal*. IBS patients who ate 10 grams of soluble fiber a day for 12 weeks reduced their symptoms by 54 percent. Insoluble fiber had about the same effect as a placebo.

"Soluble fiber may relax a person's bowel, while insoluble fiber may increase bacterial fermentation, which irritates it," says Niek de Wit, MD, the study's coauthor. If you're in pain, try eating foods high in soluble fiber, such as oatmeal, beans, and citrus.

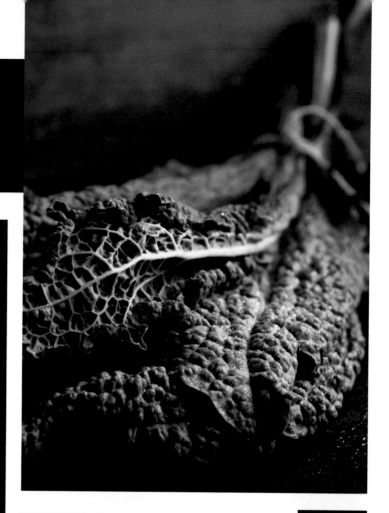

HAVE A CUP

Coffee may lower your risk of type 2 diabetes, a study in the *American Journal of Clinical Nutrition* found. People who drank five 8-ounce cups a day had less internal inflammation (a risk factor for type 2 diabetes) than those who drank no joe. Coffee may boost adiponectin, a protein that regulates glucose. Drinking fewer than 5 cups might also be beneficial, scientists say. More research is needed.

BREW UP STRONGER BONES

Green tea might help you build a strong skeleton, say scientists in China. They exposed bone cells to tea catechins, which

HARD TRUTH

325

In thousands, number of people hospitalized for food-borne illnesses each year in the United States, according to the Centers for Disease Control and Prevention

PROVE IT

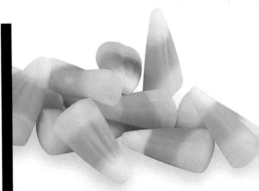

stimulated bone growth and helped slow its breakdown. One of the catechins boosted growth by 79 percent. It's not known if drinking tea does the same.

FISH FOR YOUR OMEGA-3S

People who don't want to take fish-oil supplements for their omega-3 fatty acids often turn to plant sources like flaxseed oil. But Australian researchers found that taking flaxseed oil actually increases free radicals in your body, which can lead to inflammation. When 36 men took 9 grams of a flaxseed-oil supplement every day for a month, they showed a 38 percent increase in markers of a free radical called F1-phyto-prostane. Study author Anne Barden, PhD, says your body readily oxidizes the alpha-linolenic acid in flaxseed, which creates the free radicals. Your best bet remains fish oil.

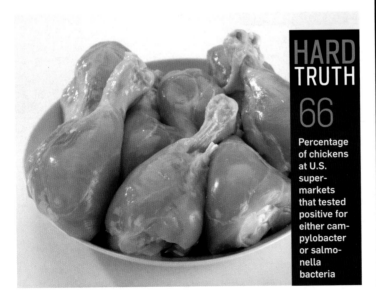

HARD TRUTH

66

Percentage of chickens at U.S. supermarkets that tested positive for either campylobacter or salmonella bacteria

FEAR YOUR SWEET TOOTH

Here's something to be afraid of: All that candy you inhale expands your waistline. In a recent Swedish study, one group of people snacked on 1,360 calories' worth of nonchocolate candy every day while another group ate the same amount of peanuts. After 2 weeks, only the candy eaters showed significant increases in body weight and waist size. They also developed higher insulin and C-peptide levels, signs of insulin resistance. The peanut eaters, on the other hand, saw a boost in resting metabolism.

"Unlike the sugar in candy, the fatty acids in peanuts elevate metabolism, protecting against weight gain and its

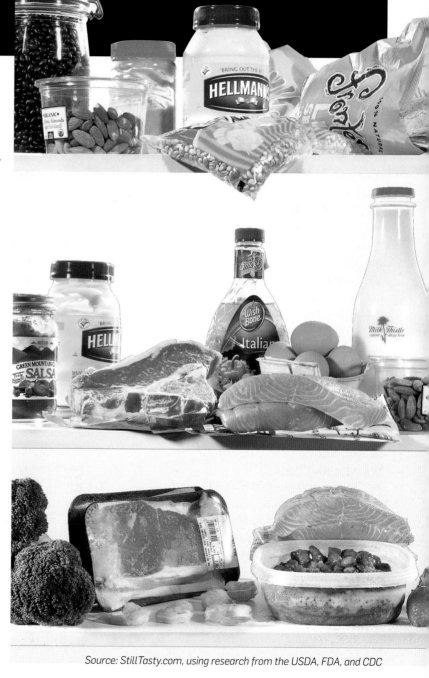

consequences in the body," says study coauthor Fredrik Nystrom, MD, PhD. So after you indulge on some sugary snacks, refill the candy bowl with dry-roasted peanuts.

DECODE YOUR FRIDGE

Use this guide to clean up your kitchen and minimize the risk of dangerous levels of bacteria.

PANTRY
Black beans, dried: 1 year
Almonds, opened: 1 month
Peanut butter, opened: 3 months
Mayonnaise, unopened: 10 to 12 months
Packaged popcorn: 1 year
Tortilla chips, opened: 1 to 2 weeks

FRIDGE
Salsa, opened: 1 month
Mayonnaise, opened: 3 to 4 months after date on jar
Beef: 3 to 5 days
Italian dressing, opened: 6 to 9 months
Eggs, raw in shell: 3 to 5 weeks
Fresh salmon: 1 to 2 days
Milk: 1 week after sell-by date
Almonds, opened: 4 to 6 months

FREEZER
Commercially frozen broccoli: 10 to 12 months
Beef: 6 to 12 months
Fresh shrimp: 9 months
Salmon: 2 to 3 months
Homemade chili: 4 to 6 months
Fresh strawberries: 10 to 12 months

Source: StillTasty.com, using research from the USDA, FDA, and CDC

YOU ASKED

Q: What's the healthiest, best-tasting chocolate?

A: Unfortunately, the "healthiest" type would also taste the worst, since the percentage of cacao in dark chocolate determines both the number of disease-fighting flavonols and the bitterness. For the best balance of flavor and flavonols, try chocolate with 70 percent cacao, says Jeffrey Blumberg, PhD, director of the antioxidants research lab at Tufts University. We tested dozens of dark chocolate brands and chose five favorites. Limit yourself to a 100-calorie serving daily (one 2-inch square) and you'll reap the health rewards without piling on the pounds, says Dr. Blumberg.

BEST BASIC BAR
Amano Madagascar (70% cacao)
Made with just four ingredients (a mild cacao bean, cane sugar, cocoa butter, and vanilla bean), this bar is a little sweet and almost creamy. $7 (2 oz), *amanochocolate.com*

BEST GOURMET BAR
Jacques Torres Midnight Soul (80% cacao)
The intense citrus-nut flavor is almost overpowering. First try it melted (in a microwave) and drizzled on fresh blueberries, cherries, and almonds. After your tongue has adjusted, savor the bar straight. $5 (2.8 oz), *mrchocolate.com*

BEST BAR WITH EXTRAS
Dagoba's Beaucoup Berries Bar (74% cacao)
Dried cranberries and dried cherries boost the sweetness, flavor, and antioxidant total. $3 (2 oz), *dagobachocolate.com*

BEST BAR WITH A KICK
Vosges Creole Bar (70% cacao)
With crushed espresso beans, ground cocoa nibs (bean fragments), and chicory coffee, it's like a Nestlé Crunch with mocha. $8 (3 oz), *vosgeschocolate.com*

BEST TOPPING
Askinosie Roasted Cocoa Nibs (100% cacao)
The nibs undergo minimal processing and are the most potent form of dark chocolate. Cut their bitterness by sprinkling them on yogurt, fruit salad, or ice cream. $11 (6 oz), *askinosie.com*

Q: What are the most nutritious mushrooms I can add to my diet?

A: The portobello is the fungus with the most firepower. Just one portobello delivers 28 percent of your daily quota of selenium and almost as much potassium as a small banana, all in a protein-packed, 18-calorie slider. What's more, portobellos contain the highest concentration of chitin, a cholesterol-lowering carbohydrate that's found in mushrooms and in the exoskeletons of crabs, lobsters, and insects.

"Chitin acts like a natural statin, binding blood lipids and reducing cholesterol in your bloodstream," says George Fahey, PhD, a researcher and professor of nutrition sciences at the University of Illinois.

Also, raw portobellos are replete with oligosaccharides, prebiotics that increase the good bacteria in your intestine. Slice your portobellos thinly and toss them into salads, pastas, and soups.

Q: What are the best ways to reduce my salt intake?

A: Home cooking—and lots of it. About 77 percent of the average man's salt intake comes from processed foods and restaurant fare, according to a Monell Center study.

"As food manufacturers and chefs cut out trans fats, they've been liberal with the saltshaker to add flavor," says Elisabeth Moore, RD, LDN, a dietitian at Beth Israel Deaconess Medical Center. To lower your intake, scan labels for the phrases "low sodium" and "sodium-free," and eat fresh produce instead of processed foods whenever possible.

At home, try other flavor enhancers—pepper, herbs, lemon juice, ginger, garlic, or wine. And when you do dine out, beware of salt bombs—cold cuts, mustard, and Parmesan cheese—and ask that any sauces or dressings be served on the side.

Aim to consume less than 1,500 milligrams of sodium daily. That's less than ½ teaspoon of salt.

Eat This, Not That! Salt-O-Meter

	Eat This	Not That!
1 BACON	**Oscar Mayer Center Cut Bacon** *90 milligrams sodium (1 slice)*	**Oscar Mayer Turkey Bacon** *180 milligrams (1 slice)*
2 DIP	**Sante Fe Packing Co. Spike's Salsa con Queso, Medium** *170 milligrams (2 tablespoons)*	**Pace Mexican Four Cheese Salsa con Queso** *430 milligrams (2 tablespoons)*
3 TOMATO SAUCE	**Amy's Low Sodium Organic Marinara** *100 milligrams (½ cup)*	**Newman's Own Tomato and Basil** *620 milligrams (½ cup)*
4 SOUP	**Amy's Organic Cream of Tomato— Light in Sodium** *340 milligrams (1 cup)*	**Campbell's Soup Creamy Tomato Soup at Hand** *940 milligrams (10¾ ounce container)*
5 FROZEN PIZZA	**Full of Life Flatbread Mushroom Pizza with Caramelized Onions & Tomatoes** *406 milligrams (142-gram serving)*	**Celeste Deluxe** *980 milligrams (167-gram pizza)*

YOU ASKED

Q: What's a good butter substitute?

A: Why bail on butter? Sure, it's high in saturated fat, but a pat here and there isn't bad for your heart. That said, if you want to improve your heart health, consider one of the following substitutes. They taste like the real thing but act like spreadable medicine.

"Spreads with plant sterols and stanols can help you slash your LDL," says Lori Mosca, MD, the director of preventive cardiology at New York–Presbyterian Hospital. "Those made with omega-3s or olive oil may lower your triglycerides."

FULL CIRCLE ORGANIC OLIVE OIL: It's what this spray doesn't have (calories, fat, sodium) that makes it a kitchen essential. Spritz to sauté vegetables, cook omelets, or grill panini. *0 calories, 0 grams fat, 0 milligrams sodium*

OLIVIO ORIGINAL: The nutty taste comes from extra-light olive oil. It's rich in mono-unsaturated fat, which studies show can reduce LDL, triglycerides, and inflammation. *80 calories, 8 grams fat (1.5 grams saturated, 3.5 grams monounsaturated), 95 milligrams sodium*

SMART BALANCE OMEGA LIGHT: This spread contains fatty acids from fish oil, the source of EPA and DHA most easily absorbed by your body. But there's nothing fishy about its airy, delicate flavor. *50 calories, 5 grams fat (1.5 grams saturated, 1.5 grams monounsaturated), 80 milligrams sodium, 32 milligrams EPA/DHA*

SMART BALANCE HEARTRIGHT: On statins? Help your heart with this smooth-tasting schmear; plant sterols, monounsaturated fat, and omega-3s cover all your cardiac bases. *80 calories, 8 grams fat (2.5 grams saturated, 2.5 grams monounsaturated), 85 milligrams sodium, 32 milligrams EPA/DHA, 1.7 grams plant sterols*

LAND O' LAKES UNSALTED WHIPPED BUTTER: If only butter will do, this creamy spread has 4 fewer grams of saturated fat per serving than stick butter. Plus, it's sodium-free to help control your blood pressure.
50 calories, 6 grams fat (3.5 grams saturated, 1.5 grams monounsaturated)

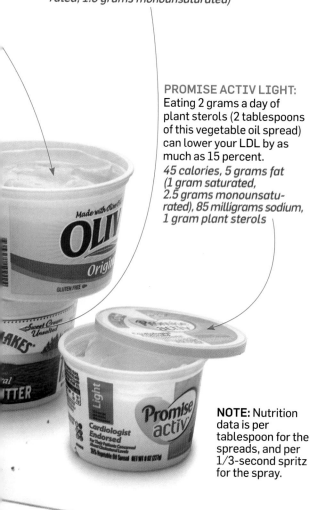

PROMISE ACTIV LIGHT: Eating 2 grams a day of plant sterols (2 tablespoons of this vegetable oil spread) can lower your LDL by as much as 15 percent.
45 calories, 5 grams fat (1 gram saturated, 2.5 grams monounsaturated), 85 milligrams sodium, 1 gram plant sterols

NOTE: Nutrition data is per tablespoon for the spreads, and per 1/3-second spritz for the spray.

Q: I use whole milk in my cereal and coffee, and I down a glass at night. Too much?

A: Actually, it's probably just enough. We've been told that whole milk is unhealthy, but that advice is based on old science that some scientists have soured on.

Q: Is it possible to wash all the pesticides off produce?

A: No amount of elbow grease, water, or suds can eliminate the chemicals from your kumquats. That's because some pesticides, instead of lingering on the skin of the produce, penetrate other parts of the plant to control pests. Residues from these pesticides cannot be washed off.

Now, if you believe the EPA, this is nothing to worry about: The agency mandates that a certain amount of time must pass between the last pesticide application and the harvest in order to ensure that any residue degrades to a safe level. But who knows what's safe?

"We can test the effects of specific chemicals on animals or on tissue samples, but no one can be certain what the effects of chemical combinations are on any one genetically unique person," says Dawn Gouge, PhD, of the University of Arizona. A recent study in *Pediatrics* linked high levels of organophosphates, one type of pesticide, in children to an increased risk of developing

YOU ASKED

attention deficit hyperactivity disorder.

The smart move: Reduce your exposure by buying organic, especially in the case of produce known to soak up the most pesticides—peaches, apples, strawberries, bell peppers, and cherries.

One exception: Don't bother lathering up your lettuce.

"Ready-to-eat salad is sanitized in a way far superior to any cleaning you can do at home," says Sam Beattie, PhD, a food safety specialist at Iowa State University. "It's washed in water and sanitizers such as chlorine compounds. Then it's rinsed thoroughly and spun dry—all at cold temperatures."

Actually, if there's a weak link in keeping prewashed greens clean, it's you.

"A leading cause of food-borne illness in the home is the norovirus, a bug transmitted by human feces on dirty hands," says Dr. Beattie. So before you stick your mitts into that bag of baby romaine, wash them with warm water and soap for at least 20 seconds. And don't ignore your nails. A British study found that 25 percent of men had harmful bacteria crawling under their claws.

Q: Other than prunes, what fruit can I eat to stay regular?

A: Melons. Cantaloupe, honeydew, and watermelon combine high water content and high fiber, says *Men's Health* nutrition advisor Jonny Bowden, PhD, CNS. "Most constipation comes from lack of water, and eating melon every day is a tasty, low-calorie way to stay on schedule."

Q: Is there a salad that can build muscle?

A: Yes, and it doesn't look like a plate of iceberg topped with creatine croutons. Picture something closer to a Cobb salad—a balanced mix of protein, fat, and carbs.

"Protein and carbohydrates work together to promote muscle synthesis," says nutritionist Alan Aragon, MS, *Men's Health*'s weight-loss expert. "Fats support testosterone production, while also keeping you satisfied."

Because the ideal muscle-building salad should contain at least 30 grams of each of these nutrients, we asked Seattle chef Tom Douglas to create a beefed-up version of the standard Cobb. This salad contains 650 calories, 49 grams of protein, 32 grams of carbs, and 35 grams of fat. When you need a break from beef, you can sub in three large shrimp or a 6-ounce salmon fillet, says Douglas.

The lettuce provides a healthy dose of folic acid, a B vitamin that enhances blood flow, according to a recent review in the *American Journal of Clinical Nutrition*.

1 strip bacon, cooked and chopped
Don't fret about the saturated fat; research shows that small amounts won't harm your heart. Plus, the pork provides choline, a

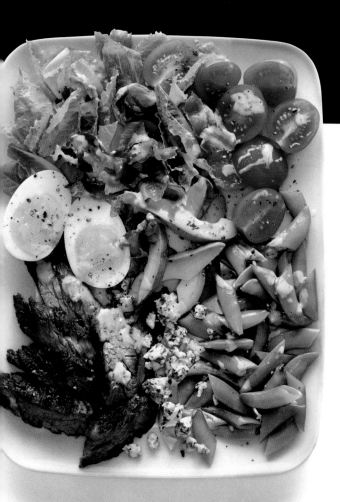

nutrient that's depleted during strenuous exercise, according to Oregon State University researchers.

1 soft-boiled egg, halved
The protein found in eggs has the highest muscle-building potential of any food—plus, the yolk contains B_{12}, which aids muscle contraction and fat breakdown.

1 hanger steak (4 ounce), grilled and sliced thinly against the grain
The creatine in beef supplies energy to your muscles, while the protein, iron, and zinc promote tissue growth.

6 cherry tomatoes, halved
Each bite-size orb contains 437 milligrams of the antioxidant lycopene, shown in a Taiwanese study to protect muscles from postexercise oxidative stress.

¼ avocado, sliced
Yes, avocados are rich in fat, but it's the heart-healthy monounsaturated kind.

1 tablespoon crumbled blue cheese
It's infused with probiotics, which may fight the immunosuppressive effects of exercise, notes a review in *Current Sports Medicine Reports*.

1 tablespoon Annie's Green Goddess dressing
Douglas makes his dressing from scratch, and includes egg yolks, champagne vinegar, and anchovies. Save time and calories with this alternative.

1 cup sugar snap peas (steamed 2 minutes, halved on the diagonal)
These power-packed pods add a shot of fiber to fill you up and help control your blood sugar.

Q: What's the healthiest beer?

A: Stout. It combines rich taste and low calories, so this dark brew is a better choice than a flavor-flat light beer. Stout also has more flavonoids, the same heart-healthy antioxidants found in wine, researchers at the University of Wisconsin report. Our favorite: Guinness Draught; a 12-ounce bottle has only 126 calories (versus Bud's 145).

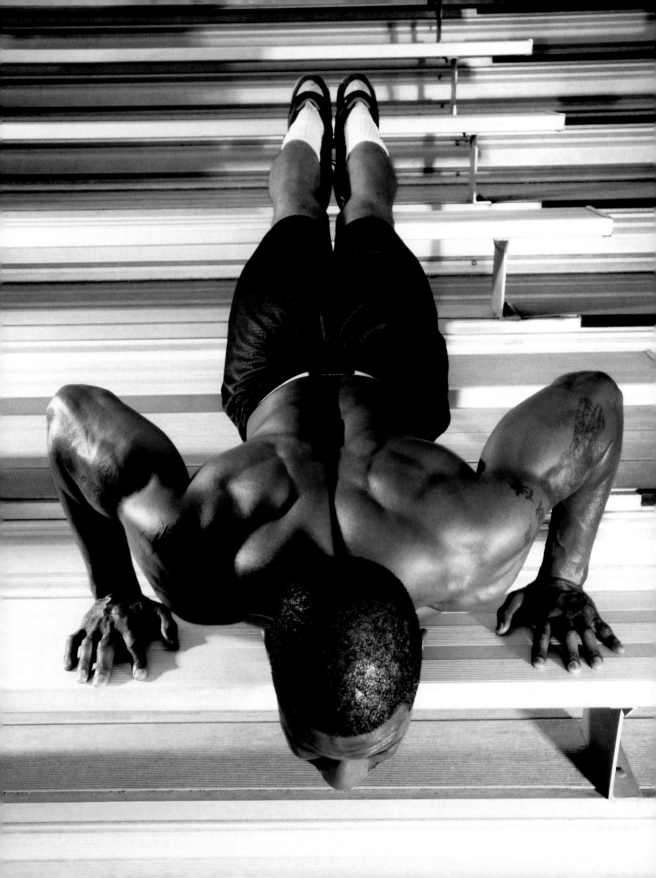

3

Muscle Up Fast

The Pushup Challenge

Take this 3-minute test to find out how fit you really are

Physical fitness isn't just about lifting. It's about how strong you are relative to your body weight, says Martin Rooney, PT, CSCS, author of *Ultimate Warrior Workouts.* That's why he has his athletes-in-training do body-weight tests. If they struggle, they need to either gain strength or lose weight. Test yourself the same way with his pushup challenge.

The Test

Do as many pushups as you can in 3 minutes.

The Rules

1. Rest whenever you want, but keep the clock running the whole time.

2. For a rep to count, you must maintain perfect form: elbows locked at the top, chest 2 inches above the floor at the bottom, hips not sagging, and knees not touching the floor.

3. Pace yourself however you'd like, but it's best not to rush, Rooney says. Take a 15-second break once you slow down after your first burst. Then take longer breaks as you become more tired, he says. Never push yourself to total fatigue.

Your Score

Here's how you did.
   < 55 pushups: Below average
   55 to 74 pushups: Average
   75 to 99 pushups: Good
   100 to 110 pushups: Excellent
   111 or more: Extraordinary

Problems to Look For

If you can't do 15 pushups with perfect form . . .
Your chest and triceps are weak. Strengthen them by doing regular high-rep (12 to 15) sets of the bench press and triceps pushdown. Also try pushups in a power rack on a barbell so you can set your body at an incline, making the pushup easier. As you improve, lower the barbell until you're doing regular pushups.

If your hips sag during pushups . . .
Your core is weak. Solution: planks and side planks. These exercises build stability and endurance in your core and mimic the movement needed to succeed at pushups. They're also great ab workouts.

If you take less than 5 seconds . . .
Your muscles and tendons already move fast, so increase the amount of weight you can lift. To do that, follow the workouts in this chart on separate days. They focus on lowering reps and adding weight. Rest 2 to 5 minutes between sets.

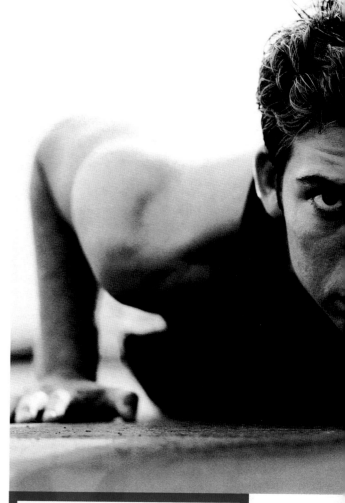

How to Boost Your Score

Add pushups to your routine twice a week for the next 4 weeks, says Rooney. Follow this pushup protocol, trying to complete each rep as quickly as possible. Then take 5 days off from pushups, and retest yourself.

Week	Sets	Pushups	Rest Between Sets
1	4	20	2 minutes
2	6	15	1 minute
3	4	25	1 minute
4	3	As many as you can	2 minutes

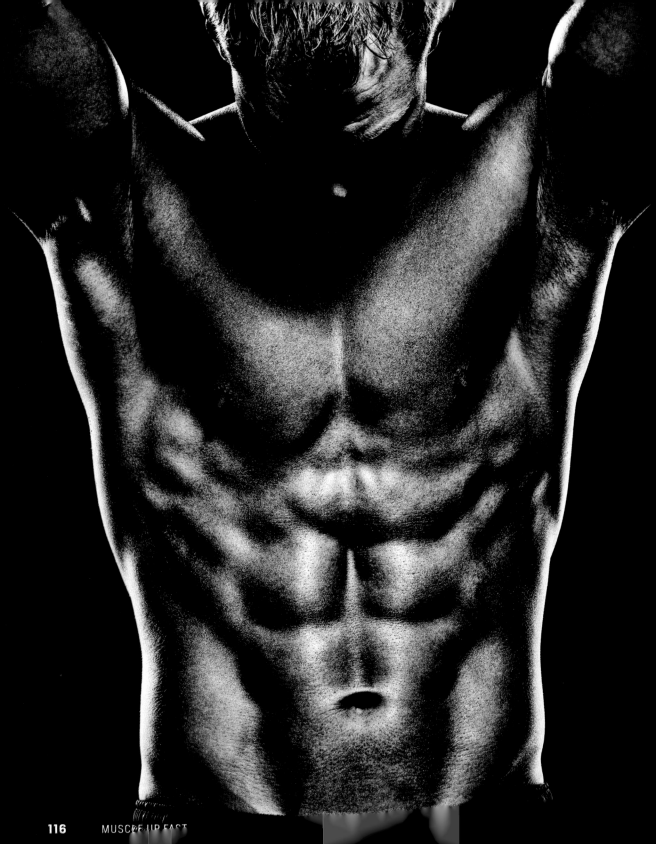

The Formula for Fat Loss

Use this cutting-edge workout to banish your belly and find your abs

This belly-busting plan from *The Men's Health Big Book of Exercises* is the last fat-loss workout you will ever need.

Created by Craig Rasmussen, CSCS, it employs the cutting-edge workout formula used at Results Fitness in Santa Clarita, California, one of America's top 10 gyms. Here, Rasmussen fills in the exercises for you. But in the book, you'll learn how to choose the moves yourself from a menu of more than 600 exercises. So anytime you want a new routine, all you have to do is plug and play—and watch your gut melt away.

WORKOUT A

1A
Barbell Rollout

Load a barbell with 10-pound plates and affix collars. Kneel on the floor and grab the bar with an overhand, shoulder-width grip. Position your shoulders directly over the barbell and keep your lower back naturally arched (**A**). Slowly roll the bar forward, extending your body as far as you can without letting your hips sag (**B**). Pause for 2 seconds, and reverse the move to return to the starting position

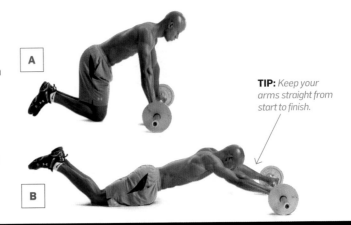

A

B

TIP: *Keep your arms straight from start to finish.*

2A
Crossover Dumbbell Stepup

Grab a pair of dumbbells and stand with a bench to your left. Place your right foot on the bench (**A**). Press your right foot into the bench and push your body up until your right leg is straight but your left foot is still off the bench (**B**). Then lower yourself to the starting position. Do all your reps on your right leg, then turn around and repeat with your left leg.

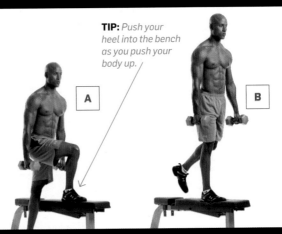

TIP: *Push your heel into the bench as you push your body up.*

A

B

3A
Barbell Front Squat

Hold a bar next to your chest with a shoulder-width, overhand grip. Raise your upper arms until they're parallel to the floor, letting the bar roll back so that it's resting on the front of your shoulders (**A**). Push your hips back, bend your knees, and lower your body until the tops of your thighs are at least parallel to the floor (**B**). Pause, and return to the starting position.

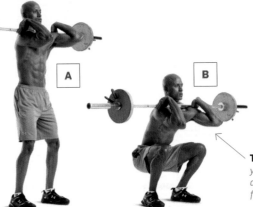

A

B

TIP: *Don't allow your upper arms to drop as you perform the exercise.*

Alternate between WORKOUT A and WORKOUT B, with a day of rest after each session. For exercise 1 in each workout, do 2 to 3 sets of 10 reps, resting 60 seconds after each set. Then perform exercises 2A and 2B as a pair. That is, do 12 reps of exercise 2A, rest 60 seconds, and do 12 reps of exercise 2B. Rest for 60 seconds again, and repeat until you've completed 3 sets of both exercises. Follow the same procedure with exercises 3A and 3B, alternating back and forth with the same sets, reps, and rest.

2B
Inverted Row

Secure a bar in a power rack at about waist height, and lie underneath it. Grab the bar with an overhand, shoulder-width grip, and hang from it with your arms straight. Your body should form a straight line from your ankles to your head (**A**). Pull your chest to the bar (**B**). Pause, and slowly lower yourself back to the starting position.

TIP: *Keep your core braced so that your body stays rigid.*

A

B

3B
Pushup

Assume a pushup position with your arms straight and your hands slightly beyond shoulder width. Your body should form a straight line from your head to your ankles (**A**). Bend your elbows and lower your body until your chest nearly touches the floor (**B**). Pause, push yourself back to the starting position, and repeat.

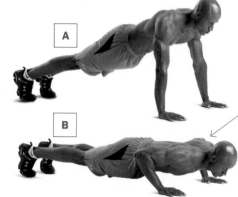

A

B

TIP: *Your shoulders should dip a bit below your elbows.*

WORKOUT B

1A
Cable Core Press

Attach a stirrup handle to the middle pulley of a cable station. With the cable taut, hold the handle against your chest with both hands and stand with your right side facing the stack (**A**). Slowly press your arms forward until they're completely straight (**B**). Pause for 5 seconds, and reverse the movement. Do all your reps, then turn around and work your other side

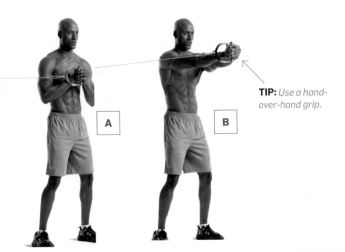

TIP: *Use a hand-over-hand grip.*

A   B

2A
Offset Dumbbell Reverse Lunge

Stand holding a dumbbell in your right hand next to your shoulder, with your arm bent (**A**). With your left foot, step backward into a reverse lunge and lower your body until your back knee almost touches the floor (**B**). Push yourself back to the starting position and repeat. Do all your reps, then switch arms and lunge backward with your right leg.

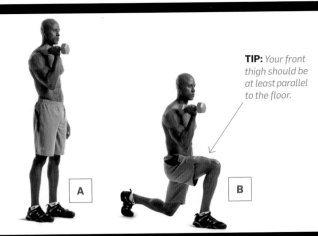

TIP: *Your front thigh should be at least parallel to the floor.*

A   B

3A
Barbell Deadlift

Load a barbell and roll it against your shins. Bend at your hips and knees and grab the bar with an overhand grip, your hands just beyond shoulder width (**A**). Keeping your lower back naturally arched, pull your torso up and thrust your hips forward as you stand up with the barbell (**B**). Lower the bar to the floor and repeat.

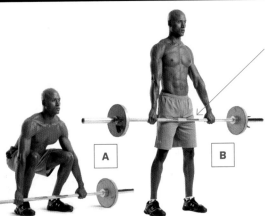

TIP: *Keep the bar close to your body from start to finish.*

A   B

This 30-minute workout will burn away your belly fat for good.

2B
Chinup

Grab a chinup bar with a shoulder-width, underhand grip, and hang at arm's length (A). Now squeeze your shoulder blades down and back, bend your elbows, and pull the top of your chest to the bar (B). Pause, slowly lower your body back to the starting position, and repeat.

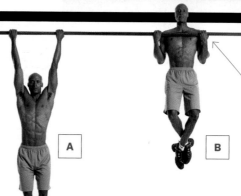

TIP: *Aim to touch your collarbone to the bar.*

3B
Dumbbell Push Press

Stand holding a pair of dumbbells just outside your shoulders, with your arms bent and palms facing each other. Your feet should be shoulder width apart and your knees slightly bent (A). Dip your knees (B), then explosively push up with your legs as you press the weights straight above your shoulders (C). Lower the dumbbells to the starting position and repeat.

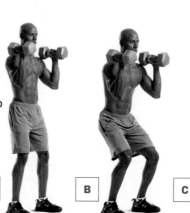

TIP: *Keep your wrists straight and press the weights directly above each shoulder.*

121

The Power

Within

Writer Grant Stoddard explores the untapped energy source
that's completely green, highly sustainable, and 100 percent free.
And right now, it's probably covering your abs.

As soon as Mike Taggett realizes I don't know the first thing about electricity, he insists on helping me set up the Human Dynamo 4.2 in person. And who better? After all, the HD 4.2 is Taggett's invention, and I'm more than eager to have it installed in my home. That's because the Human Dynamo is the first commercial exercise machine that converts human effort into usable electricity. And, I'm hoping, it's also a great tool I can use to burn the lingering belly flab I can't seem to lose. In fact, if this machine works, I'll be able to illuminate my house using energy generated from my own body fat. So I'll reduce not only my carbon footprint but my pants size, too. Now that's a green movement anyone can support. But is it too good to be true?

Mike Taggett's electro-ergonomic innovation was first inspired by high-level athletes. The engineering researcher observed that these powerful creatures waste a lot of energy—their own. That's when he set out to build a machine that could use this untapped energy to power any number of devices.

"I believe I've found the best way to produce usable power with the human body," says Taggett, who built the prototype in his El Paso workshop. "It's all about moving your legs and arms in unison." Taggett points out that one version of his machine, called Team Dynamo, is already in use at the Green Microgym in Portland, Oregon. Picture four exercise units, each resembling a stationary bike, linked together by a shared driveshaft. The upshot: Club members help power the facility's lighting and sound systems as they build fitness and shed fat. It could be a blueprint for the gym of the future.

As we assemble the Human Dynamo 4.2 in my New York apartment, Taggett surveys the room.

"I see you have a few human-powered machines in here already." He points to an antique hand-cranked gramophone and an old Singer sewing machine with a manual foot pedal, curios my girlfriend picked up. Both items speak of a historical continuum of human power, one that stretches from the Bronze Age potter's wheel to the 21st-century hand-cranked laptop.

Now I'm becoming one of Tagget's turbines, and it's not a moment too soon. At 32, I've noticed a deterioration in my body composition, so I've added a 6-mile run to my daily workout. As a result, I burn 500 or so calories exercising each morning, which is enough for me to stay in reasonable shape. Yet I'm expending most of those calories for no greater purpose than to propel myself around a golf course. Running my circular route is tantamount to being a hamster on a wheel. Shouldn't my sweat equity offer a greater return? That's the promise of Taggett's machine.

To understand how the Human Dynamo 4.2 works, you have to start with the name. A dynamo, of course, is a generator. But "4.2" isn't the current version of the machine. No, those digits describe the number of kilocalories (or simply "calories") that equal about 1 watt of electric power. (It's actually closer to 4 than 4.2.) Put in context, the 500 calories I expend during my daily run is equivalent to wasting about 125 watts. Until now.

This isn't to suggest that I can simply muscle my way to energy independence. Taggett claims, though, that with the help of his invention, I can run a significant percentage of my electrical appliances on self-generated electricity—if I'm willing to do the work. It's like going back decades in time, before the conveniences of the modern world made us such a sedentary— and fat—society. (See "The Rise of the Machines" on page 126.)

And that's what really interests me. Research shows that in your third decade, the metabolic storm of youth begins to drop about 1 percent every 4 years. The Human Dynamo 4.2 could help me combat this age-related decline—and protect my abs from a future blanket of fat.

A man's metabolism is generally described in one of two ways: fast or slow. A fast metabolism, of course, suggests that you can eat to your belly's content with little regard for the calorie load of your meals. A slow metabolism, on the other hand, supposedly means that just

glancing at a deep-dish pizza can cause your fat cells to swell. But, scientifically speaking, there's a much more concrete definition. In simple terms, your metabolism is the sum total of chemical reactions that break down fats, carbohydrates, and proteins in order to liberate the energy they contain, says Alex Koch, PhD, an exercise scientist at Truman State University. These metabolic reactions can be divided into three categories.

First is your basal metabolic rate. "This is the energy required to sustain life," says Dr. Koch. Remarkably, 60 to 70 percent of the daily calories your body burns are spent just keeping your vitals signs vital. This number includes the amount of energy needed to keep your heart pumping, lungs breathing, liver functioning, and hair growing.

So you can't really control that part of the metabolic formula. "It's highly related to your body mass," says Jeff Volek, PhD, RD, an exercise and nutrition scientist at

The Myth about Muscle

Ever hear that a pound of muscle burns 50 calories a day? Forget that stat: It's a myth. When we asked Jeff Volek, PhD, RD, to roughly estimate the metabolic activity of muscle, his ballpark figure surprised even us. Dr. Volek's calculations: One pound of skeletal muscle burns about 6 calories a day, while 1 pound of fat burns about 2 calories a day. ("Many factors are at play, so call this my best educated guess," says Dr. Volek.) Here's the good news: Even though muscle tissue itself doesn't provide much of a metabolic boost, the physical work you need to do to build and maintain new muscle can have a dramatic effect on your overall metabolism. What's more, research shows that a single weight-training session can spike your calorie burn for up to 39 hours after you lift. And finally, the more muscle you have, the better your body's ability to use the nutrients you eat—instead of storing them as fat.

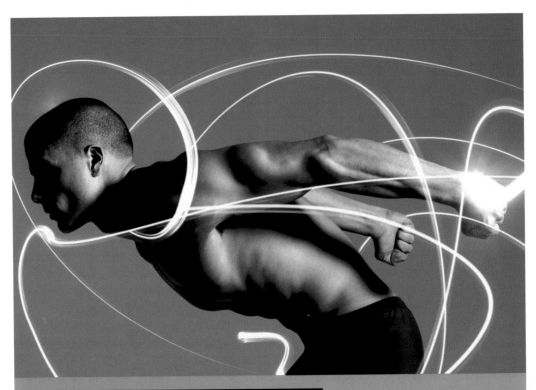

The Rise of the Machines

In a Dutch study, researchers compared the activity levels of modern office workers with those of actors mimicking the daily lives of 19th-century Australian settlers. The findings: The actors' activity levels were 1.6 times higher—the equivalent of walking 3 to 8 more miles a day. The scientists published the "logically intuitive" graph below in the *International Journal of Sports Medicine;* it shows how technological advances over the past 100 years have contributed to decreased physical activity—and coincided with the obesity epidemic.

USE OF TECHNOLOGY AND CHANGE IN ENERGY EXPENDITURE

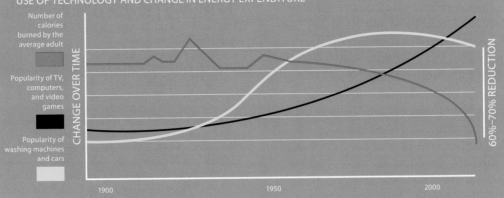

Number of calories burned by the average adult

Popularity of TV, computers, and video games

Popularity of washing machines and cars

CHANGE OVER TIME

60%–70% REDUCTION

1900   1950   2000

the University of Connecticut. So the more you weigh—whether you're built like a bodybuilder or a sumo wrestler—the higher your basal metabolic rate. It makes sense: If your body is bigger, there are simply more total cells and tissue it has to maintain. And that requires energy.

The second part of the equation is one you can influence a little more.

"Metabolic rate goes up with ingestion of food," says Dr. Volek. "This is called the thermic effect of food, or TEF." The TEF of protein is about 25 percent, meaning a quarter of the calories this nutrient provides are burned during digestion and processing. Carbohydrate has a TEF of 8 to 10 percent, and fat's TEF is 3 to 5 percent. "This is why consuming several small protein meals over the day can help keep your metabolism elevated," says Volek.

The third component of metabolism is physical activity. The energy you use to haul yourself around falls into two subcategories, each with a convenient acronym: EAT and NEAT. "Exercise-activity thermogenesis, or EAT, is the amount of energy expended by your muscles during planned exercise, like when you lift weights or go for a run," explains Dr. Koch. "NEAT, or nonexercise-activity thermogenesis, is the amount of energy expended by your muscles during any incidental movement." Not everyone exercises, but everyone expends energy through physical activity. Walking through the grocery store, opening a bag of pretzels, and even flipping through the channels with your thumb involve muscular activity that expends energy.

This is where a contraption like the Human Dynamo can really help.

Say your gym time is fixed. Maybe you have time for only three 30-minute workouts a week. And let's also assume that you're closely watching what you eat. If you want to lose body fat faster, there's seemingly only one other option. You have to increase your NEAT, the activity you do that's not part of an actual workout, but just part of your life.

"If this machine works, I'll reduce my carbon footprint and my pants size, too."

Enter the Human Dynamo 4.2. If I want to watch TV, I have to start moving. It's like a chore. I hold the power of choice: Catch the new episode of *Friday Night Lights*—or sit on the couch and stare at the wall. It's not planned exercise; it's more like using a washboard to clean my shirts.

This burns calories, of course, but there's a surprise benefit, too. Boosting my metabolism by increasing my NEAT also allows me to boost my metabolism with something much more pleasurable: food. Confused? Let me explain.

During the 2008 Olympics, it was widely reported that gold-medal swimmer Michael Phelps consumed some 12,000 calories a day while he was training. Yet Phelps was as lean as a dolphin. This is what's known as "high-energy flux": a lot of calories in and a corresponding amount of calories out. Because Phelps was burning so many calories, he could eat an enormous amount

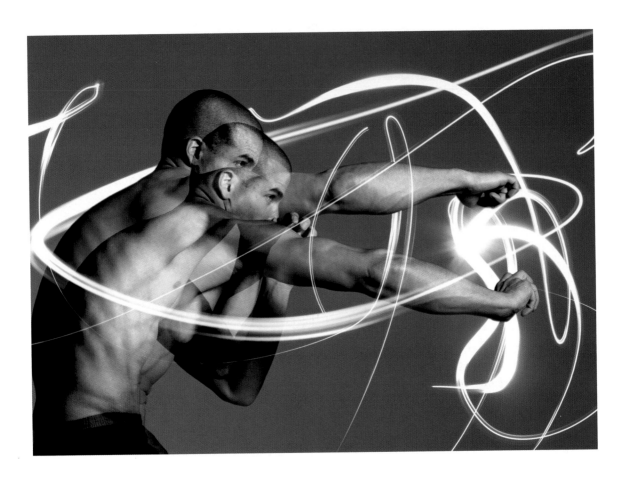

Metabolism slows a little each year.

of grub. And digesting all that food led to an even greater total calorie burn. So as it turned out, Phelps had a fast metabolism because, well, he made it fast. You can do the same.

While high-energy flux will push metabolism into overdrive, people's metabolic rates do go through stages as they age. In children and adolescents, a significant proportion of food intake is channeled into growth. As that growth slows, so does metabolic rate. By your mid-20s, your body doesn't process pizza and soda in quite the same way it did

when you were a kid.

And while it's been documented that metabolism slows a little more each year until death, the good news is that it appears this process can be thwarted. When researchers at the University of Colorado compared older and younger people doing the same amount of exercise and eating the same number and quality of calories, they found no difference in metabolic rate. This suggests that the most important factor isn't age, but lifestyle.

The frame of the Human Dynamo 4.2 is stylish and simple: a V shape nestling up to an orange flywheel that drives a motor. The position of the foot pedals is fixed, but you can adjust the rotating handles for "sprinting" in an upright climbing position. A knob on the console lets you add torque to the resistance and hence increase the amount of power you generate as you pump. My sweat will charge a battery that's hooked up to a DC-to-AC power inverter to run my appliances.

"Okay," says Taggett. "Hop on!"

I begin pedaling with my arms and legs at a fair rate, with the dial up at 100 percent resistance. Within a few minutes, I've produced more sweat than I do on my daily run.

"Watts, by definition, are by the hour," says Taggett. "If you keep this up for an hour, you will have created about 160 human watts."

"Human watts?" I manage to say between huge gulps of air. "As opposed to…?"

"Well, the amount of human watts and the amount of usable watts are two different things," explains Taggett. "There's energy loss from the bike to the battery. There's further loss from the battery to the inverter. So the power you'd end up with is a little over half the power you would actually generate."

Because I'm already nearing utter exhaustion after just minutes on the bike, it sucks to hear that I'm losing 40 percent of my power. But locomotive inefficiency and power-transfer loss are the bugbears of any engineering project. I decide to focus on a different number: 3,500, or roughly the number of calories in a pound of body fat. In electrical terms, that's 875 watts. I'm enthralled at the idea of turning a pound of something I don't want into power I need.

"Okay, so what stuff do you want to run with this?" asks Taggett. "Everything," I reply, giving my "stored energy" a pat.

Taggett raises an eyebrow and produces a small electrical metering device from his backpack. The Kill-A-Watt plugs

Weight Loss Made Simple

Yes, you know you should use the stairs, not the escalator. But while this kind of advice may prompt you to roll your eyes, heeding it can have a significant impact on your daily energy expenditure. Case in point: the five simple strategies below. Infuse them into your life and you can instantly—and almost effortlessly—burn about 10 percent more calories a day.

+ Do This	− Not This	= Equals
Go for a brisk 20-minute walk	Sit for your entire lunch hour	49 extra calories burned
Stand during three 10-minute phone calls	Put your feet up on your desk	33 extra calories burned
Play vigorously with your kids or pet for 15 minutes	Watch TV before dinner	82 extra calories burned
Spend 15 minutes washing the dishes	Head straight to the couch	27 extra calories burned
Take 10 minutes to straighten up one room	Go right to bed	21 extra calories burned

Total extra calories burned: 212
Metabolism boost: about 10 percent

into an outlet and displays the wattage of any appliance you choose to plug into it. With a knowing grin, he begins pointing at things in my apartment.

"The blender?" he asks.

I quickly learn that, depending on the setting, the blender draws between 260 and 365 watts; the TV requires 160 watts; my laptop, 20 watts; my alarm clock, 4 watts; the dryer sucks an incredible 4,000 watts; an LED reading lamp needs just 6 to 7 watts. We go through several other appliances and gadgets until I have a fairly good idea of what I can power myself. I revise my expectations somewhat, and decide that starting the next day, I will attempt to power my TV, charge my laptop and cell phone, and provide the juice for my

The Truth about Calories

You may be burning fewer calories than you think. That's because the "calories burned" stat on a treadmill display (or in a magazine!) includes the amount of energy you expend when you're just sitting around, says Alex Koch, PhD.

"For example, depending on your size, you burn about 1.2 calories a minute while you're sleeping," says Dr. Koch. "So to know how many extra calories you're burning with exercise, you have to subtract that number from your total." For instance, a 180-pound guy might burn 120 calories while mowing his lawn, but that's not 120 additional calories; it's 120 calories total. Turns out, it'd be just 60 more calories than what he'd expend while surfing the Web. The same rule applies to your workout. To know your true bonus burn, use this chart to calculate the calories you would have expended had you not exercised—and then subtract them from your total.

Activity	Calories per Minute
Watching TV	1.4
Typing on a computer	2.5
Driving a car	2.7

reading lamp. If I still have energy after that, I'll try to make some toast.

Twenty-four hours later, my apartment door flies open. "I want to watch the news," my girlfriend declares as she arrives home from work. I've been using the bike intermittently for 20 minutes every hour since she left, and I'm confident my sweat has bought oodles of time in front of the tube. Katie Couric has barely finished reading the headlines, however, when the inverter starts beeping. Seconds later, the TV shuts off.

"Hey," my girlfriend says indignantly. "I was watching that!"

I dutifully straddle the bike and begin pedaling again. Two minutes of hard work charges up enough watts to turn the TV back on, but we soon hear the pre-shutoff warning and I have to pedal like hell to avoid interrupting Ms. Couric further.

Despite what it might sound like, I'm not in too bad shape. But my maximum, gut-busting sprint on the HD 4.2 could scare up only about 250 average watts for a matter of several seconds. For perspective, Taggett estimates that during a 4-to-6-hour race stage, an oxen-hearted specimen like Lance Armstrong could average 250 to 300 watts.

But even if a competitive cyclist—someone who could produce serious wattage—were using the Human Dynamo to power a decent proportion of his household, it would be misleading to think of the device as an entirely green energy solution. In order to power a few gadgets, I was expending an extra 1,000 calories a day. Good for my metabolism, but good for the planet? Consider: Unless I planned to

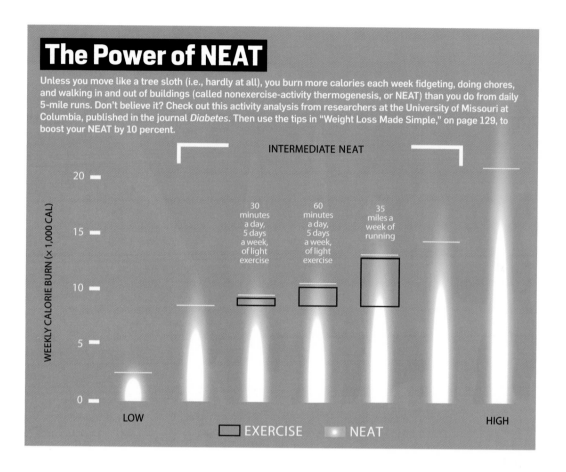

The Power of NEAT

Unless you move like a tree sloth (i.e., hardly at all), you burn more calories each week fidgeting, doing chores, and walking in and out of buildings (called nonexercise-activity thermogenesis, or NEAT) than you do from daily 5-mile runs. Don't believe it? Check out this activity analysis from researchers at the University of Missouri at Columbia, published in the journal *Diabetes*. Then use the tips in "Weight Loss Made Simple," on page 129, to boost your NEAT by 10 percent.

INTERMEDIATE NEAT

WEEKLY CALORIE BURN (× 1,000 CAL)

20

15

10

5

0

30 minutes a day, 5 days a week, of light exercise

60 minutes a day, 5 days a week, of light exercise

35 miles a week of running

LOW

HIGH

☐ EXERCISE   ● NEAT

wither away completely, I'd have to up my food intake. That food would in turn have to be planted, irrigated, fed, harvested, processed, and transported hundreds or even thousands of miles to my local store. And if I'm going to eat more food, I'll need to produce more energy to cook it.

My week of generating my own power was a revelation. The Human Dynamo 4.2 opened my eyes to the power demands of both my body and every gadget I possess. During my experiment, television was a rare treat. I became far more discerning with my viewing choices, given the effort

I'd have to expend to keep the thing on. I'd guess that reality TV might cease to exist if its fan base were asked to sweat for it.

Though the duration of my experiment was too short for me to note giant physiological changes, it did imbue me with a better understanding of how to impact my metabolic rate. As with a fireplace, keeping your metabolic flames roaring requires adequate fuel, oxygen, and a good poke at regular intervals. Done right, there's no reason the fire should die out. Remember that, and you have the foundation for stoking your own eternal flame.

The Gut Buster

Use this metabolism-boosting workout to transform your body faster than ever

This program uses the latest training techniques to torch belly fat. Instead of running, you'll do total-body exercises at a fast pace. After all, whether you're running or lifting, your muscles require energy to help you move. And this workout forces more of your muscles into action than you'd ever use while jogging for the same duration. Not convinced? Just try it once.

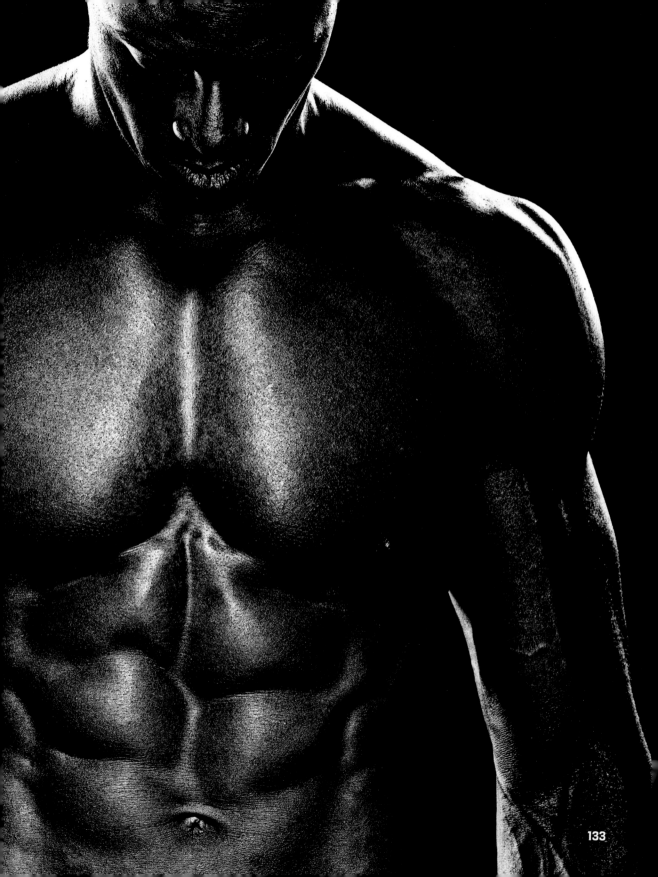

Perform each workout once a week, resting at least 1 day between sessions. So you might do WORKOUT A on Monday, WORKOUT B on Wednesday, and WORKOUT C on Friday.

WORKOUT A

Complete these exercises back-to-back, using a technique known as countdowns. Do 15 reps of swings, followed by 15 reps of burpees. Without resting, do 14 reps of swings and then 14 reps of burpees. Continue this pattern until you do only 1 rep of each exercise.

WORKOUT B

Perform these four exercises as a circuit, doing one after another in succession. Do 10 repetitions of each movement, and rest for no longer than 20 seconds between each exercise. Complete the entire four exercise circuit a total of 10 times.

WORKOUT C

Perform the exercises as a circuit. Do 6 reps of each movement, and cycle through all four exercises as many times as possible in 20 minutes. Rest as needed.

WORKOUT A

1
Dumbbell Swing

Bend at your hips and hold a dumbbell between your legs (**A**). Thrust your hips forward and swing the weight to shoulder height (**B**).

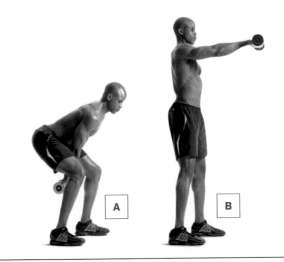

> **TIP:** *Keep your lower back slightly arched as you swing the dumbbell back and forth.*
>
> *Your arm should swing up from the momentum of your body.*

2
Squat Thrust

Stand with your feet shoulder width apart (**A**). Bending at your hips and knees, lower your body until you can place your hands on the floor (**B**). Kick your legs backward, then perform a pushup (**C**). Reverse the move and stand up. That's 1 rep.

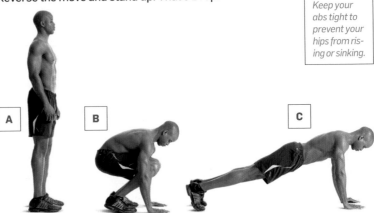

> **TIP:** *Place your hands on the floor in front of you, shifting your weight onto them.*
>
> *Keep your abs tight to prevent your hips from rising or sinking.*

WORKOUT B

1
Overheader's Walk

Grab a pair of dumbbells and press them over your head, your palms facing each other. Walk forward—each step is 1 rep.

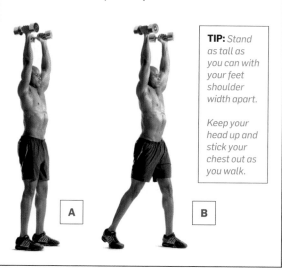

TIP: *Stand as tall as you can with your feet shoulder width apart.*

Keep your head up and stick your chest out as you walk.

A

B

2
Pushup-Position Row

Place a pair of hex dumbbells on the floor and set yourself in pushup position with your hands on the dumbbells (**A**). Pull the right dumbbell up to the side of your chest (**B**). Pause, then lower the dumbbell; repeat the move with your left arm. That's 1 rep.

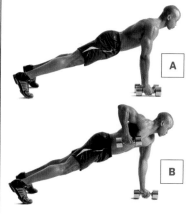

TIP: *The dumbbells should be set slightly beyond shoulder width.*

Don't allow your upper body to rotate as you row the dumbbell.

A

B

3
Thrusters

Hold a pair of dumbbells next to your shoulders (**A**). Squat down (**B**), and as you stand back up, press the dumbbells overhead (**C**).

TIP: *Keep your torso as upright as possible through-out the movement.*

The tops of your thighs should be parallel to the floor when you squat.

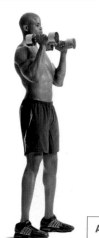

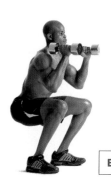

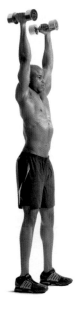

A

B

C

4
T-Pushup

Do a pushup with your hands on a pair of hex dumbbells (**A**). As you push up, rotate your right arm toward the ceiling (**B**); return to the starting position. That's 1 rep. Repeat to the other side.

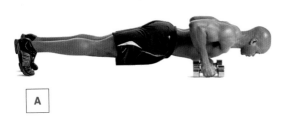

A

TIP:
(**A**) *The dumbbells should be set slightly beyond shoulder width. With your feet hip width apart, lower your chest to the floor.*

(**B**) *Raise the dumbbell and rotate your body in one fluid motion. Your arms should form a T with your body.*

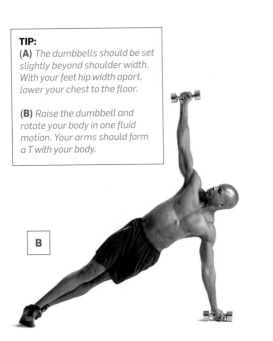

B

WORKOUT C

1
Lateral Shuffle

Stand in an athletic stance (**A**). Shuffle to your left by moving either foot and then the other (**B**). That's one step. Take three steps to your left, six steps to your right, and three steps back to your left. That's 1 set.

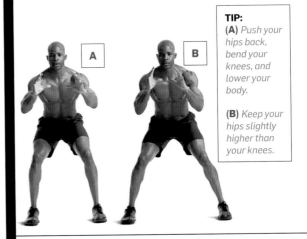

A   **B**

TIP:
(**A**) *Push your hips back, bend your knees, and lower your body.*

(**B**) *Keep your hips slightly higher than your knees.*

3
Dumbbell Reverse Lunge

Grab a pair of dumbbells and hold them next to your sides, your palms facing each other (**A**). Step backward with your left foot and lower your body until your front knee is bent at least 90 degrees (**B**). Return to the starting position, and step back with your right leg. That's 1 rep.

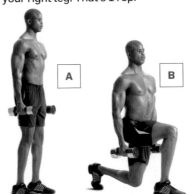

A   **B**

TIP:
(**A**) *Brace your core and hold it that way for the entire exercise.*

(**B**) *Keep your torso upright during the move.*

2
Pushup and Row

Place a pair of hex dumbbells on the floor and set yourself in pushup position (A). Perform a pushup (B), but once you return to the starting position, row the dumbbell in your right hand to the side of your chest (C). Lower the dumbbell and repeat with your left arm. That's 1 rep.

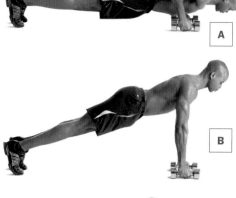

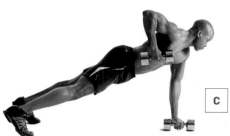

This 4-week plan can turn your body into a **fat-burning machine.**

TIP:
(A) *Your body should form a straight line from your ankles to your head.*

(B) *Lower your body to the floor, pause, and then push yourself back up.*

(C) *Your torso shouldn't rotate as you row.*

4
Dumbbell Getup

Lie faceup and hold a dumbbell in your left hand with your arm straight above you (A). Roll onto your right side and prop yourself up (B). Stand up while keeping the dumbbell above you at all times (C and D). Once standing, reverse the movement. Do all 6 reps, then switch arms and do another 6.

TIP:
(A) *Lock your elbow and keep your legs straight.*

(B) *Place one foot flat on the floor and don't take your eyes off the dumbbell at any time.*

(C) *Push yourself to a kneeling position.*

(D) *Stand tall before reversing the movement.*

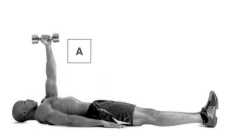

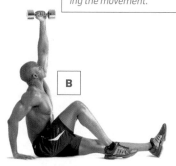

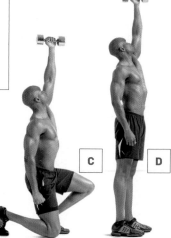

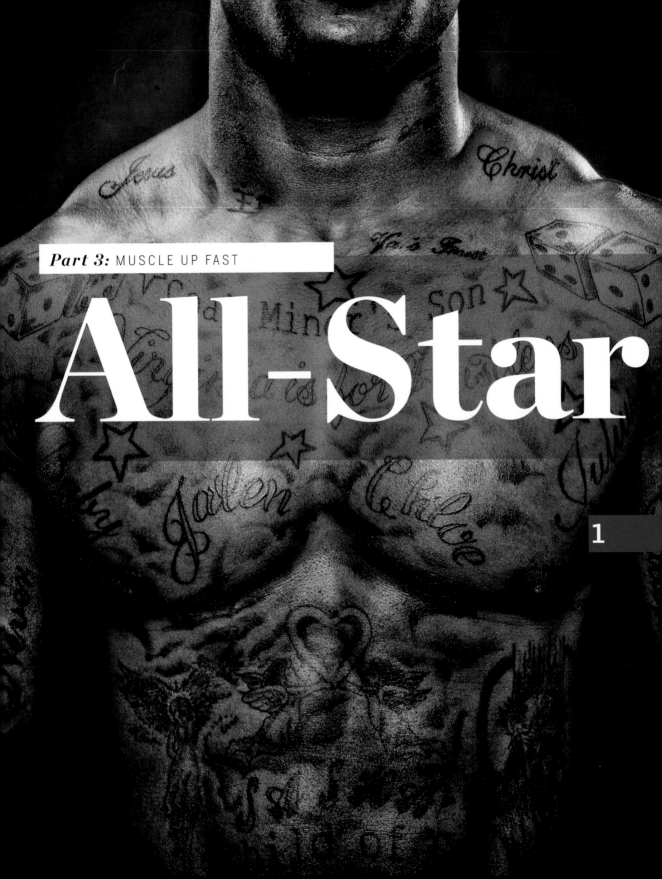

All-Star

1

Sure, you don't have a cadre of trainers, chefs, and personal assistants. Nor do you have 6 hours a day to train. But with the help of these trainers, you can build the abs you want.

Abs

How do men create camera-ready cores? We asked their trainers.

1 THOMAS JONES
Kansas City Chiefs running back
SECRET: small muscles

Most men perform crunches because they think they can "feel" their abs working. The reality: Your abs will pop and you'll be a stronger athlete if, like Jones, you also work the smaller stabilizer muscles in and around your core.

"Your pelvis and spine are subject to lots of movement when you play sports, so it's important to learn how to stabilize your body," says Pete Bommarito, CSCS, Jones's trainer when he was with the Jets. Here are two exercises he uses.

Prone Arm Lift
Begin in a pushup position, your body forming a straight line from shoulders to ankles. Lift your right hand and extend your arm overhead with your thumb pointing up. Slowly lower your arm back to the starting position, and repeat the move with your left arm. Do 6 repetitions on each side, and try to avoid any rotation in your hips and lower back.

Hip Rotation
Lie on your back with your arms outstretched, legs together, knees bent, and feet on the floor. Raise your feet off the ground so your hips and knees are at 90-degree angles, then rotate your knees to the right until your right knee is about 2 inches above the floor. Pause for 3 seconds, then repeat in the other direction. Complete 8 reps to each side.

2 BRADLEY COOPER
Actor
SECRET: cross-training

"Combine cardio, strength training, and core exercises into one workout," says trainer Ramona Braganza. That way you burn fat while building strength and targeting your core.

With Cooper, she uses a method she calls "321": three cardio circuits, two strength-training circuits, and one core circuit, each 10 minutes long. Your workout is finished in an hour. Start with a cardio session, then do a weight-training circuit of three multimuscle exercises (such as squats, bench presses, and pullups). Next, do high-intensity cardio intervals, like sprints. Follow that with three more full-body exercises. Next up: one final cardio session, followed by 10 minutes of core exercises, such as V-ups and planks.

3 HASHEEM THABEET
Houston Rockets center
SECRET: power diet

"Don't skip meals, and don't eat less. The more you eat, the more you'll burn—if you're training and eating right," says Tom Vachet, CPT, who prepped number-two pick Thabeet for his rookie season.

High-intensity training revs metabolism, and you need the right calories to fuel your transformation. Vachet recommends snacking about 30 minutes before a workout; aim for a 60/40 carb/protein mix, with only trace amounts of fat. (Try 16 ounces of juice with 3 ounces of chicken breast, or juice with a scoop of whey protein isolate.) Immediately after your routine, down a meal that's 50 percent carbs, 25 percent protein, and 25 percent fat— a banana, 16 ounces of chocolate milk, and a tablespoon of peanut butter, for example.

4 GERARD BUTLER
Actor
SECRET: heavy weights

"Moving heavy weight and engaging your core, as with squats and deadlifts, is one of the best ways to help build your six-pack," says trainer Joe Dowdell, CSCS. (And multimuscle exercises burn more calories, to melt the fat that hides your abs.)

Dowdell also challenges Butler with direct core moves, such as hanging leg raises, front planks, and side planks; these work your abs from many angles. At the end of a workout, do 3 sets of 10 to 15 reps of hanging leg raises, and 3 sets of planks that you hold for 30 seconds to 2 minutes.

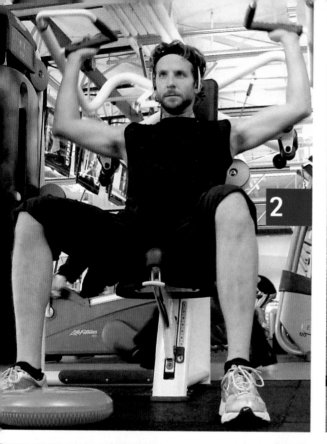

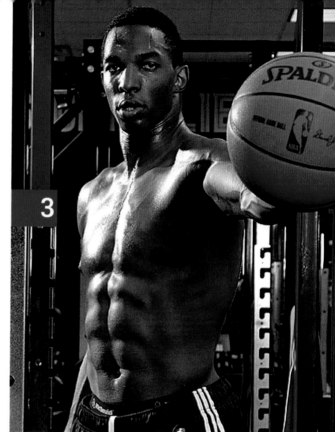

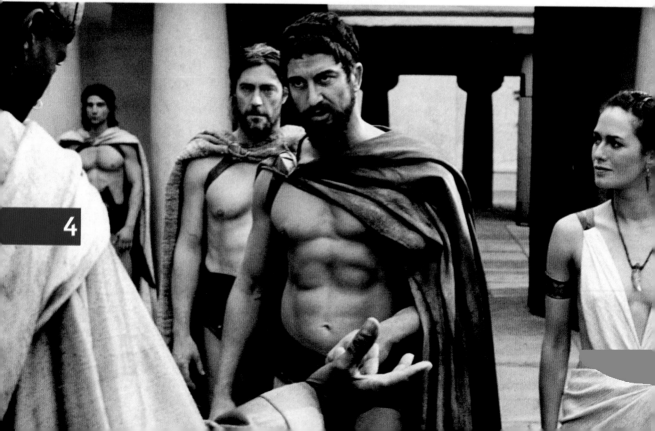

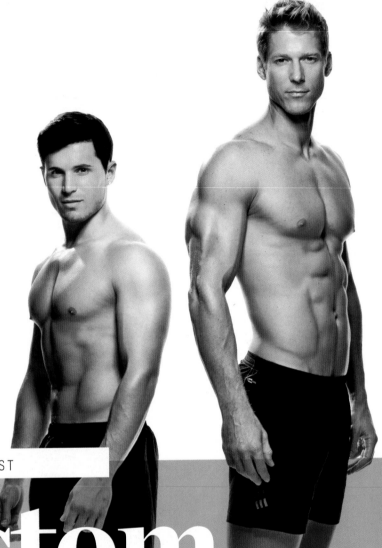

Custom Body Plans

Don't let your DNA ruin your chance to build muscle, strength, and power

Here's a guaranteed motivation killer: After months or years of dedicated lifting, you realize that you'll never bench your body weight, jump high enough to reach the rim, or hit double digits on pullups. It's just not in the cards. You start to wonder why you even bother.

It might seem unfair, but there will always be guys—some of whom inevitably find their way to the bench or squat rack next to yours—who seem born to excel at certain exercises. The truth is, they were. And you weren't. But that's no excuse to cancel your gym membership.

"Even if your body proportions aren't ideal, you can still perform exercises that maximize your body's potential," says Todd Durkin, CSCS, the owner of Fitness Quest 10 in San Diego.

So don't give up. Instead, sack up and tackle the problem head-on. Here are some common traits that can lead to frustration in the weight room, and ways to make the most of what you have to build a better body.

THE PROBLEM
Long Arms

The bench press may be a barometer of masculinity, but it discriminates against long-limbed lifters. While the distance the bar travels does limit both performance and results, long arms can also set you up for injury. A tall man's ball-and-socket shoulder joint—the place where his upper-arm bone meets his shoulder blade—is more vulnerable than a shorter man's.

"You actually drive your arm bone into the joint, setting yourself up for rotator-cuff injuries down the road," says Martin Rooney, PT, CSCS, of the Parisi Speed School.

THE WORKAROUND

With medicine-ball throws, you can focus on speed instead of on lifting weight.

"You'll work more of the fast-twitch muscle fibers that come into play during quick movements," says Durkin. No medicine ball? Do 3 to 5 sets of as many pushups as you can in 30 seconds.

Lying Medicine-Ball Throw

Lie on your back, using both hands to hold a heavy medicine ball against your chest. Push the ball just high enough into the air that it leaves your hands. Catch it, and immediately bring it back to your chest for the next throw. Do as many as you can in 30 seconds. Rest, and do 4 more sets.

THE PROBLEM
Short Arms

"Most of the big powerlifters you see have a short, stocky build," Rooney says. It serves them well on squats and bench presses. But when the bar starts on the floor, as with the deadlift, short arms force you to drop into a lower starting position. That changes your leverage and adds strain to your back.

THE WORKAROUND

"With a sumo deadlift, placing your legs farther apart helps your hands start closer to the ground," Rooney says. It also allows you to begin with a more upright torso, taking stress off your lumbar spine.

Sumo Deadlifts
Stand with your feet about twice shoulder width apart and your toes pointed out. Squat and grab the center of the bar using an overhand grip, with your thumbs 12 inches apart and your torso almost perpendicular to the floor. Without allowing your back to round, thrust your hips forward and stand up with the barbell. Then lower it, keeping it as close to your body as possible. Do 3 sets of 8 to 10 reps.

THE PROBLEM
Small Hands

Short-armed men tend to have smaller mitts; this makes holding the bar harder for them. A small hand's grip gives out faster, reducing the amount of work you can do on pulling exercises, says Rooney.

THE WORKAROUND

Because you can't grow longer fingers, focus on your forearm endurance with grip training, Rooney says. Add these exercises to the end of any workout.

Farmer's Walk
Grab a pair of heavy dumbbells and let them hang naturally at arm's length next to your sides. Walk forward as long as you can, then put the dumbbells down and rest. (If you last longer than 1 minute, use heavier weights.) Do this 3 to 5 times.

Towel Bar Hang
Wrap a towel around a pullup bar. Grab the towel using an overhand, shoulder-width grip. Hang for 20 seconds, rest, and repeat.

THE PROBLEM
No Butt

If you rolled a quarter off the back of your head, would it hit anything on the way down? If not, you have a flat back, most likely caused by a pelvis that's tilted backward at the top. A tilted pelvis puts your lower back in a vulnerable position, setting you up for spinal injuries.

THE WORKAROUND

Strengthen your hip flexors. Once they're in shape, they'll pull your pelvis back to neutral and improve your posture, says Eric Cressey, CSCS, cofounder of Cressey Performance, in Hudson, Massachusetts.

Lying Psoas March
Lie on your back with your right leg on the floor and your left leg off the floor and bent 90 degrees. Loop an exercise band under your right foot and over the top of your left foot. (You can also use a low-pulley cable with an ankle strap, looped around your left foot.) Keeping your right leg steady, pull your left knee toward your chest without your lower back tucking beneath

you. Pause, and return to the starting position. Do 10 to 12 reps; switch legs and repeat.

THE PROBLEM
Long Legs

Long legs can place your lower back at risk when you perform squats.

For tall men—basically anyone over 6 feet—the back squat can present two problems, says Durkin. The first involves physics: The longer the bones in your legs, the farther the bar has to travel on each rep and the harder your muscles need to work to lift it. Even with perfect form, you'll have a tougher time adding size and strength. Men with shorter bones can do more reps with heavier weights.

The second problem is that your form is probably flawed. Longer bones have more opportunity to make false moves. You might struggle to keep your lower back in a neutral position (slightly arched) throughout the full range of motion. Or you might lean forward as you tire, putting stress on your lower back.

THE WORKAROUND

Choose leg exercises that achieve more with less weight, such as the stepup. "You can work your legs hard but with potentially less back strain," says Bill Hartman, PT, CSCS, co-owner of Indianapolis Fitness and Sports Training.

Dumbbell Stepup

Holding a pair of dumbbells at arm's length next to your sides, stand in front of a step or bench that's about 18 inches high. Place your left foot flat on the step; your left knee should be bent 90 degrees. Push your left heel into the step

and lift yourself up until your left leg is straight and you're standing on one leg on the bench. Lower yourself to the starting position. Do 8 to 10 reps and switch legs. To make it harder, place a barbell across your back.

THE PROBLEM
Flat Feet

Everyone is born with flat feet, but most people develop their shock-absorbing arches in childhood. Sometimes, however, the arches never form properly, or they fall from repeated stress, injuries, or some combination of the two. Either way, you end up with feet that can pronate—roll inward—when you walk, run, or jump.

Flat feet can also limit your strength and power in the weight room. "When you pronate, you're in deceleration mode," says Cressey. "Your foot needs to roll in the opposite direction to push off." That affects your strength on squats and deadlifts, and acts like ballast when you jump.

THE WORKAROUND

Your glutes and hamstrings act as "anti-pronators," Cressey says. Strengthen them and you can compensate for the loss of power caused by your feet.

Hip Raise

Lie faceup on the floor with your knees bent and feet flat on the floor. Raise your hips off the floor by flexing your glutes so your body forms a straight line from shoulders to knees. Pause, and lower your hips. Do 3 sets of 15 reps; when it becomes too easy, lift one foot off the floor and do a single-leg hip raise. Start with your weaker leg and repeat the set with your stronger leg.

Custom-Made Muscle

Modify any exercise to suit your fitness level with these simple adjustments. All exercises are from Todd Durkin, CSCS, owner of Fitness Quest 10, in San Diego.

SQUAT

Make it easier
Band-Assisted Squat

Place a stretchable band around a chinup bar and stand just behind the bar. Hold the band with both hands as you squat until your thighs are parallel to the floor. Stand back up.
Why it works: The band lends stability as you squat, and assists your legs as you press back up to the starting position.

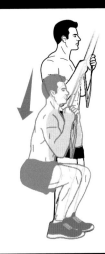

DEADLIFT

Make it easier
Elevated Straight-Leg Deadlift

Stand between two 6- to 12-inch-high boxes with your knees slightly bent, holding a barbell with an overhand grip. Bend at your hips and lower your torso until the barbell touches the boxes. Pause, and return to an upright position.
Why it works: The box limits your range of motion, helping you master the deadlift.

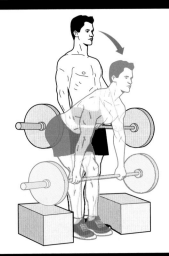

Make it harder
Box Squat

Stand 4 to 6 inches forward of a knee-high bench or box. With a barbell loaded onto your upper back, squat and sit on the bench for a moment. Keeping your heels pressed into the ground, stand back up.

Why it works: When you sit, you kill the weight's momentum; to rise again, you need to use your lower-body muscles more. That teaches your body to move explosively.

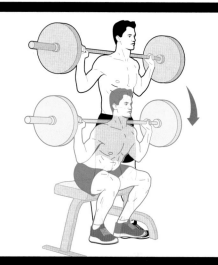

Make it harder
Straight-Leg Deadlift with Shrug

Hold a barbell at arm's length in front of your hips, using an overhand grip as shown. Bend at your hips and lower your torso until it's almost parallel to the floor. Pause, then come back up and shrug your shoulders.

Why it works: You're emphasizing your hamstrings, glutes, and lower back, which are typically weaker than your quads.

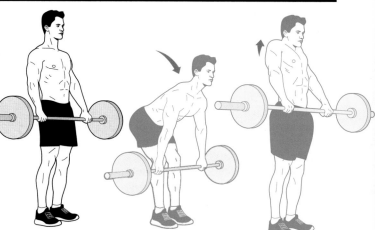

147

CHINUP/PULLUP

Make it easier
Negative Chinup/Pullup

Stand on a box beneath a pullup bar. Jump up, pulling your chest to the bar. Then take 6 to 10 seconds to lower yourself until your feet touch the box. Repeat.

Why it works: Slowly lowering your body can help build your upper-body muscles and increase the pulling power you need for chinups or pullups.

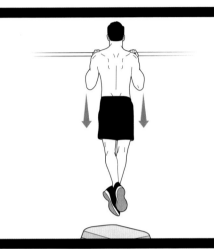

BARBELL BENCH PRESS

Make it easier
Negative Pushup

This isn't a bench press, but it provides the same benefit. Perform a pushup, and take 6 to 10 seconds to lower your body as you keep your core tight. Once you're an inch above the ground, explosively push your body back up.

Why it works: When you slowly lower your body, you activate more muscle fibers, increasing your chest, back, and triceps strength.

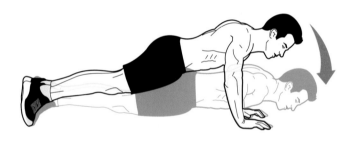

PLANK

Make it easier
Kneeling Plank

Assume a pushup position, but rest on your forearms and your knees. Your body should form a straight line from shoulders to knees. Brace your core and hold the position as long as you can.

Why it works: Bending your knees reduces the weight your core has to support. Also, if you feel back pain when you do regular planks, this eases tension.

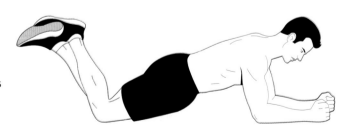

Make it harder
Commando Pullup

Instead of facing the bar, stand as if you're looking down its length. Grab it with one hand in front of the other, your palms facing inward. Now pull up and lean to the right so your right shoulder touches the bar. Repeat on the left.

Why it works: This kind of pullup causes an imbalance of weight and forces you to work your back and arms more as you pull your body up on each side.

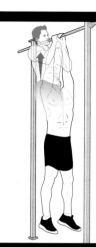

Make it harder
Cage Bench Press

Lie on a bench inside a power rack with the barbell resting on safety bars 3 to 6 inches above your chest. Press the bar off the rack until your arms are straight. Then lower it.

Why it works: You're starting from your weakest position in the bench press, with no momentum to help out. This forces your chest to work harder and improves your ability to bench more weight.

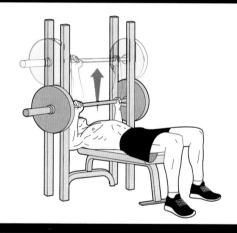

Make it harder
Plank with Opposite Arm and Leg Lift

From the plank position on your elbows, lift your left foot and right arm off the floor for 5 to 10 seconds. Switch sides and repeat.

Why it works: By adding movement and instability, you force your body to work harder to keep your core tight and stable.

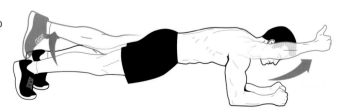

PROVE IT

LIFT TO LOSE WEIGHT

A new study from the College of New Jersey confirms that pumping iron can make your cardio workout more effective. Participants who performed an intense weight workout before riding a stationary bike burned more fat during their cardio session than those who pedaled but skipped the weights. The weight training may trigger fat-burning hormones, scientists speculate.

The best form of cardio may require weights. University of Wisconsin researchers found that kettlebell snatches can burn 20 calories a minute. See how this exercise stacks up against other forms of activity.

In 1 minute, the number of calories a 180-pound man will burn . . .

SPINNING	ROWING (vigorously)	ELLIPTICAL TRAINING	STAIR STEPPING	RUNNING (7-minute-mile pace)	SWIMMING (laps)
14.3	11.5	9.8	12.2	19	13.6

TRAIN YOUR BRAIN

A tough day can lead to a blah workout. In a study by McMaster University, people who took a difficult test that taxed their self-control exercised at a lower intensity than those who were given an easy test. Study author Kathleen Martin Ginis, PhD, says we all have a limited amount of willpower.

"If you're rigorous about sticking to a deadline at work, you may not have enough willpower left to exercise," she says. The good news is that willpower is like a muscle: The more you use it, the stronger it becomes.

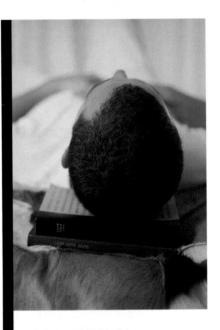

REST LESS

Are you new to lifting? Don't turn your gym time into social hour. Beginners can increase their strength with shorter rest periods, according to American and Brazilian scientists.

"Beginners can't activate as many muscle fibers, and they often train with less exertion," says study author Jeff Willardson, PhD. Seasoned lifters need 3 minutes of rest to build strength, while beginners need only 1 to 2 minutes.

GET STRONGER, FASTER

You can use supersets for supergains. Researchers in Australia and Canada have found that alternating between a back exercise and a chest exercise boosts strength more than working just one muscle group at a time does.

Although the researchers aren't sure why this approach yields better results, they're quick to point out another benefit: It saves you time. Because one muscle group rests while the other works, you can use shorter rests between sets while giving each muscle time to recover.

Here's how to try it: Do 6 repetitions of a dumbbell row, rest for 60 seconds, and then do 6 repetitions of a dumbbell bench press. Rest again and repeat the sequence.

WORK IT OUT

Here's a new use for dumbbells: pain relief. Exercise can speed shoulder recovery better than shock-wave therapy can, say researchers in Norway. When study participants performed range-of-motion shoulder movements and rotator-cuff exercises, their pain subsided more and they returned to activity sooner.

MASTER YOUR BENCH

If you're ready to conquer the bench press, remember this tip: Push the weight quickly. Researchers in Norway found that if your speed in pressing the bar slows, your strength slips.

"Decreased acceleration limits the amount of force you create," says study author Roland van den Tillaar, PhD. A simple technique to produce more power: Pull your elbows in toward your sides as you lower the weight, then press the bar straight up from your sternum.

HARD TRUTH

43

Percentage increase in leg-muscle activation doing free-weight squats instead of using a Smith machine, according to a study in the *Journal of Strength and Conditioning Research*

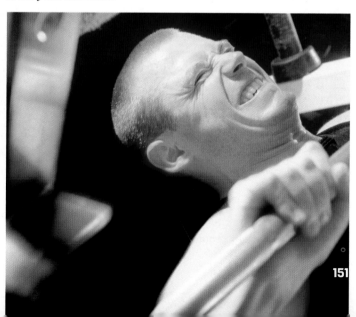

YOU ASKED

Q: Is the pec deck an effective way to build my chest?

A: True to its name, the pec deck does target your pectorals. However, there's a price for this pump.

"The pec deck's design, with the handles far away from your shoulders, increases the likelihood of injury because it stresses the small muscles in your shoulders, including your rotator cuffs," says Mark Peterson, PhD, CSCS, an exercise physiologist at the University of Michigan. A faster, safer strategy for adding inches to your chest is to do more pressing exercises, such as the dumbbell or barbell bench press. These moves target the pecs, but also recruit other major muscle groups as you lift and lower the weight, so you'll build more overall strength in your arms, shoulders, and chest.

Q: What's the best way to increase my bench press?

A: Squeeze. Just before you lift the bar off the rack, squeeze the metal as if you were trying to crush it in your bare hands.

"You will 'lock up' proximally, meaning the center of your body will reflexively activate to give you more trunk stability," says Eric Cressey, CSCS, a Boston-based strength and conditioning coach who works with many pro athletes. This, in turn, will enable you to lift more weight. Maintain your clench throughout the whole set.

Q: What's the best way to build bigger forearms?

A: Ignore them and focus on your back instead. When you perform pulling exercises, like pullups and rows, your back (and biceps) help with the heavy lifting, forcing your forearms to handle more weight than they would with isolation exercises.

"Pulling up your entire body requires shifting significantly more weight than the 20 pounds you'll use on a wrist curl," says Nick Tummi-

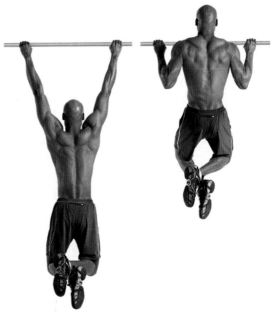

Imagine that you're pulling the bar to your chest, instead of your chest to the bar.

Hold the up position for 7 seconds. This improves grip and activates the muscles in your forearms.

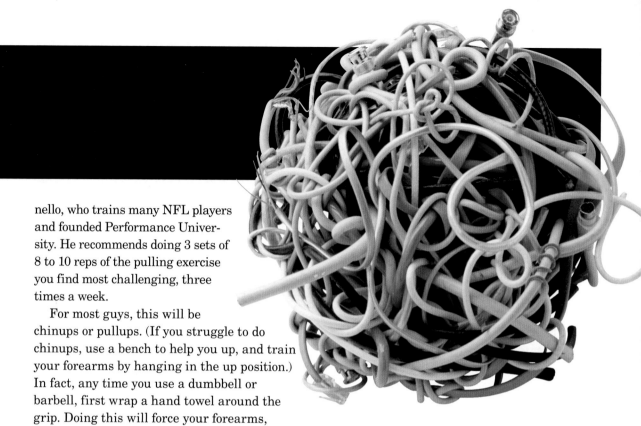

nello, who trains many NFL players and founded Performance University. He recommends doing 3 sets of 8 to 10 reps of the pulling exercise you find most challenging, three times a week.

For most guys, this will be chinups or pullups. (If you struggle to do chinups, use a bench to help you up, and train your forearms by hanging in the up position.) In fact, any time you use a dumbbell or barbell, first wrap a hand towel around the grip. Doing this will force your forearms, wrists, and fingers to work harder, so you'll end up activating more muscles and adding size faster.

Q: What's the benefit of warming up before working out?

A: Viscoelasticity. Not only are you pumping blood into the nooks and crannies of your muscle fibers, priming them for activity, but you're also warming up your tendons.

"This heat makes you more pliable, so you'll perform better and decrease your risk of injury," says Nicholas DiNubile, MD, a clinical assistant professor of orthopedic surgery at the University of Pennsylvania and the author of *FrameWork for the Lower Back*. The key is to break a sweat, whether it's by jogging or doing light drills that replicate the activity you're about to do.

Q: What's the best exercise to target love handles?

A: You can't spot-reduce fat, but those handles will be history if you slim down all around and then build up your obliques. Start off with one of the fastest fat burners known to man: the metabolic circuit. Once you shed your spare tire, add the full-contact twist to your workout.

"It's a hybrid between a plank and a crunch performed standing up," says Alexander Koch, CSCS, PhD, an associate professor of exercise science at Truman State University.

All you need is a towel, a regular 45-pound barbell, and the corner of a room. Remove all the weight plates from the barbell, place the towel over one end, and then wedge that end into the corner. Next, hold the other end of the barbell at a 45-degree angle from the floor, with your arms extended straight out in front of you. Now swing the bar to the right side of your body in a fast rotation (stop before it goes behind your body) while pivoting with your left foot. Then twist back to the left side while pivoting with your right foot. That's 1 rep. Aim for 3 to 5 sets of 10 to 20 reps.

Q: **My back and leg muscles are tighter these days. What's a good way to test my lower-body flexibility?**

A: If you're parked at a desk all day, your body stiffens up. Sitting shortens your hip flexors, the group of muscles that originates on each side of your spine and pelvis and connects to your inner thighs, says Bill Hartman, PT, CSCS, co-owner of Indianapolis Fitness and Sports Training.

"Tight hip flexors can limit your range of motion and are frequently the cause of lower-back pain." He recommends this simple test: Start out by sitting on the foot of a bench. Now recline on your back, bring both knees to your chest, and hold them there. Then lower your left leg, return to the starting position, and repeat with your right leg. If your thighs don't lie flat against the bench, your hip flexors are too tight. To fix the problem, do Bulgarian split squats three times a week, he says. Assume a wide stance with your back to a bench. Place the top of your left foot behind you on the bench and lower your body until your left knee is just above the floor. Hold this position for 30 seconds, and return to the starting position.

Switch legs, and repeat. That's 1 set. Aim for 3 sets with 30 seconds of rest after sets 1 and 2.

Q: **I have chicken legs. What's the best way to build my calf muscles?**

A: The same way Arnold built his: isolation. Before he was Mr. Olympia, Schwarzenegger cut the legs off his sweatpants and targeted his skinny calves until they looked as buff as his upper body. In your case, skip the scissors and just do standing and seated calf raises at a slow tempo.

"Most guys blow through sets and move too quickly to improve the soleus and gastrocne-

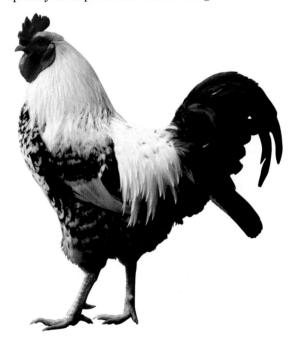

mius, the two muscles that make your calves look meaty," says Mike Robertson, CSCS, co-owner of Indianapolis Fitness and Sports Training. "Slowing the exercise minimizes contributions from other muscles and places the stress on the muscles in your calves."

Aim for 2 sets of 20 reps of both seated and standing calf raises three times a week. (For a full description, see MensHealth.com/calves.) Take 2 seconds to raise the weight and 2 seconds to lower it, and hold the bottom position for 2 seconds.

Q: What's the fastest way to cool down after a lunchtime workout?

A: We threw this question out to Sam Cheuvront, PhD, a research physiologist at the U.S. Army Research Institute of Environmental Medicine, who recommended the old standby: a cold shower. Before you cringe, don't worry—cool water is also effective, Dr. Cheuvront says.

You'll feel better instantly, but your body needs 5 minutes to cool down internally. Afterward, towel off and rub on a tonic spiked with menthol, such as Friction de Foucaud Energizing Body Tonic ($30, bigelowchemists. com) or Jack Black Cool Moisture ($22, getjack-black.com). The menthol aids evaporation and stimulates the cooling receptors in the skin, creating a refreshing chill. Next, drink a slushie. (Make it by pouring a sports drink over shaved ice.) Australian research reveals

that this lowers your core temperature faster than sipping cold water does.

However, if your head is still spraying sweat like a sprinkler, consider the BEX Runner ($50, betterexerciseexperience.com). It's a gel pad that you freeze and then strap to your palm during or after exercise. We were skeptical, but this doohickey works by chilling your hand's blood vessels, gradually cooling the blood that pumps through them.

Q: I'm too busy to work out. When will my muscle loss begin?

A: "You will notice some lack of muscle tone and strength after 3 to 4 weeks. To maintain muscle, you need to strength-train 3 days a week for 45 minutes. That said, a week off every 4 months can actually help your training efforts," says David Pearson, PhD, CSCS, a professor of exercise physiology at Ball State University.

Q: My wife has noticed that I snore more on days I work out. What's going on?

A: "Exercise, over time, will decrease snoring. It also increases sleep quality and produces deeper sleep," says W. Christopher Winter, MD, the medical director of the sleep medicine center of Martha Jefferson Hospital, in Charlottesville, Virginia. Try sleeping on your side.

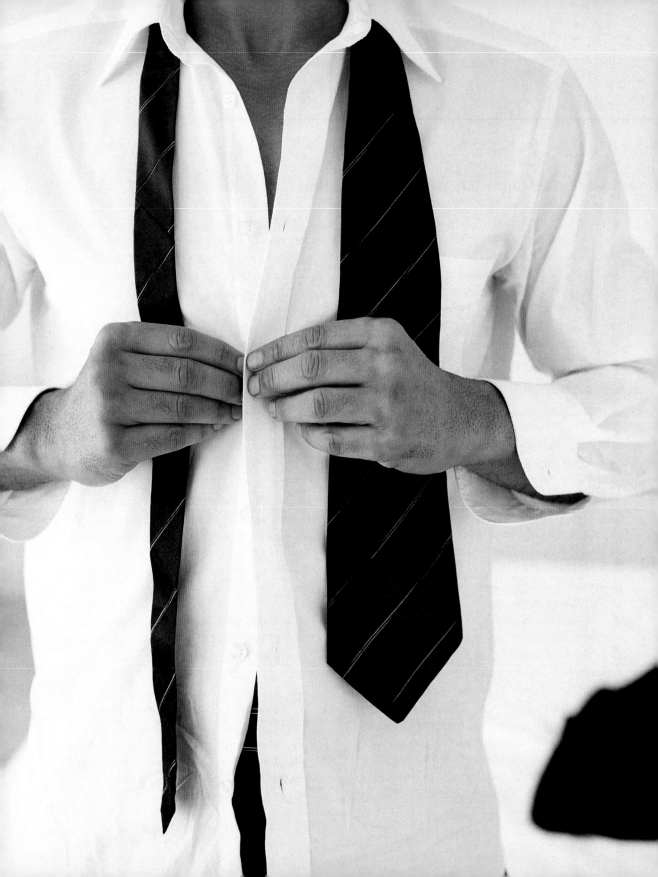

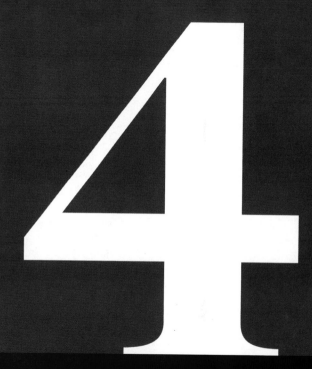

Look Better Instantly

100 First Dates

Within 5 minutes of meeting you—and sometimes sooner—a woman knows whether she's interested or not. Are you making the most of that time?

The *Men's Health* Girl Next Door, Carolyn Kylstra, set out to meet 100 men and see how they used the opportunity. Learn from them.

Last summer I had a date with a prison guard named Shawn. He had tattoos on his neck: "Alisha" and "Jasmine." The names of his daughters, it turned out—not ex-lovers sharing everlasting real estate on the banks of his carotid artery.

I have no desire to speak with Shawn again, for reasons unrelated to his all-too-visible life decisions. What disqualified the guy was his earnest, unending, obvious monologue about the importance of family. Blood runs thick, you know. Loyalty, fraternity, on and on, for what felt like eternity.

But it was only 5 minutes. Then the bell rang, and Shawn moved on to the next woman.

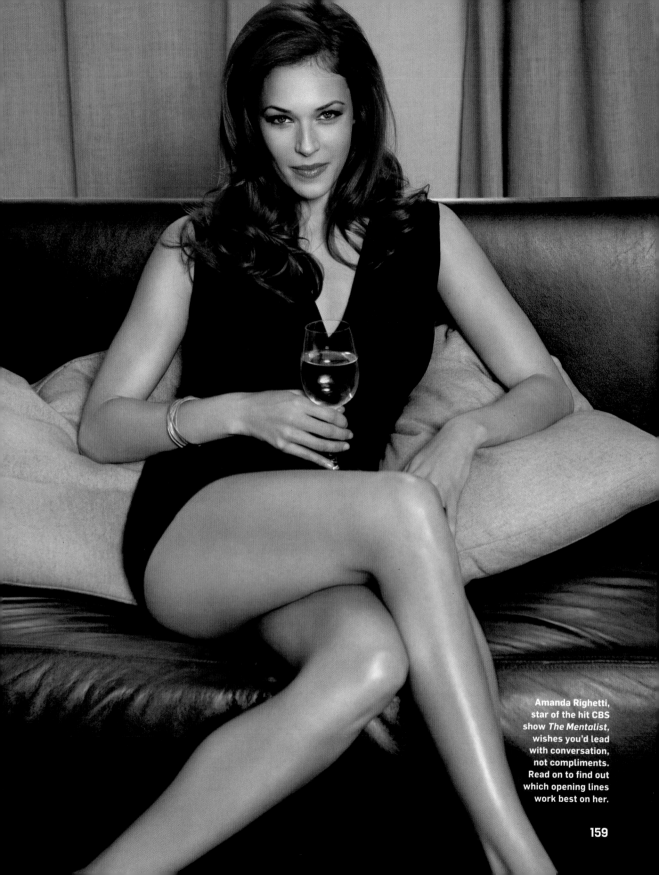

Amanda Righetti, star of the hit CBS show *The Mentalist*, wishes you'd lead with conversation, not compliments. Read on to find out which opening lines work best on her.

159

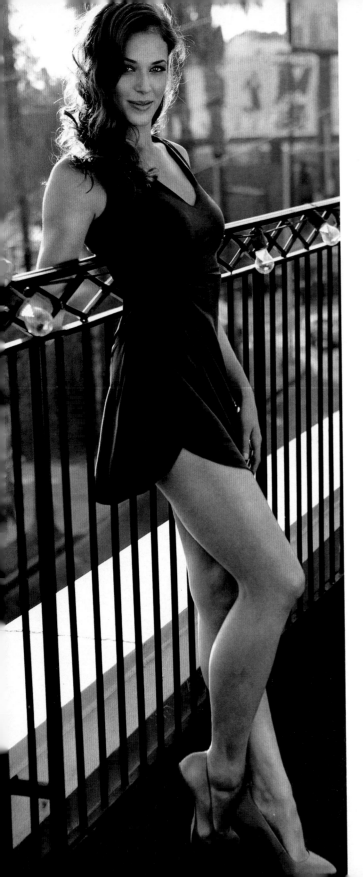

I went on 100 first dates last year. Fifteen dates one night, 12 another, and more the next. The typical setup: A speed-dating company rents out a room in a bar and sells seats for about 30 bucks a pop. Usually, more women than men show up. The women stay seated while the men rotate through.

For 2 to 6 minutes, we meet, greet, bedazzle, or bore one another, and decide, Yes, I'd like to see more of this one, or Next, please. Please, please. Then we stand, shake hands, switch partners, and repeat. At the end we turn in a sheet indicating which ones we'd like to see again. When two people show mutual interest, they receive contact info. And a beautiful love is born.

That's the idea, anyway.

My mission was to meet 100 men and assess their first-impression skills. It was efficient, and it felt legit. Relationship researchers are now using speed dating in their laboratories o' love.

Like Paul Eastwick, PhD, an assistant professor of psychology at Texas A&M, who says speed dating has real-world parallels: "Everyone goes to parties or bars and has brief conversations with people they've never met before. The lessons apply to all initial romantic encounters." Fair enough.

Let's look at a few of the men I met, and see what I learned about first impressions.

Insight 1
We don't know what we want.

Call him: The Total Package

First noticed: Sharp clothes, great smile

Thought to myself: Stop flirting with her! Look at me!

His name was Jake. Really. Chiseled

jaw, broad shoulders, big brown eyes. Swoon. He was smart, driven, and thoughtful. We liked the same music, we'd read the same books. On paper, perfect.

He was also arrogant as hell, and boring. Afterward I did not mark "yes" next to his name.

Ask a woman about the traits she looks for in a boyfriend or husband, and she'll rattle off a list of requirements strict enough to make you surrender your man-card on the spot. My advice: Just ignore the damn list. It means next to nothing.

In one study of more than 10,000 members of the speed-dating service HurryDate, researchers from the University of Pennsylvania and Arizona State University found that, aside from race, a woman's list of preferred characteristics didn't correlate much with the men she actually liked.

We all have misconceptions. A study of 163 college speed daters conducted by Dr. Eastwick and Eli Finkel, PhD, of Northwestern University, found that men, contrary to their stated assumption, care just as much about a mate's earning potential as women do.

And women are just as motivated by attractiveness as men are. "People have these elaborate theories about the qualities they're looking for in a partner, but ultimately they have little real insight into themselves," Dr. Eastwick says.

YOUR MOVE

Don't try to be the man she wants you to be.

"Being too agreeable and connected actually hurts you," Dr. Eastwick says. "If you agree with everything she says, you come across as submissive or weak. You're not her best friend yet; you're still trying to establish yourself as someone unique and interesting." Throw in some lighthearted teasing or a contrasting viewpoint. We like the give-and-take, and you'll stand out from the spineless, personality-less crowd.

Insight 2

You can't really read her.

Call him: Presumptuous Peter

First noticed: Graying hair, refined; coat and tie

Thought to myself: Loosen up—this is pleasure, not business.

Peter looked about 15 years older than I am—fine by me, as long as the gent makes me laugh and treats me as an equal. We chatted amicably, and I asked him what he did for a living.

He paused. "I'd rather save that information for the next date, sweetheart."

What next date, hotshot? The condescending "sweetheart" was bad enough, but in my mind, playing coy about his employment implied that he thought I was interested in his money. He wasn't being friendly, so he never had a shot.

The cold truth is that we sometimes make up our minds within 5 minutes of meeting someone. The scarier truth is that the criteria we use to judge strangers are often skewed and irrelevant.

Psychologists classify personalities in five dimensions: agreeableness, extroversion, conscientiousness, openness, and emotional stability. Upon meeting someone, we most often judge their agreeableness, researchers from Columbia University found. But the same research also shows that this is precisely the dimension we're least accurate in judging.

YOUR MOVE

Smile. Make good eye contact. Smile some more.

Be as friendly as possible. No posing, please. Researchers from Texas State University at San Marcos surveyed speed daters' "thin-slice judgments," based on 30 seconds of interaction. Women who had positive first impressions gave five reasons. Three of the five: The man communicated well, had a great smile, and acted friendly. Do you notice a trend?

Insight 3
We can be as shallow as men.

Call him: Ugly Owen

First noticed: Wonky teeth and worse hair—wispy and thinning and wild, like a meth-head clown

Thought to myself: No, thank you.

Owen was from London. He was delightful, a music producer and a fascinating conversationalist. A friend and I agreed: Owen is awesome. Just, not for us. "I almost want to mark 'yes' next to his name so that we can hang out and be friends," my friend said. Talk about the kiss of death.

Beauty rules early on, says Shanghong Luo, PhD, an assistant professor of psychology at the University of North Carolina at Wilmington, who conducted a speed-dating study testing the principles of attraction. "In the first 5 minutes, you don't have that much other information about the person besides what he or she looks like."

Great news for men like Jake. But what of the others? Dr. Eastwick weighs in: "You might not be the most attractive person in the room, but some people in that room are going to think you are."

YOUR MOVE

Sell yourself.

In that thin-slice judgment study, women listed attractive traits. "Tall" and "handsome" were there—but so were "clean-cut," "neatly groomed," and "stylish clothing." So packaging matters. I might have marked "yes" if Owen had tamed his mane. A close cut is superior to the circus look.

Insight 4
You can play the odds.

Call him: Card-carrying Kevin

First noticed: His stack of notebook cards

Thought to myself: I'm curious.

Kevin fanned the cards in his large hands and then asked me to pick one and read it. "If you could have dinner with three people, living or dead, who would they be?" His answers: Barack Obama, Martin Luther King Jr., and Britney Spears.

This guy was good. By the time the bell rang, I was smitten. Then Kevin sat down with the woman to my left, and out came the cards and canned answers. I pouted as I erased the "yes" by his name.

Mine was a typical reaction: According to Luo's research, people are attracted to those who like them (big surprise), but only if the interest seems unique. Poor Kevin was a perfect example. I loved our connection, but then felt slighted when I saw I wasn't the only queen in his deck.

YOUR MOVE

Be an open book.

If you're jonesing for pretty lady number 9, make it clear how you feel, says Dr. Luo. Compliment her, but drop in a line about how great it is to meet someone you can connect with. Singling her out as above the rest will make her remember you.

Insight 5

You can connect in 5 minutes.

Call him: Barbecue Ben

First noticed: He looks like Michael from *Lost*.

Thought to myself: Great smile!

Ben did everything right. He said he'd seen me from across the room before the event and was eager to talk to me—a textbook "you're special" ego boost. Within 30 seconds, we learned that we were both from North Carolina, and a lively conversation about NC barbecue commenced. My energy was higher than it had been with any of the dozen or so guys who came before him. Our back-and-forth made me laugh and I was eager to hear what he'd say next. When the bell rang, we were shocked—5 minutes was up already?

Ben received a definite "yes."

YOUR MOVE

Have a conversation.

Dr. Eastwick's research reveals that both men and women say the best dates have a 60-40 split. You talk about the other person 60 percent of the time, and yourself 40 percent. So ask questions, listen, and respond accordingly. You want to focus mostly on her while still communicating information about yourself. Easy enough, right?

One last point. Just be polite. Remember: You only have to keep it up for 5 minutes.

Leave a Lasting Impression

Sorry, guys: Amanda Righetti, star of the hit CBS series *The Mentalist*, is married. She's also beautiful, so she's fielded plenty of come-ons in her life. Here are her three rules on how to leave a woman wanting more.

Skip the Bar

"A bar is the worst place to ask a woman out on a date," Righetti says. For starters, drinking doesn't help you put your best foot forward. "Men who hit on women in bars tend to be obnoxious. It comes off as desperate." Try the bookstore, Righetti says. The conversation can let you flex your intellectual muscle.

Be Positive

Laughter works, but a lighthearted attitude is what matters most. "A sense of humor is great, but if you're trying too hard, it's off-putting," Righetti says. "Don't take yourself too seriously. Have fun."

Turn Off the Charm

Open with conversation, not compliments. "Some men think paying a compliment will open a door for them, but in my experience it never really does," Righetti says. Conversation, not flattery, is what will really make you stand out from the guys who are always trying out lines.

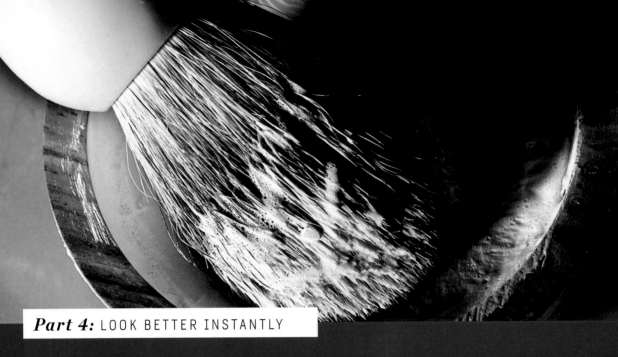

65 Instant Grooming Upgrades

You want to look sharper, cleaner, and sleeker—and there are grooming products for all of that. Hundreds of new ones each year, in fact. But you don't need them all. Here are the best, and tips from the experts on how to make them work for you.

In simpler times, men scraped by each morning with soap, shampoo, and shaving cream. But we've evolved, and so has our routine. The majority of men spend 20 to 30 minutes a day in the john, trying to look better.

We surveyed more than 1,000 *Men's Health* readers to learn what bugs guys most about getting ready. And because 96 percent of men say they groom for women, we asked women to chime in on how we're doing. Then we gathered all the latest lotions, soaps, gels, serums, and pastes we could find and turned loose our panel of grooming experts, editors, and everyday guys. After much lathering, slathering, shaving, sniffing, splashing, rinsing, and repeating, we have your results: the *Men's Health* Grooming Awards.

HARD TRUTH

52

Percentage of men who are worried about sun damage, but only 22 percent used sunscreen in the past month; 54 percent of women surveyed said a man's sun-damaged skin is a turnoff.

Face

Oily skin: Surprise: Oily skin needs moisture.

"The right moisturizer will actually balance your skin, leading to less oil production," says Stuart H. Kaplan, MD, a dermatologist in Beverly Hills, California. Stay away from heavy creams and opt for a lightweight, oil-free moisturizer, like Neutrogena Men Sensitive Skin Oil-Free Moisture SPF 30 ($7, neutrogena.com). A lotion or serum with hyaluronic acid penetrates to help skin retain its natural moisture balance. Peter Thomas Roth's viz-1000 ($65, peterthomasroth.com) is one good option.

Breakouts: Be gentle with tough skin.

"Using a harsh scrub is the same as picking at your skin," says Dr. Kaplan. "You'll cause more inflammation and irritation." Keep skin clean with a mild cleanser that contains salicylic acid or benzoyl peroxide, or their natural alternatives, salix alba bark extract and farnesol.

One we like is Billy Jealousy White Knight Gentle Daily Facial Cleanser ($20, billyjealousy.com). Dr. Kaplan also suggests using a gentle exfoliant three times a week to lift dead cells that can clog pores. We like Eyre BioBotanics Triple Action Facial Scrub ($50, eyrebiobotanics. com). When breakouts occur, continue tender treatment with Dr. Dennis Gross Skincare Trifix Acne Clearing Lotion ($30, dgskincare.com), which contains anti-inflammatory and antibacterial compounds.

Tidy up, too. Change your pillowcase once a week so your freshly washed face is not resting on a buildup of your hair's oil. Use a disinfecting wipe on all your phones to reduce breakouts by your ear and jawline.

Under-eye circles: Blame your parents: A lot of pigmentation is genetic. And as you age, the quality of your collagen diminishes, and blood vessels become prone to breaking. Also influencing under-eye circles are lifestyle factors, which include late nights, smoking, drinking, and

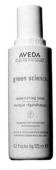
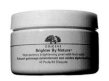

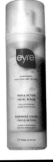
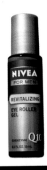

The Best

Here are the best products for your face.

TONER
Aveda Green Science Replenishing Toner
Large pores and oily skin? This toner, used after cleansing, gently exfoliates and provides extra moisture. $40, aveda.com

PEEL
Origins Brighter by Nature
The fruit acids in these pads made testers' skin feel smooth and refreshed without drying or redness. $40, origins.com

MASK
Kiehl's Rare Earth Deep Pore Cleansing Masque
Oily skin and blackheads? This mixture of white clay, bentonite, and oat-kernel flour can extract the gunk that clogs pores. Testers said it rinsed off easily. $23, kiehls.com

FACE SCRUB
Eyre BioBotanics Triple Action Facial Scrub
This organic product from Australia is gentle enough for all skin types. For a closer shave, use it first. $45, groominglounge.com

EYE MOISTURIZER
Nivea for Men Revitalizing Eye Roller Gel Q10
Studies show that coenzyme Q10 fights wrinkles. Our test panel loved the roller-ball applicator. $9, niveaformenusa.com

caffeine. Fight the hangdog look with Anthony Logistics for Men Continuous Moisture Anti-Aging Eye Cream ($30, anthony.com), which boasts vitamins A, C, and E—ingredients that build collagen back up.

Sun damage: Decades of neglect can lead to skin cancer. If that threat is hard to picture, then look in the mirror at the surface damage from the sun: deep crevices on your forehead and creases around your eyes. In sunny weather, apply sunscreen 15 to 20 minutes before you go out.

"Application in the sun leaves you exposed for more time than you realize," says Dennis Gross, MD, a Manhattan dermatologist. And make sure you're liberal with it. "To be truly protected, we need to use a lot of sunscreen—about 2 to 4 ounces to cover your face and body, depending on your size," he says. Reapply every 3 to 4 hours, no matter how high the SPF level, because it's easy to sweat off. Better yet, even if you don't plan on swimming, wear a sunscreen that's waterproof so it lasts longer as you perspire.

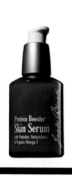
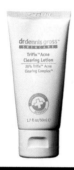
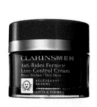
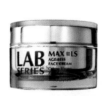
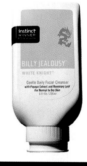
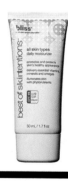

SERUM
Jack Black Protein Booster Skin Serum
Use after shaving. It has protein and antioxidants to fight aging. Testers swore it worked. $60, getjackblack.com

ACNE TREATMENT
Dr. Dennis Gross Skincare Trifix Acne Clearing Lotion
Colloidal sulfur treats blemishes and eliminates oil; willow bark extract calms inflammation; and farnesol kills bacteria. $30, dgskincare.com

MOISTURIZER
ClarinsMen Line-Control Cream
Fights wrinkles with shea butter and paracress, which nourish skin and increase firmness. $50, clarins.com

ANTIAGING MOISTURIZER
Lab Series MAX LS Age-Less Face Cream
Restores firmness and repairs damage with whey, protein, and rice and leaf extracts. $65, labseries.com

FACE WASH
Billy Jealousy White Knight Gentle Daily Facial Cleanser
Use a mild cleanser like this on your face. Testers loved the rich texture and smell—peppermint, rosemary, and eucalyptus. $20, billyjealousy.com

MOISTURIZER WITH SUNSCREEN
Bliss Best of Skintentions All Skin Types Daily Moisturizer, SPF 15 UVB/UVA
It's lightweight and loaded with vitamins A, C, and E to help improve the appearance of sun-damaged skin. $35, blissworld.com

Shave

Close shave: The average guy shaves in a hurry, somewhere in between showering, dressing, vacuuming down breakfast, and checking his BlackBerry. Pirooz Sarshar, owner of the Grooming Lounge, suggests that you take a breath. "The shaving process should take between 10 and 15 minutes. You can't expect great results by rushing."

Dirt and dead skin cells can form a barrier between your skin and the razor, so start with a well-scrubbed face. "When you scrub, move your fingers in a circular motion to get a sense of your direction of growth while allowing your beard to stand at attention," Sarshar says. A preshave oil like Molton Brown Re-charge Black Pepper Shave Oil ($29, moltonbrown.com) creates a smooth surface so your razor can glide without slipping or dragging.

Which direction? "The trick is to go with the grain first, and then go cross-grain as an in-between step, before eventually graduating to against-the-grain shaving," says Sarshar.

Our survey shows that 36 percent of men are using razors of three blades or

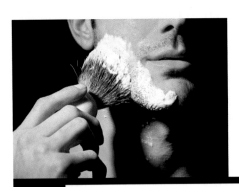
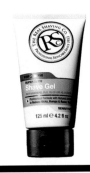
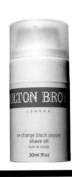
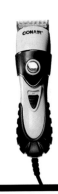

The Best

Here are the best products for a close shave.

SHAVE GEL
The Real Shaving Company Super Slide Shave Gel
It's alcohol-free, so it won't dry your dermis. Almond oil lubricates the blade, and aloe and vitamin E condition your skin. $6, realshaving.com

SHAVE OIL
Molton Brown Re-charge Black Pepper Shave Oil
This oil protects skin with natural oils, including those of the gymestra sylvestra leaf, which have antimicrobial properties. $29, moltonbrown.com

ELECTRIC RAZOR
Panasonic Wet/Dry Shaver ES-LA93-K
A linear system shaves side to side and up and down. The head pivots to match the curves of your face. $400, panasonic.com

fewer. For some, a razor like the Schick Hydro 5 ($9, schickhydro.com) might improve the quality of their shave. Over a third of men use a blade more than 10 times before changing it. Ouch. Even in ideal conditions, a blade should be used no more than five or six times before it's replaced, says Sarshar.

Razor burn: Feeling the burn? Examine your technique. Always cleanse or exfoliate to remove dead-skin buildup, which can lead to bumps and ingrown hairs. Then, "keep your skin in kind of a neutral position when you shave so you don't stretch the skin too tightly," says Kathleen M. Welsh, MD, a dermatologist in San Francisco. "Don't tilt your head back too far or you'll stretch the skin on your neck and cut it too closely. Ease up on the pressure as well."

Body hair: When trimming body hair, shoot for a little longer than half an inch. With clippers, find the ideal setting and test a patch first. Or use scissors: Comb up a section of hair, and hold the ends between your middle and index fingers, with your thumb underneath them to keep the ends in place. Then cut away the excess.

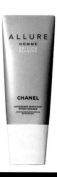 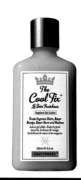 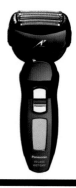 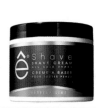 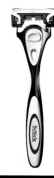

POSTSHAVE LOTION
Chanel Allure Homme Edition Blanche, Anti-Shine Moisturizing After Shave
A dab offers a subtle scent and quenches freshly shaved skin. Testers liked the texture and said it left their skin soft but not greasy. $50, chanel.com

POSTSHAVE SOLUTION
Shaveworks The Cool Fix
Glycolic and phytic acids help dissolve dead skin cells that can lead to nicks and razor bumps. $25, sephora.com

TRIMMER
Conair Chopper 2-in-1 Custom Styler
More than a dozen attachment combs take care of everything from sideburns to chest hair. It comes with barber scissors, cleaning brush, and cape. $30, conair.com

SHAVING CREAM
eShave Verbena Lime Shaving Cream
It's free of parabens, preservatives that can irritate skin. Testers liked the citrus scent and creamy texture. $20, eshave.com

RAZOR
Schick Hydro 5
Testers say it gave them a close shave while sparing their face. Shave guards control the amount of skin trapped between each blade. $9, schickhydro.com

Body

Excessive sweating: You produce two types of sweat: one when you're hot and the other when you're stressed. The latter, produced by your sympathetic nervous system, is more likely to smell, says Dr. Welsh.

She suggests an antiperspirant with a 12 percent concentration of aluminum chloride, such as Certain Dri ($6, certaindri.com). Use this antiperspirant at night, when your skin is dry and the ingredients can be absorbed. No need to reapply in the morning; you're covered. Or try a deodorant with 18 percent aluminum zirconium, such as Gillette Odor Shield Antiperspirant/Deodorant ($5, gillette.com); apply morning and night.

Body odor: If tenacious stink is an issue for you, try an antibacterial soap—body odor can be a product of bacterial growth on the skin. And skip the Indian buffet at lunch—odors from onions, garlic, curry, and spicy foods are excreted in sweat glands. Finally, do the laundry. Bacteria from sweat can cling to fabrics; the heat from your body acts like a plug-in scented warmer, but in this case it activates offending odors.

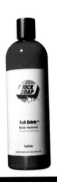 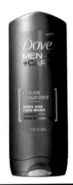 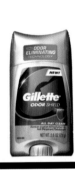 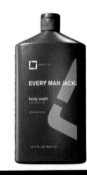 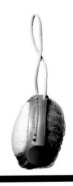

The Best

Try these best-for-your-body products.

MOISTURIZER
Jock Soap Tall Drink Body Hydrator
This complex formula of natural moisturizers includes shea butter and cane sugar. And there's no scent and no greasy film. $22, getjock.com

BODY WASH
Dove Men+Care Clean Comfort Body and Face Wash
Combining moisturizers with a light, appealing scent kept our testers using this wash long after the testing was done. $5, dovemencare.com

DEODORANT
Gillette Odor Shield Antiperspirant/Deodorant
An 18 percent aluminum compound (just 2 percent less than prescription strength) kept testers' pits dry. The subtle scent was popular, too. $5, gillette.com

BODY SCRUB
Every Man Jack Citrus Scrub
Natural oils give it a clean, citrusy smell; coconut derivatives slough off the grime; and glycerin keeps skin soft and moisturized. $6, everymanjack.com

BODY TOOL
Dove Men+Care Active Clean Dual Sided Shower Tool
Our testers wondered why they'd stayed with washcloths so long. Build lather with one side of this tool, polish your skin with the other. $4, dovemencare.com

Form, Meet Function

Look better, faster, with these design upgrades to must-use products.

THE DILEMMA:
You're still sweating in the office from your lunchtime workout.

THE SOLUTION: Dermalogica Skin Purifying Wipes
Dabbing your brow with a deskside towel doesn't scream professional. Instead, swipe with these one-use wipes, to remove sweat, oil, and dead skin. $17 for a pack of 20 wipes, dermalogica.com

THE DILEMMA:
Morning shaves scorch your face.

THE SOLUTION:
Eyre BioBotanics Absolute Shaving System
Your mug needs moisture before you shave, says dermatologist Zoe Diana Draelos, MD. This double-barreled bottle stores both shaving oil and cream. $45, eyrebiobotanics.com

THE DILEMMA:
Your travel razor didn't survive the trip.

THE SOLUTION:
eShave Travel Razor
The plastic protector on a travel razor can pop off when your bag is jostled. This razor comes with a protective canister for storing the removable razor head and handle. Your digits will thank you. $75, eshave.com

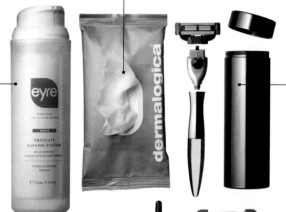

THE DILEMMA:
There's barely room left in your bathroom cabinet for anything.

THE SOLUTION:
Kevin.Murphy Night. Rider Matte Texture Paste
Most hair product packages are cylindrical, so they're hard to store. With this slim, rectangular one, it's easy to save space by stashing it sideways. $22, kevinmurphy.com.au

THE DILEMMA:
Your last cologne bottle broke open in your gym bag.

THE SOLUTION:
Victorinox Swiss Army Swiss Unlimited Eau de Toilette
Toss your bag without worry—the protective rubber case surrounding this cologne's glass bottle keeps the fresh, woodsy scent from spilling. $55, swissarmy.com

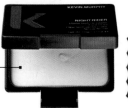

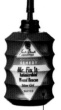

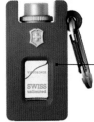

THE DILEMMA:
You cut yourself at the gym.

THE SOLUTION:
Jack Black Mr. Fix It Antimicrobial Wound Rescue Silver Gel
The oilcan-type packaging allows you to apply germ-killing solution directly to your cut, rather than using your finger and potentially infecting the wound. $20, getjackblack.com

Fragrance

Scent overload: Avoid nose fatigue. That's what happens if you try more than three scents at the store, says Mary Ellen Lapsansky, vice president of the Fragrance Foundation. When applying fragrance, spritz your favorite scent on your pulse points (like your wrists and the base of your neck) and wait 10 to 12 hours before reapplying, if you want a refresher.

Accidental overdose? Use a wet wipe (or a cotton ball dipped in alcohol) on the spot to lift off some of the scent. "This should take the strength of the fragrance down a notch or two," Lapsansky says. But don't even think about forgoing cologne altogether; 93 percent of women surveyed say a man seems sexier when he wears a subtle scent.

Hair

Styling: Fine, limp locks were a complaint of 42 percent of the men we surveyed. Some styling tricks can help—starting with never putting product on wet hair, says Erica Fleischman, owner of Erica Fleischman: A Men's Salon, in Manhattan. Grooming paste, such as Redken for Men Forming Paste Mint Shape ($14, redken.com), can add texture and girth to fine follicles. Use a small amount of product and work it into the palms of your hands before applying in order to achieve even distribution and avoid clumping.

Almost a third of men surveyed have trouble managing their curly, dry, or coarse hair. Fleischman suggests washing it less often to allow the scalp's natural oils to coat

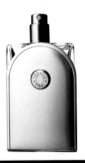 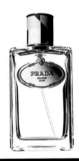 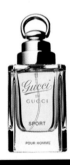 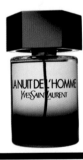

The Best

Here are the best fragrance products around.

ADVENTUROUS
Voyage d'Hermes
Share this with the woman in your life, or wear it to attract one. Equal parts fresh, musky, and peppery. And the bottle is a work of art. $90, hermes.com

SOPHISTICATED
Prada Infusion de Vetyver
A limited edition with a rich, warm blend of vetiver, tarragon, and pepper, accented with the zing of ginger. $75, prada.com

EVERYDAY
Gucci by Gucci Sport
An initial rush of cypress, grapefruit, cardamom, and juniper berry gives way to warmer notes of patchouli and vetiver. "Luxurious but masculine," said one tester. $55, gucci.com

EVENING
Yves Saint Laurent La Nuit de L'Homme
Our test panel was addicted to the unique combination of woody and floral notes in this sophisticated, bold scent. $55, ysl.com

the strands. Try rinsing your hair with conditioner instead of washing sometimes.

"It will keep the hair hydrated and make it smell and feel clean without the drying effects of shampoo," she says.

Eyebrows: Speed your brow trimming like this, says Patrizi of Halo [for Men]: With a fine-toothed or mustache comb, brush the hairs of your eyebrows upward. Take a pair of nose-hair or baby scissors (with protective tips) and trim the tops of the hairs on a downward angle. "Never do them straight across. They'll look choppy when you brush them back down, which is a sure sign of botched grooming," he says. Next, use tweezers to pluck any thick hairs between the eyebrows, leaving the smaller, finer hairs so you won't look overgroomed.

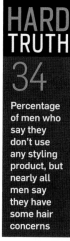

HARD TRUTH

34

Percentage of men who say they don't use any styling product, but nearly all men say they have some hair concerns

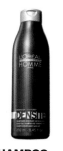

The Best

Here are the best hair products for men.

POMADE
Axe Smooth and Sophisticated Look Shine Pomade
A little shine without that shellacky, gluey feel. Our testers said their hair felt polished but not weighed down. $7, theaxeeffect.com

SHAMPOO
L'Oréal Professionnel Homme Densite Shampoo
It contains polymers, which add luster and smoothness, according to a study in the *International Journal of Cosmetic Science.* $15, us.loreal professionnel.com

HAIR PASTE
Redken for Men Forming Paste Mint Shape
Consider this fresh-smelling paste a scaffold for fine hair. It rinses out easily, testers said. $14, redken.com

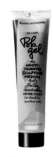

VGEL
Bumble and bumble Bb.gel
Didn't leave sticky hands or "hair-helmet" syndrome, and a tousle kept hair flexible but styled. $24, bumbleandbumble.com

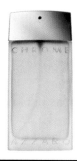
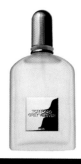
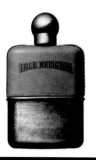

FRESH
Azzaro Chrome Sport
It's more sophisticated than many fresh, sporty scents, thanks to a layer of aquatic and woody notes. Blends grapefruit, bergamot, mandarin, and white musk. $50, azzaroparis.com

CLASSIC
Tom Ford Grey Vetiver
Traditional vetiver is updated with orange flower, grapefruit, warm amber woods, and oakmoss. The bottle is quintessential Tom Ford—both cool and minimalist. $85, tomford.com

MODERN
True Religion for Men
Like the denim brand that inspired this scent, True Religion is versatile and easy to wear, mixing fresh, herbal, and woody elements. $60, truereligionbrandjeans.com

Mouth

Bad breath: It starts with oral hygiene. "Think of your gums as a turtleneck collar that hugs each tooth," says Sally Cram, DDS, a periodontist in Washington, DC. You have to get under the collar to remove bacteria. Brush for at least 2 minutes; Dr. Cram prefers a sonic toothbrush, like the Supersmile LS45 Advanced Sonic Pulse Toothbrush ($100, supersmile.com). Its 45-degree angle is ideal for removing debris.

Floss that has tiny grooves, like Reach Total Care ($3, reachbrand.com), might remove gunk better. To rout bacteria, scrub your tongue with a Supersmile Tongue Cleaner ($4, supersmile.com), suggests New York City dentist Thomas Connelly, DDS. That, plus some oxygenation with a toothbrush, will eliminate odors.

Yellow teeth: Our survey showed that whitening pastes, gums, and rinses are popular. Too bad they can't really do much. For real results, Jennifer Jablow, DDS, a Manhattan-based dentist, suggests

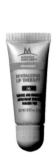 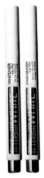 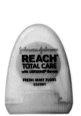 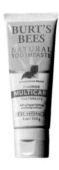 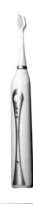

The Best

Try these products for oral hygiene.

LIP TREATMENT
Mission Skincare Revitalizing Lip Therapy Gel
Developed with input from Carmelo Anthony and Serena Williams, it earned accolades from our mortal testers, too. $4, missionskincare.com

WHITENER
IntelliWhite Pro Whitening Kit
Its pen system keeps chemicals away from your gums. Users liked the no-mess experience and 7-day results. $80, rxbright.com

FLOSS
Reach Total Care Floss with Listerine Flavors
One tester said, "Flossing can be easy and fun. Who knew?" Others thought the springy texture and thicker ribbon did a better job than thinner standard floss. $3, reachbrand.com

TOOTHPASTE
Burt's Bees Natural Toothpaste Multicare with Fluoride
Natural and effective. Fluoride and cranberry extract inhibit bacteria and fend off gingivitis. $5, burtsbees.com

BRUSH
Supersmile Series II LS45 Advanced Sonic Pulse Toothbrush
It helps you maintain an ideal 45-degree angle while providing 30,000 strokes per minute. Comes with a 2-minute timer. $100, supersmile.com

professional in-office bleaching. "It should be done only once or twice a year, but everyday upkeep is incredibly important," says Dr. Jablow.

If you don't have the bucks (up to $1,000) for treatment at your dentist's office, try a professional fix at home, such as Dr. Jablow's IntelliWhite kit ($80, rxbright.com). This product features whitening pens that target the teeth and keep chemicals off gums. Steer clear of generic trays that can make gum tissue sensitive. Before you try anything, consult with your dentist so your expectations are realistic.

Chapped lips: Stick to unscented, flavorless balms. Fragrances can irritate inflamed skin. (And you'll be less tempted to lick your lips.) Reapply at night, when the oils can sink in and fissures can fuse. In extreme cases, Dr. Welsh suggests using 1 percent hydrocortisone cream.

Sleep with This

AN EXTRA PILLOW.
As you sleep, fluid can pool around your eyes, leading to baggy skin in the morning. An extra pillow under your head can prevent fluid buildup, says dermatologist Neal Schultz, MD. Also try sleeping on your back; side sleeping can create sleep lines from the stress of your skin pressed against a pillow.

A HUMIDIFIER.
Yes, it works. Even in the spring, this simple device (or just a bowl of water in the room) adds moisture to the air, which your skin then absorbs, Dr. Schultz says. Once summer arrives, though, put it away. Too much humidity can promote the growth of bacteria and mold allergens.

Wake Up Looking Great

Blood flow to your skin is higher while you sleep. The advantage: Active ingredients in grooming products can work more effectively. Add these to your bedtime routine.

DRYNESS
While you sleep, you're not exposed to daytime drying agents like wind or pollution, so it's a great time to let lotion soften wrinkles and reduce dryness, says dermatologist Ariel Ostad, MD. Look for a product with hyaluronic acid, which bonds moisture to skin without leaving it feeling greasy. **Try:** Mario Badescu Hydrating Moisturizer with Biocare & Hyaluronic Acid ($20, mariobadescu.com)

SKIN DAMAGE
During the day, your skin broils as it absorbs ultraviolet rays. For defense, it needs antioxidants. Many creams and tonics contain antioxidant-rich green tea or berry extracts. Applying them at night helps your skin replenish antioxidants for the day ahead, according to a 2009 study in *Skin & Aging* magazine. **Try:** Kiehl's Açaí Damage-Protecting Toning Mist ($26, kiehls.com)

CRACKED LIPS
Even if you use lip balm during the day, all your talking and eating keeps cracks from healing. But at night, a coating of balm allows your skin to swell with moisture and fuse the cracked sides together, says Manhattan dermatologist Neal Schultz, MD. **Try:** Neosporin Overnight Renewal Therapy lip protectant ($5, drugstore.com)

RAZOR BUMPS
Scrubbing your skin just before scraping a razor blade across it can lead to ingrown hairs and razor bumps. Instead, exfoliate at night and then shave in the morning. Look for a product that contains 1 to 2 percent salicylic acid, says Dr. Schultz. **Try:** Every Man Jack Face Scrub Skin Clearing ($6, everymanjack.com)

Perfect Hair Solutions

The carefully coiffed, clean-shaven look is so pre-recession. You can now let it grow, but that's not license to become Teen Wolf. Follow these rules.

Is your hair unruly? "Don't obsess about changing or struggling against what you have," says stylist Antonio Prieto, owner of Antonio Prieto Salon in Manhattan. Instead, learn to work with it.

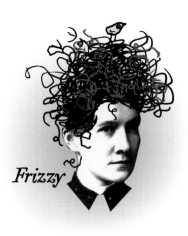

Frizzy

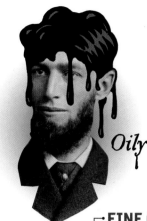

Oily

OILY HAIR

Known enemies: Over-exposure to blow-dryer heat, and vigorous brushing or combing. "That triggers more oil production on the scalp," says Craig Whitely, owner of the Grooming Concierge in Los Angeles.

Secret weapon: Use fewer brushstrokes, to reduce the amount of oil you distribute from your scalp. If you want to be creative, squeeze a lemon into 1 cup of water and use it to rinse your hair after shampooing, Whitely says. The acid strips away excess oil buildup. (The fresh scent is a bonus.)

BEST FIX:
Phyto Phytopanama+ Intelligent Shampoo

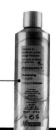

DRY HAIR

Known enemy: Frequent shampooing in hot water.

Secret weapon: Wash your hair in lukewarm water twice a week—max. That way you won't scald already dry ends or scrub away your hair's natural oils with detergents. Then style it using a natural boar-bristle brush. The bristles spread the oil from your scalp to parched strands down the length of the hair shaft. "This creates more evenly moisturized hair and a healthier scalp," says Whitely.

BEST FIX:
Bumble and Bumble Quenching Shampoo

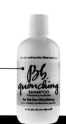

FINE OR THINNING HAIR

Known enemies: Thick, moisturizing conditioners and styling products. A heavy coating of moisture weighs your strands down and makes them clump, exposing your scalp.

Secret weapon: Have your hair cut every 3 to 4 weeks. "Don't try to compensate with extra length—it only makes you look like you're trying to hide something," says Prieto. If balding is your challenge, have the thinning areas cut slightly shorter than the fuller parts so they blend seamlessly with the rest of your hair.

BEST FIX:
Bosley Professional Strength Nourishing Shampoo

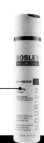

DANDRUFF

Known enemies: Rushed rinsing. Daily shampooing and conditioning is important for removing flakes and keeping your scalp clean and moisturized, but be sure to rinse your hair thoroughly. It's vital to clearing residue from your hair, Whitely says.

Secret weapon: Sunshine. Ultraviolet light can be effective in resolving many flaky-skin conditions. Try a noontime run outdoors to help clear dandruff.

BEST FIX:

Molton Brown Anti-Dandruff Jackberry Hairwash

Head & Shoulders Classic Clean Shampoo

CURLY OR FRIZZY HAIR

Known enemies: Frequent washing, which can turn your natural curls to frizz, and vigorous towel drying, which makes the frizziness even worse.

Secret weapon: Don't dry your hair aggressively; just blot it, says Erica Fleischman, owner of Erica Fleischman: A Men's Salon, in Manhattan. "Blotting reactivates the curls without shocking them," she says. The way you dry your hair sets the stage for how it behaves the rest of the day.

BEST FIX:

Aveda Be Curly Shampoo

DULL HAIR

Known enemies: Styling products applied to wet hair. Since many pomades and volumizers are water-based, adding a dab to wet hair just dilutes the effect. "The product will work best with a dry base," says Fleischman.

Secret weapon: Beer. Just take one into the shower and massage it into your hair a few times a week after shampooing. Then rinse. The hops may help coat your hair and add volume, Fleischman says. Is your hair completely normal? In that case:

BEST FIX:

Intelligent Nutrients Harmonic Shampoo

Axe Heat Igniting Citrus 2 in 1 Shampoo + Conditioner

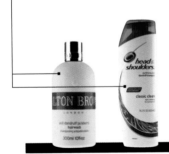
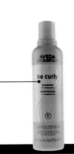
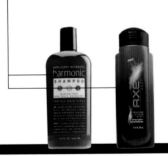

Whatever your hair type, there are ways to make it look great.

Snip Tips

A little scruff is good; too much is, well, not so much.
Here are some hints to heed.

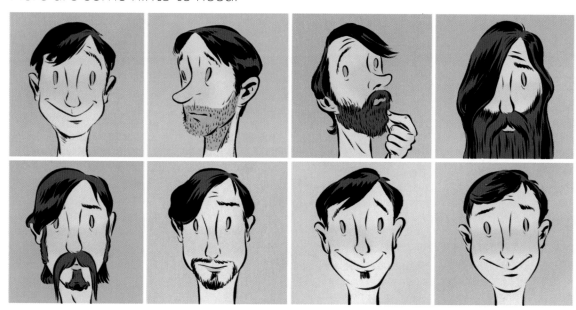

BEARD

Consider the chin. The longer your face is, the shorter your chin hair should be. Otherwise the beard will exaggerate your features, says Grooming Concierge owner Craig Whitely.

Fade it out. You can just trace your jawline and shave below it. But for a more casual look, Whitely says, create a fade. Use the shortest clipper setting on the bottom quarter inch of your beard; go a bit longer every quarter inch up your neck. Adjust the blade settings to blend any lines.

Clean regularly. Each time you shower, shampoo your beard and rub in a dime-size dollop of moisturizing conditioner, Whitely says. Rinse after 10 seconds.

HAIR

No 'fro. As curly hair grows out, thin the sides every 3 to 4 weeks, but barely trim the top, says Danny Kerr, head stylist at Spiff in New York City. Until your hair's weight controls your curls, tame them with a molding product like Bumble and Bumble's Sumotech.

Neaten your neck. "As long as you clean the back of your neck, you'll look like you've had a haircut," Whitely says. If you have a wide neck, round the edges of the neckline. Otherwise, trim straight across. Every 6 weeks, ask your barber to take off a quarter inch and thin your hair.

SIDEBURNS

Check length. Let your face shape be your guide. If your face is round or your chin isn't very pronounced, keep 'burns at mid-ear or shorter. If you have an oblong or rectangular face, keep them a little longer—mid-ear to earlobe length.

Keep 'em narrow. Don't let them grow wider than about an inch or you'll need a sequined jumpsuit to match, says Whitely. Keeping them that way is easy: Buy a comb as wide as your 'burns, hold it up against them, and follow its smooth edge with a trimmer.

Avoid fluff. Watch the edges and puffiness of your sideburns. If you have shaggy hair, keep your sideburn hair short, around an eighth of an inch.

The Great Shave-Off

Are the new razors true innovations, or gimmicks? Skin-care expert Tony Sosnick, creator of Anthony Logistics, tests the latest crop using his own product: Action 2-in-1 Shave Cream

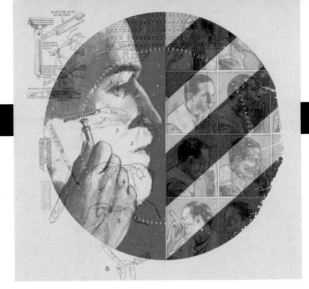

BEST OF THE BUNCH
Gillette Fusion ProGlide Power Razor ($11)

The claim: A tiny "microcomb" fluffs scruff into slicing position for the five blades, which have low-resistance coatings. Slots in the head let shaving gel rinse out.

Sosnick's shave: It provided the smoothest result of all the razors, and he raved about the sturdy handle. Cream built up despite the slots, but a rinse took care of that.

THE BARGAIN
Bic Flex4 ($6 for three)

The claim: This four-blade disposable has a sturdy, pivoting handle and a lubricating strip containing aloe and vitamin E.

Sosnick's shave: He was surprised. The razor glided with impressive ease. But he did have trouble reaching under his nose. "There could be a better pivot," he says. Also, the conditioning strip didn't last for many shaves. Disposable indeed.

THE TRAVELER
FaceBlade Folding Travel Razor ($7, headblade.com)

The claim: It's light, collapsible, and designed to be easy to stash, with room to store an extra blade inside. Raised plastic on the handle improves grip.

Sosnick's shave: It pivots well, making it better than the average disposable. But the design was perhaps too lightweight: "I didn't feel 100 percent safe," he says.

THE STYLIST
King of Shaves Azor Hybrid Synergy System Razor ($9, shave.com)

The claim: Its Y shape is made to be ergonomic, and the razor has a built-in conditioning strip.

Sosnick's shave: The handle is light yet sturdy enough for a serious grip. But the head is so bulky he had trouble navigating his face. "They were trying too hard to be different," he says.

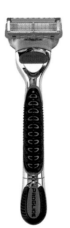

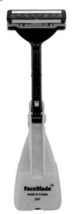

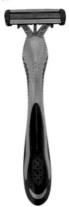

Clean-shaven or scruff, **whatever your look,** you can plus it up.

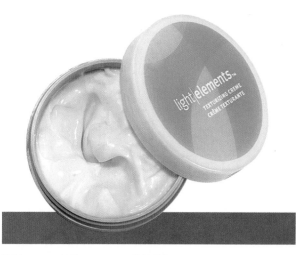

THE GLIDER
Schick Hydro 3 Razor System ($9)

The claim: A hydrating gel reservoir releases water-activated gel with every stroke; skin guards protect your skin from irritation.

Sosnick's shave: It slid more smoothly than any of the others, and kept delivering after multiple shaves. But the reservoir blocked the blades from reaching the corners of his face. You can flip it open, but who has time for that?

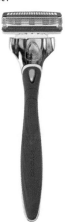

Mess Yourself Up

"You can create that second-day unwashed look without actual second-day greasiness," says Seattle stylist Jake Gravbrot. Just use a product like Aveda Light Elements Texturizing Creme ($24, aveda.com). No matter what your hair length, just rub a small amount between your palms and then use your fingertips to work the cream evenly through the ends of your hair, Gravbrot says. It'll leave your hair soft and movable, but still properly mussed.

Clean Up That Beard

Neaten it with help from Manhattan master barber Diane Wood.

MAINTAIN A 1:1 RATIO OF BEARD TO HAIR LENGTH. In general, your beard should not be any longer than the hair on your head. If you're closely cropped up top, your beard hair should be just about the same length.

CUT BELOW THE JAW. Don't shave at the jawline; it looks awkward and abrupt. End your beard an inch above your Adam's apple. Best move: Create a natural fade there by setting a trimmer to 2 or 2.5.

CLEAN IN THREE STEPS. Use a mild, non-lathering face wash. Apply conditioner to your beard. If you've trimmed enough to see skin through your beard, exfoliate.

Adam Eskin, 28, CEO of The Pump Energy Food, dropped 22 pounds by tweaking his diet and doing body-weight exercises.

Part 4: LOOK BETTER INSTANTLY

Great Looks at Any Age

The way you age is determined by more than just your DNA.
The latest research reveals that exercise can help delay and even reverse aging's debilitating effects on your muscles, heart, and brain.
The only side effect? You will also look your best.

Men's Health talked to the world's leading cardiologists, neuroscientists, nutritionists, and trainers to create this master plan for your 20s, 30s, 40s, 50s, and beyond. It can help you anticipate your body's physiological shifts, then guide you through critical adjustments to your workout and diet to match them. Yes, you will grow older, but you'll also grow stronger and even smarter

20s: Power + Agility

In your 20s, you have a wonderful ability to execute intense, heavy, frequent exercise," says Alexander Koch, PhD, an associate professor of exercise sciences at Truman State University. "Don't blow the opportunity."

The reason for that ability: a high tide of human growth hormone (HGH) and testosterone—currents that spur growth of the muscle fibers that ignite explosive lifts, sprints, jumps, and swings.

"A man's HGH levels drop from 6 nanograms per milliliter when he's 20 to 3 nanograms per milliliter when he's 40," says Dr. Koch. Your 20s represent the best time to build muscular power, which consists of generating maximum force as quickly as possible. (Muscular strength, by contrast, consists of force with no regard to time.) To exploit this moment, you should head straight for the heavy weights, says Mike Boyle, ATC, the elite trainer who created the exclusive decade-by-decade workouts for this chapter.

"You don't need much cardio because your metabolism still vaporizes pizza on contact. And you don't have to worry about flexibility because your joints are healthy and your range of motion doesn't need priming—yet."

How Do You Measure Up?

Vertical jump is a good way to measure lower-body power, and it peaks during your 20s. For details on self-testing, go to MensHealth.com and search "Are You MH Fit?"

The average guy's vertical jump

Age	Height
20–29	19.7"
30–39	16.9"
40–49	13.8"
50–59	11.0"

The *Men's Health* fit standards = 22"
To boost your hops, says Kelly Baggett, the author of *Vertical Jump Development Bible,* stand at the edge of a 12- to 18-inch-high box. Step down, landing squarely in front of the box, then jump as high as you can. Do 3 sets of 5, pausing 10 seconds between reps and 2 minutes between sets. Do this routine 3 times a week before your workout.

The Big Small-Business Man

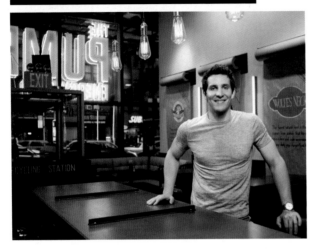

Adam Eskin, 28, CEO, The Pump Energy Food

Like many guys, Adam Eskin graduated from college in his physical prime. "I played hockey and rugby and lifted weights," says the 6'1" Eskin. Then he stepped onto the Wall Street treadmill and began grinding out 90-hour workweeks. Crunching numbers replaced crunches. After a few years, his bank balance was bulging, but his strength was sagging. In 2006 Eskin escaped the investment-banking fire for the frying pan—or, more accurately, the grill. He led a group that took charge of The Pump, a New York City health-food chain. At the same time, he streamlined his diet and made a pact with his buddies to work out 4 days a week. By combining weights, racket sports, and bodyweight drills, he slimmed from 212 to 190 pounds. "Now I feel more energetic than ever," he says.

Busy-Man Fitness Secrets

Simplify your diet. Working with The Pump's in-house nutritionist, Nicole Garfield, RD, Eskin used the chain's healthy eating philosophy to remodel his own diet into key groups that he hits at every meal: lots of lean protein (poultry, grass-fed bison and beef, and fish), lots of nutrient-dense vegetables (sweet potatoes, spinach, beans, and lentils), and small amounts of good fats (from avocados, hummus, and Cheddar cheese).

Master the muscle trinity. There's no faster way to build muscle than with low-rep, heavy-resistance routines based on the fundamental strength exercises: the squat, the bench press, and the deadlift, says Mike Robertson, CSCS, an Indianapolis-based trainer. Use these tips to do each exercise better.

Squat: Keep your chest up and back naturally arched, and turn your knees out during the movement.

Bench press: As you push the weight up, keep your shoulder blades back and down, and tighten your leg muscles. Tuck your elbows close to your sides.

Deadlift: Keep your chest up and back flat, squeeze your glutes, and push from your heels on the lift.

Accelerate strength gains. Power is a function of strength and speed working in concert, so when you're in your 20s, your training should also include plyometric exercises, or explosive movements.

"Jumps allow strength to be converted to power," says Boyle. "Think of it this way: Jumps train mainly your nerves, while weights train your muscles." In fact, along with helping you gain speed and power, doing plyometrics also builds new muscle, according to a 2008 Danish study published in the *Journal of Strength and Conditioning Research*.

Build a body she'll desire. Don't deny your vanity; just remember who you're trying to impress. In a landmark Harvard study, male undergraduates were asked to choose which bodies they wanted to have from a range of composite images. On average, the guys chose bodies with 30 pounds more muscle. By contrast, when women were asked to select men's bodies they found attractive, they chose guys with 15 to 30 pounds less muscle than the male participants had selected.

"The ideal is closer to Derek Jeter's body than that of Barry Bonds," says Roberto Olivardia, PhD, a clinical psychologist and co-author of the study.

Fuel up on supper. Protein is the key nutrient for building muscle. And all men, especially guys in their 20s, should take in at least 30 percent of their total calories from high-quality protein sources like lean meats, fish, dairy, and poultry, says Susan Bowerman, MS, RD, an assistant director of UCLA's Center for Human Nutrition. Eat 1 gram of protein for each pound of your target weight. For instance, if you weigh 200 pounds but want to weigh 180, eat 180 grams of protein a day. To speed recovery from power workouts, drink a shake made with at least 20 grams of whey protein powder, ⅓ cup milk, 1 cup cranberry juice, and 1 cup frozen mixed berries (which are inflammation fighters).

THE 20s WORKOUT: POWER + AGILITY

The Look-Great Formula: "Ultimately, to become fit you need three ingredients," says trainer Mike Boyle, ATC: "resistance training, cardiovascular training, and flexibility training." Boyle divides his 60-minute workouts into three parts to achieve whole-body strength and fitness. "The ingredients don't change decade by decade, but the amount of time you dedicate to each phase does, to counteract aging." For workout descriptions, videos, and PDFs, visit MensHealth.com/lookgreat.

Do this whole-body workout 3 days a week. Use the heaviest weight that allows you to complete the prescribed repetitions. The lifting tempo is 2 seconds up, 4 seconds down. Rest 2 minutes between the short sets and 1 minute between the longer sets.

FLEXIBILITY: 5 MINUTES
Start with 2 minutes of foam rolling (see page 194) over any areas that feel tight. Then do 10 kneeling hip flexor stretches and 10 lateral squats (like a lateral lunge, but with your feet wide apart).

STRENGTH: 40 MINUTES
MONDAY:
Squats: 3 sets of 5
Bench press: 3 sets of 10
Deadlifts: 3 sets of 10
Ab-wheel rollout or barbell rollout: 3 sets of 15

WEDNESDAY:
Bench press: 3 sets of 5
Squats: 3 sets of 10
Deadlift: 3 sets of 10
Ab-wheel rollout or barbell rollout: 3 sets of 15

FRIDAY:
Deadlifts: 3 sets of 5
Incline bench press: 3 sets of 10
Single-leg straight-leg deadlifts: 3 sets of 10
Ab-wheel rollout or barbell rollout: 3 sets of 15

CARDIO: 15 MINUTES
Outdoors or on a treadmill, run 15 sprints of 15 seconds each, with 45 seconds active recovery (jogging at a pace at which you can easily hold a conversation).

30s: Strength + Stamina

The 30-something man can have it all. With his judgment now enhanced, he can compensate for the slight decline from his physiological peak in his 20s. And if he trains the right way, he can still whip the whippersnappers.

That's why the 30s are often the prime years of professional sports stars and, in particular, endurance athletes. For instance, a 2007 analysis of marathon times by German researchers revealed that runners don't slow down at all in their 30s—even though their hearts start losing stroke volume and their VO_2 max levels begin to even out. One reason: You can still extend your lactate threshold (LT), says Andrew Doyle, PhD, an associate professor of kinesiology at Georgia State University.

"LT is the point when your muscles pump out fatigue-producing lactate faster than the blood can clear it and the muscles start burning more carbohydrates than fat. By extending your LT, you can exercise at a higher intensity, burn more calories, and better control your weight."

Supercharge your turbo. The shortcut to fitness is interval training, says Robertson. Brief, intense bursts of exercise at 80 to 95 percent of your maximum heart rate, interspersed with recovery interludes during which your heart rate returns to normal, burn more calories than steady, less intense efforts do. They also improve performance. For instance, cyclists doubled their endurance after just 2 weeks of sprint interval training, according to a study in the *Journal of Applied Physiology*. Interval-training principles also apply to running, stair climbing, rowing, and circuits.

Hit your fighting weight. In this decade, your metabolism slows and your body-fat percentage creeps up. It's critical to keep that number below 22 (18 is optimal); research shows that doing this reduces your risk of high blood pressure, diabetes, and heart disease, says Heidi

How Do You Measure Up?

More than any other measure, your body-fat percentage indicates your overall health. From this decade on, the average guy adds on the adipose (a.k.a. flab).

The average guy's body-fat percentage

Age	Body Fat
20-29	14.1–17.4 percent
30-39	17.5–20.5 percent
40-49	19.6–22.5 percent
50-59	21.3–24.1 percent

The *Men's Health* fit standard = 11%–18%
Use this simple strategy to maintain a healthy weight: Stand on a scale every day. More than 44 percent of dieters who've kept pounds off for at least 5 years weigh themselves daily, according to a National Weight Control Registry study. The WifiBody Scale ($160, withings.com) measures your body fat and lets you track your weight loss and muscle gains from any Web browser or your smartphone.

Skolnik, CDN, nutritionist for the New York Giants.

"The two biggest diet saboteurs for busy men are calories from drinks and binge eating sessions caused by staying late at work," she says. Solution: Find a low-calorie drink you can sip all day. Skolnik recommends green tea, because it also revs your metabolism. Also, stock your desk drawer with healthy, filling snacks, such as instant oatmeal, beef jerky, dried fruit, cans of tuna, and wholegrain crackers.

Make training more fun. The most effective and enjoyable way to prepare for an endurance event is to join a group training program. Canadian research shows that you're more likely to stick to a workout program if you train with others rather than going solo. British researchers note that you're also more likely to push yourself much harder. Team in Training, for example, specializes in taking people from the couch to a marathon, triathlon, or century bike ride in a 5-month training program run by certified coaches. Along the way, you raise money for the Leukemia & Lymphoma Society and meet fitness-minded, charitable women: Nationwide, 73 percent of TNT participants are female.

Prevent back pain. Boyle tailored the 30s strength segment to focus on body-weight exercises that develop endurance and coordination. That means replacing high-weight, low-rep lifts with lower-weight, higher-rep sets, and doing some exercises on one leg.

"As you grow older, you should begin to decrease spinal loading," he says.

The Brothers Trim

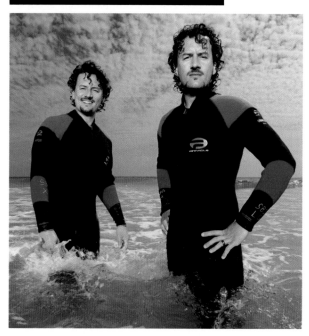

Nicola and Fabrizio Carro, 34, chefs, Quattro Gastronomia Italiana, Miami and New York City

As chefs, marathoners, and scuba divers, twin brothers Nicola and Fabrizio Carro know a bit about pacing. Whether it's searing tuna, churning out 8-minute miles, or slowing their breathing for a wreck dive, they've learned to move with greater efficiency in every aspect of their lives. And it's working. The brothers (both are 5'9", and Nicola weighs 170 pounds and Fabrizio 180) helm Miami's successful Quattro Gastronomia Italiana, and this year they opened a New York arm of the restaurant and ran the Rome Marathon.

"We're not ready to slow down," says Fabrizio. "Now that we're in our mid-30s, it just means we need to train better. Not harder; smarter."

Busy-Man Fitness Secrets
Find the exercise yin to your work yang. Fabrizio is in charge of a kitchen that's 15 people strong. "I work with a team all day," he says. "When I exercise, I want a break: I love the rhythm of running and diving. All I have to think about is breathing."

"Lifting higher reps with a lighter load still yields benefits, but with less structural stress." Boyle's workout also includes Swiss-ball rollouts, which help you build core strength and endurance. In fact, men with poor muscular endurance in their lower back are three times as likely to develop back pain than those with fair or good endurance, according to a study in *Clinical Biomechanics*.

THE 30s WORKOUT: STRENGTH + STAMINA

Do this whole-body workout 3 days a week. Use the heaviest weight that allows you to complete the prescribed repetitions. The lifting tempo is 2 seconds up, 2 seconds down. Rest 1 minute between sets.

FLEXIBILITY: 10 MINUTES
Start with 5 minutes of foam rolling (see opposite); pay special attention to your back. Then do 5 kneeling hip flexor stretches and 5 lateral squats.

STRENGTH: 25 MINUTES
Pushups (elevate your feet on a 12-inch-high bench): 3 sets of 10
Single-leg or split squats (add dumbbells when you're ready): 3 sets of 10
Single-leg straight-leg deadlifts: 3 sets of 10 (each leg)
Inverted rows (add a weight vest if you can): 3 sets of 10
Core: 3 sets of 15 Swiss-ball rollouts

CARDIO: 25 MINUTES
Stick with interval running (if you have no knee pain) or ride a stationary bike. Add a 5-minute warmup, or spin and then do 15 sprints (15 seconds each) with 45 seconds active recovery. Finish with a 5-minute cooldown jog.

40s: Flexibility + Strength

Your 40s mark the decade when you shift to caring for your body in the gym, inste ffectiveness, which diminishes coordination, says Doyle. Your heart beats more slowly, cutting down the blood flow that delivers nutrients to and removes waste from joints and muscles. And you're losing about 0.5 percent of your muscle mass a year. To reverse these processes and stretch peak performance, your workouts now emphasize flexibility.

Roll out your kinks. Every workout you do should now start with 10 minutes of targeted self-massage using a foam roller, says Boyle. Like a steamroller smoothing out a road, this device alleviates knots and tangles that constrict blood flow and hinder elasticity in your muscle tissue. Place your body on the foam and roll up and down for 10 to 15 seconds on the muscles you're targeting. Rollers are especially useful for soothing back pain, stretching tight hamstrings, and relieving shoulder tension. We like the Grid ($40, tptherapy.com), which has three density zones. Research from Japan shows that people whose bodies are more limber have about 5 percent less arterial stiffness—a marker for heart disease.

Stuff your face. "Men in their 40s should try to eat 10 servings of fruit and vegetables daily," says David L. Katz, MD, an associate professor of public health at Yale University and a *Men's Health* weight-loss advisor. "They need the antioxidant protection, and it's a proven way to stay lean."

How Do You Measure Up?

The number of pushups you can bang out without stopping is a good test of your upper-body strength and endurance. This is the kind of muscle you need to ferry groceries or carry an exhausted toddler. In his 40s, the average guy's total drops to 60 percent of its peak in his 20s.

The average guy's pushup total:

Age	Total
20-29	25
30-39	19
40-49	15
50-59	11

The *Men's Health* fit standards = 30
Here's how to avoid joining the ranks of the sparrow-chested: Determine your pushup max (the number you can do without stopping while maintaining perfect form). Now divide that number by 2 to determine your number of reps per set. Start with 3 sets, resting 1 minute between each. Each week for 6 weeks, shave 10 seconds from your resting period until you eliminate it entirely, says Alwyn Cosgrove, MS, CSCS.

If 10 seems too hard, try 7. Studies suggest that diversity is as important as volume, and Bowerman advises trying to hit 7 different food colors to provide a wide shield of protection from heart disease and common forms of cancer. To help you hit your quota, Dr. Katz recommends including produce with every meal and eating it first, because the fiber

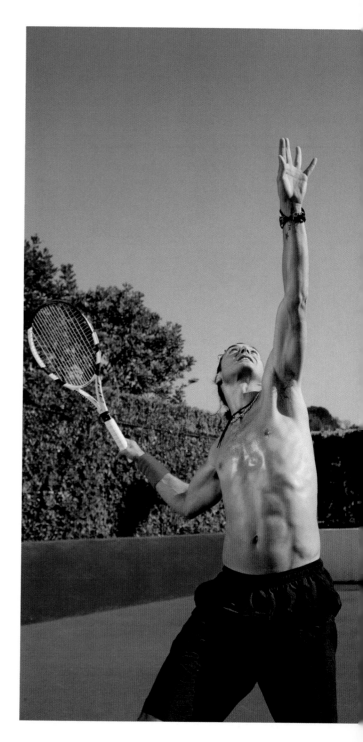

The Shot Caller

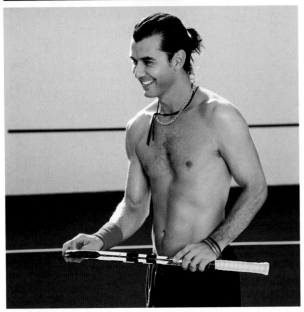

Gavin Rossdale, 44, musician, former frontman of Bush

"'Stay positive.' Roger Federer gave me that advice. It's made the game more fun and made me a stronger player," says Rossdale, who tested out the tennis circuit as a junior. "If you believe you're going to hit a great shot, you play looser and more aggressively. More than winning or losing, I care about whether I played my game—did I go for my shots?"

The 5'10", 170-pound Rossdale is finding his sweet spot these days. He's working on a new solo album while sharing child-rearing duties with wife Gwen Stefani. (The couple's second son was born in 2008.) His tennis game is sharper than ever as well, thanks to a new stretching regimen that includes Bikram yoga and those tips from his friend and coach Roger.

Busy-Man Fitness Secrets
Stay sharp on the road. Rossdale travels close to 100 days a year and always takes two fitness tools with him: a tennis racket and a jump rope. "I've developed a network so I can find a hitting partner anywhere," he says. "Jumping rope fires my leg muscles. I do it to warm up and to stay sharp."

will satisfy hunger. Also, try making all your snacks vegetables and/or fruit.

Be a little selfish. You deserve it. Inhale and focus on yourself. "Yoga is especially beneficial for men in their 40s, because that's when flexibility declines more," says Mehmet Oz, MD, a professor of surgery at Columbia University and coauthor of *You: The Owner's Manual.* New science shows that doing yoga can improve flexibility, relieve back pain, and reduce stress. Oh, about that yoga glow: Boston University researchers report that people who did yoga weekly boosted levels of the brain chemical GABA by 27 percent. Low levels of GABA have been linked to anxiety. Practicing yoga can also help your body maintain its antioxidant levels, which get depleted when you're rundown, report Indian researchers.

Extend your range. Your new focus on flexibility is actually a three-pronged effort that also encompasses building mobility and honing balance. Boyle's workout includes a strength-training component: full-body, complete range-of-motion exercises that stress your muscles enough to build or maintain mass but not enough to burden your joints.

THE 40s WORKOUT: FLEXIBILITY + STRENGTH
Do this workout 3 days a week. Master your form before you add weight. The tempo is 2 seconds up, 2 seconds down. Do the strength-and-cardio part as a circuit: Perform 1 set of each of the 6 exercises (resting 30 seconds between exercises), and rest 1 minute. Then repeat 2 more times.

FLEXIBILITY: 15 MINUTES
Foam rolling: 10 minutes before stretching
Kneeling hip flexor stretches: 10
Lateral squats: 10
Wall hamstring stretches: 10
Doorway pec stretches: 10
Bridges: 3 (hold for 10 seconds each)

STRENGTH: 25 MINUTES
Pushups (elevate your feet on a 12-inch-high bench): 3 sets of 10
Rear-foot elevated single-leg squats: 3 sets of 8 each leg
Inverted rows: 3 sets of 8
Split squats: 3 sets of 8 each leg
Core: planks, 3 reps (hold for 30 seconds each)
Side planks: 3 reps (hold for 10 to 30 seconds each side)

CARDIO: 20 MINUTES
Alternate between running, rowing, and biking intervals. Start at a pace at which you can sustain a conversation for 5 minutes. Then do five 60-second sprints with 2 minutes active recovery.

50s: Balance + Mobility

A certain urgency permeates your workouts now: You still want to look good, but you're also training to stay alive. Exercising regularly is your strongest medicine. In fact, according to a recent commentary in the *Archives of Internal Medicine*, "Physical activity may be the most effective prescription physicians can dispense for the purposes of promoting successful aging."

The evidence keeps accumulating: Exercise protects your heart, relaxes your arteries, makes your erections harder, builds muscle, strengthens your bones, fights cancer, boosts your immune system, and, perhaps most inspiring, it's one of

the best ways to rewire your brain.

"If you don't exercise, it's like your brain is in a cast. Your brain cells and networks atrophy," says John Ratey, MD, an associate clinical professor of psychiatry at Harvard Medical School and the author of *Spark: The Revolutionary New Science of Exercise and the Brain.*

Recharge your brain. Adults who devoted 4 days a week to an hour of moderate aerobic exercise (running, stair climbing, or riding a stationary bike) had more blood flow in their dentate gyrus, the area of the brain where memories are formed, according to a 2007 Columbia University study. Increased blood flow may signal the growth of new brain cells, a process known as neurogenesis, says Adam M.

How Do You Measure Up?

The sit-and-reach test measures flexibility, which declines by about 25 percent from your 20s to your 50s.

The average guy's sit-and-reach:

Age	Reach
20-29	15"-17"
30-39	15"
40-49	13"-15"
50-59	11"-13"

The *Men's Health* fit standard = 17"
To improve flexibility, hold a barbell at arm's length, your grip slightly wider than shoulder width. Bend forward from your hips with your knees slightly bent and your back straight, until your torso is almost parallel to the floor. Pause 2 seconds before returning to the starting position. Do 3 sets of 15 reps, 2 to 3 times a week, says Bill Hartman, PT, CSCS.

Brickman, PhD, a neuropsychologist and coauthor of the study. It's also possible, he says, that exercise stimulates the release of a growth factor in the brain tied to neurogenesis. Another study found that people who did resistance training once a week saw a 12.6 percent jump in a performance on memory tests.

Slow your cells' aging process. The cells of people with high omega-3 levels age more slowly, according to research from the University of California at San Francisco. Researchers aren't sure why, but it may have to do with the anti-inflammatory properties of omega-3 fatty acids.

"Many of the conditions associated with aging—arthritis, cardiovascular disease, Alzheimer's—are related to chronic inflammation," says Bowerman. She advises eating cold-water fish (mackerel, salmon) twice a week, and taking 2 grams of a fish-oil supplement a day. Our favorite: Nordic Naturals Omega-3D, which delivers 550 milligrams of EPA and DHA and 1,000 IU of bone-strengthening vitamin D.

Relax your arteries. Regular aerobic exercise can delay and may even reverse aging in your arteries, concluded a 2008 review in the *Journal of Applied Physiology*. Study coauthor Douglas R. Seals,

PhD, a professor of kinesiology and applied physiology at the University of Colorado at Boulder, explains how: Exercise boosts your heart rate, which increases blood flow. Better blood flow creates more friction on the blood vessels' inner lining (a.k.a. the endothelial layer), which, in turn, stimulates the production of nitric oxide. This improves the ability of your arteries to dilate and confers other benefits as well, like reducing inflammation and oxidative stress, protecting your arteries from developing disorders.

New research indicates that high-intensity aerobic intervals appear to deliver greater endothelial benefits than steady-state aerobic training, according to a study published in the *Journal of the American College of Cardiology*.

Fight age with muscle. After 50, the sedentary man's muscle loss speeds up and he then loses about 10 percent of his muscle mass every decade. This leads directly to osteoporosis. If you've been lifting weights, keep it up. If you haven't, start now; it's not too late. American College of Sports Medicine guidelines cover strength training for people over 65. Your workout should involve more balance moves to strengthen your feet, ankles, and core and to straighten your posture.

Exercise protects your heart, relaxes your arteries, makes erections harder, builds muscle, strengthens bones, fights cancer, and rewires your brain.

THE 50s WORKOUT: BALANCE + MOBILITY

Complete this workout 3 days a week, but do the flexibility training every day. The tempo is 2 seconds up, 2 seconds down. Do the strength-and-core part as a circuit: Perform 1 set of each of the 6 exercises (resting 30 seconds between exercises), and rest 1 minute. Then repeat 2 more times.

FLEXIBILITY: 20 MINUTES
Foam rolling: 10 minutes
Kneeling hip flexor stretches: 10
Lateral squats: 10
Wall hamstring stretch: 10
Doorway pec stretches: 10
Bridges: three 10-second holds
Bosu-ball drills: progress to one leg

STRENGTH: 20 MINUTES
Pushups: 3 sets of 10 to 20
Split squats: 3 sets of 12; add dumbbells when you master the form
Split lunges: 3 sets of 12
Front pulldowns: 3 sets of 12
Core: planks, 3 reps; hold for 30 to 60 seconds
Side planks: 3 reps; hold for 10 seconds on each side

CARDIO: 20 MINUTES
Alternate running, rowing, and bicycling intervals. Start with a 5-minute warmup; then do five 60-second sprints, with 2 minutes rest. Mix in steady-state days during which you just bicycle, row, or run for 20 minutes at a pace slower than 70 percent of your maximum heart rate.

The Energizer Buddy

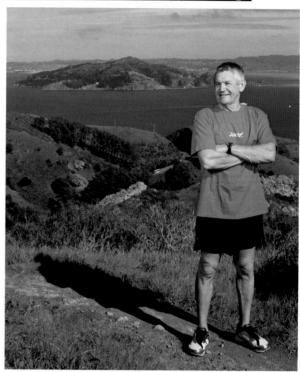

Vito Bialla, 61, CEO, Bialla & Associates

To mark turning 60, Vito Bialla swam in a relay across the English Channel with four friends. It's just the latest challenge for the 6'1", 190-pound dynamo. He's a decorated Vietnam veteran and was the first man to complete back-to-back Ultraman races (think an Ironman times five). He does 300 situps a day, chased with either a circuit of bench presses, pullups, and pushups, or some jogging, cycling, or swimming. He also runs a successful headhunting firm based in Sausalito, California. His pet project: making wine. The Bialla winery's 2006 Cabernet Sauvignon scored a 94 from *Wine Spectator.*

Busy-Man Fitness Secrets
Play mind games (on yourself). Make the halfway mark of a race or training run your goal. "It's always uphill to that point, but then you're on top and you start heading for home," says Bialla. "Every step, stroke, or pedal becomes successively easier because you're closer to the finish."

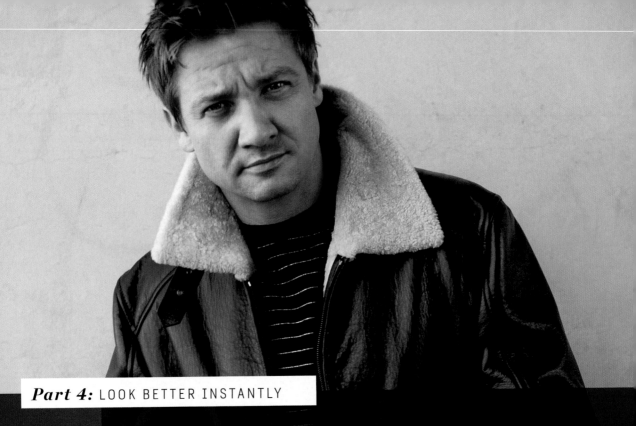

The Fit Man's Perfect Fit

You work out to look and feel your best, so don't hide the results

Clothes that fit well draw attention to your best attributes—and disguise the rest. Accessories help you to emphasize that too. Use this guide to show off in style.

Sculpt Your Suit

Choose a suit that follows the outlines of your body while masking imperfections. Then let a tailor have at it. "It's the tailor's job to take a mere mortal and sculpt a suit around him to give him the body of a Grecian statue," says James Sherwood, author of the new book *Bespoke: The Men's Fashion of Savile Row.*

The precise fit that tailoring provides can make a moderately priced suit look expensive. (Conversely, an expensive suit will look cheap if it doesn't fit well.) "A gym-toned body is the enemy of off-the-rack suits," says Sherwood, because a jacket for a big-shouldered man won't always come with the right size trousers. When you try on a jacket, lift up your arms just an inch or two. If the coat rides up, the jacket is perfect—for comedy. But it's too tight for normal use. A well-fitting shoulder is the starting point for an off-the-rack suit. A tailor can't save a shoulder that doesn't fit.

Then check the jacket at your waist; you want it snug when buttoned. Sherwood says the waistline of the jacket should be cut high, around the narrowest part of your waist. As for the pants, avoid puddling at your feet; the hem should fall gracefully on the shoe. And go with a tight four-in-hand knot for your tie. "It will always be in proportion and subtle, rather than shouting out loud," says Sherwood.

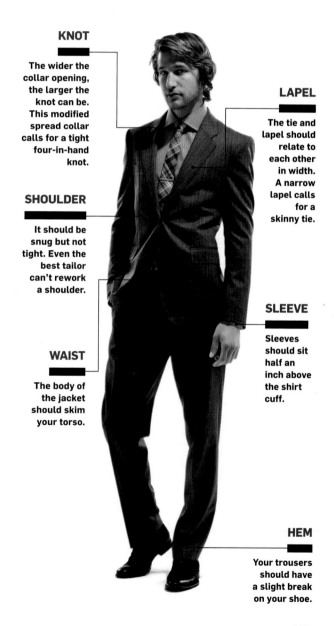

KNOT
The wider the collar opening, the larger the knot can be. This modified spread collar calls for a tight four-in-hand knot.

LAPEL
The tie and lapel should relate to each other in width. A narrow lapel calls for a skinny tie.

SHOULDER
It should be snug but not tight. Even the best tailor can't rework a shoulder.

SLEEVE
Sleeves should sit half an inch above the shirt cuff.

WAIST
The body of the jacket should skim your torso.

HEM
Your trousers should have a slight break on your shoe.

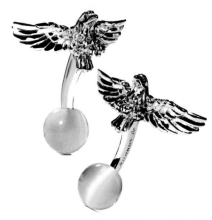

Final Touches Matter

Even an expensive suit can look like a uniform. Let your personality shine with accessories that say something about you.

Watch: Wearing a cheap watch with a suit is like drinking single-malt Scotch from a paper cup. A basic stainless-steel watch is usually fine, but the detail-oriented man should opt for a dressier timepiece with a thin case and leather strap. Match the leather of its strap to your belt and shoes.

Tie bar: Don Draper has made it safe to wear a tie bar again, which should be simple and understated silver or gold. (Simply wearing one is statement enough.)

The bar should also be slightly smaller than the width of the tie. Where does it go? Between the third and fourth shirt buttons.

Cuff links: Your cuffs, not your tie, are the place to reveal your interests. Cuff links that look like fly-fishing reels are much cooler than a necktie emblazoned with jumping trout. If your tastes fall somewhere between basic and novelty, opt for cuff links with color or unique shapes.

Rules of Matching Shirts and Ties

Some men become paralyzed when they try to match ties with shirts. But different patterns and textures can look knowingly stylish—if you follow this guide.

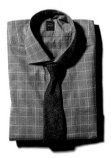

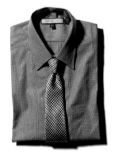

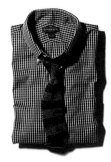

SOPHISTICATED
Why it works: The dominant colors in both shirt and tie are the same tone, but not a perfect match. The flecked texture of the wool tie provides a contrast with the shirt's classic windowpane.

CONSERVATIVE
Why it works: Stripes and checks can work when the shirt and tie share a common color. Make sure one of the two (in this case the tie) is bolder than the other.

CASUAL
Why it works: The bigger the checks, the more casual the shirt. Match that feeling with a textured tie in a loose knot. To make it more formal, switch the tie for a silk one, and tighten the knot.

Rules for Buying a Great Suit for Under $500

You can look sharp on a budget. "As a general rule, most people will not be able to tell how expensive your clothes are if they fit you perfectly," says Clinton Kelly, host of TLC's *What Not to Wear*. "I'm fooled all the time." Even if you have only $200 to spend on a suit, take it to a tailor and it will look like it was made for you.

A long crotch reveals a poorly made suit. "It looks like you bought it at a big-and-tall warehouse sale," says Kelly. The crotch should fit comfortably close without hugging your equipment.

Lesser suits have wider armholes. Sloppy, says Kelly.

Whenever possible, opt for wool. Synthetic fabrics can make you sweat, and they don't have the staying power of wool.

Classic styles always seem more luxurious. You can't go wrong with a two-button notch lapel and side vents.

If workouts have given you a chest and shoulders much larger than your waist, try suit components. Buying the pants and jacket separately makes it easier to achieve a good fit. Try: Banana Republic, J.Crew, Alfani, Calvin Klein, Topman, Express, and Club Monaco.

Expensive Isn't Always Best

Buying the best is a safe bet, but it's not always necessary. Besides, saving money on your work wardrobe will leave you with more cash to spend on fun.

SAVE ON:
BASIC DRESS SHIRTS
Baggy shirts can look cheap even when they're not. If you have a slim or muscular build, a slim-fit white shirt from Banana Republic or Club Monaco will look much better than a pricier but more blousy version. Even a bigger man can look slimmer if he wears a well-tailored shirt instead of a tent.

Thicker buttons indicate quality. If you have a good-looking shirt with shoddy buttons, have a tailor swap in better ones.

Look for better fabrics—you shouldn't see the nub of cotton or any errant threads. Shirts with stretch tend to look more expensive because they fit so well and the fabric looks smoother.

SAVE ON:
SOLID OR CLASSIC TIES
You can spend less on a basic solid tie, but make sure it has a lining. Without it, a tie looks less substantial and won't lie correctly. Beyond solids, stick with traditional patterns, like stripes or checks. Interesting textures and sheens appear richer than flat weaves. Try brands like J.Crew, Express, and Topman.

Cuffs: Trouser cuffs are appropriate only if your pants have pleats and you're over 5'9". Flat-front trousers call for an uncuffed leg. No exceptions.

Tie length: The tip of your tie should hit the top of your trousers. Go a little shorter for a retro look, but never go longer. Ever.

Reveal Yourself with a Pocket Square

A loud shirt is no way to announce yourself. Try using a pocket square to inject some flair, says Kelly.

"It's a nice opportunity to subtly add a pattern or print to a look without going overboard," he says. Three of his favorite folds are the conservative three-point, the easygoing rounded puff, and the classic square (or TV) fold.

THREE-POINT

What: This is for the man who's bolder than most. It's elegant and precise, but you never want to look like you've spent a lot of time on it.

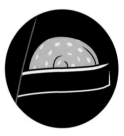

How: Fold a silk square as if you're making a triangle, but don't fold it exactly in half. Instead, make two side-by-side "peaks." Now bring the left side of the folded edge up and to the right of your peaks, to make a third peak. Then bring the right side of the folded edge across to the left.

Wear: Always wear this formal and conservative style with a tie.

Difficulty: High

ROUNDED PUFF

What: It's a stylish way to wear a pocket square, but more carefree than the three-pointed look.

How: Fold it in half and round the folded edge over so it looks like a half-moon. Tuck and go.

Wear: This is more casual than other folds, so add this to a sport jacket. Because the puff is soft, use a silk or soft cotton fabric.

Difficulty: Medium

SQUARE OR TV FOLD

What: The classic midcentury pocket square. Think *Mad Men*.

How: Use a stiff cotton or cotton/linen square. Fold it in half and then in half again, ironing the edge of the fold with each crease. Wear it straight across or tilted diagonally with about half an inch of material peeking out.

Wear: You can add this to everything from a sharp, well-tailored suit to a tuxedo.

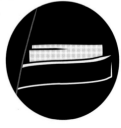

Difficulty: Low

Show Off Your Body

A dress shirt should make you look good and flatter the body you've worked hard to build—not hide it with a tent. Darlene DeAndrade, an expert tailor in Manhattan, explains how to find the right fit.

A shirt that's too large can make a big guy look bigger, a small guy look tiny, and any guy look sloppy.

Neck: When your shirt is completely buttoned, you should be able to stick one or two fingers in your collar comfortably. If you can turn your head without choking, it's a good fit.

Shoulder: The seam should sit at the shoulder; it can be half an inch over, but never under. If it's more than half an inch over, the body may be too loose or boxy. Too much under and the armhole will be uncomfortable.

Body: You should be able to pinch an inch of fabric on each side of your body. Any more and the fit will be too loose. Look for darting (that sewn-in shaping), which indicates a slimmer fit. The shirt should fall at least 7 inches below your waist; you should be able to lift your arms without the shirt coming untucked.

Sleeves: A shirt cuff should sit 1 to 1½ inches above your thumb joint. If you can slide your hand through a cuff without unbuttoning it, the cuff's probably too big.

Sweat a lot? Choose a dark hue, like navy or black, to hide unsightly perspiration stains.

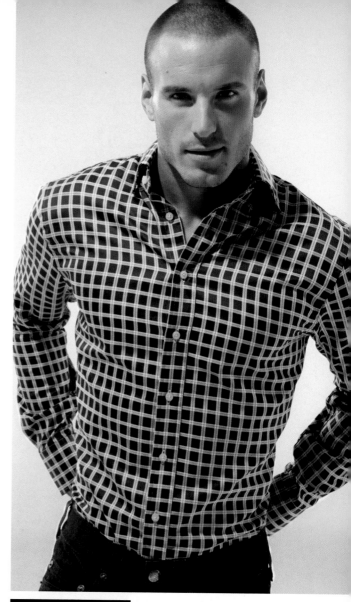

Tuck It In

"Untucking your office shirt on the way to happy hour won't cut it. The classic dress shirt is made to be tucked in. Untucked, it's too long and boxy. The cut and fabric don't translate to a casual setting. If you want to look relaxed, I recommend a more casual shirt rendered in checks, stripes, or solids. It should be short enough to hang right over the waist of your pants and just rumpled enough to convey that you're officially off the clock."

—*Steven Alan, designer*

Four Sweaters You Should Own

A good sweater can last years. You can take it almost anywhere and wear it layered or solo. The thinner the knit, the closer it should fit your frame.

V-neck: If you own only one, make it fine-gauge and solid, in either merino wool or cashmere. When you wear it with a collared shirt, keep the collar tucked in. T-shirt underneath? Make that a V-neck as well.

Sweater jacket: Relaxed peacoat-style sweaters are great for outerwear. Since you'll wear layers under it, the fit should be roomy.

Crewneck: Solids are the foundation, but patterns add texture. Nonbanded bottoms are more forgiving on heavier midsections.

Cardigan: The ultimate multipurpose knit. Dress it up with a shirt and tie for the office, or go casual with a T-shirt and jeans.

Keep It Natural

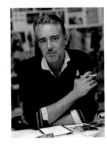

"There's less of a distinction between casual and formal clothes today, so there are more opportunities to discover the versatility of sweaters. You can wear a thin crew or V-neck to work, substitute a heavy sweater for a coat, or wear a zipped cardigan instead of a jacket. My one rule is to always stick to natural fibers, because you get the most wear out of them, they're the most comfortable, and they let your body breathe no matter what the temperature." —*Michael Bastian, designer*

Thin Knits Are a Fit Man's Friend

If you're in good shape, wear a thin sweater or knit instead of a run-of-the-mill collared shirt under a tailored jacket. The result is more casual, flatters a fit body, and pairs well with jeans or chinos.

Don't hide behind a bulky sweater. A fine-gauge knit or sweater—cardigan, crew, or V-neck—offers a better fit than a thick one does. With just a T-shirt underneath, you'll look both sleek and relaxed, and feel more comfortable.

Necklines: Match the neck of your T-shirt to the neck of your sweater. Wear V-neck T-shirts and sweaters together; the T-shirt can have a higher neck. A cardigan works with any style. But a crewneck T-shirt with a V-neck sweater is okay only if Captain Kirk is your style icon.

Everyone Notices Your Watch

Don't undermine a carefully crafted look by wearing a plastic watch, says Andrew Block, executive vice president of Tourneau, a nationwide specialty watch retailer.

"One of the watches you own should be a classic design," Block says. "There's a subtle elegance to a classic watch that makes it versatile." It'll look good with whatever you wear, whether it's a tuxedo or jeans and a sport coat. Look for a watch that has emotional impact for you. "Make a statement," says Block. "For the most part, men don't wear jewelry, so the watch is really the only thing a man can wear to show his accomplishment."

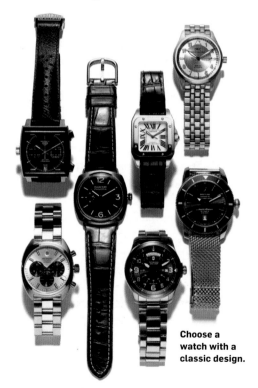

Choose a watch with a classic design.

The Accessory Rule

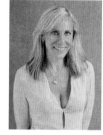

"Women notice everything, especially when it comes to a man's style. Get noticed the right way simply by adding a subtle accent to your usual attire. Whether your style is bold or understated, a vintage watch, unusual cuff links, or a colorful pair of socks can add just the right touch. Think of them as conversation starters."
—*Jan Leslie, accessory designer*

A Fat Wallet Is Ugly

It's bad for you, too. Sitting on a thick wallet can stress your back and cause pain.

"You're elevating your pelvis on one side, which bends the spine," says Stuart McGill, PhD, a professor of spine biomechanics at the University of Waterloo, Ontario. "You're also compressing the sciatic nerve, which runs behind your hip." Move the wallet from your back pocket, or switch to one of these slimmer versions. It'll force you to edit the cards, cash, and trash you're carrying now.

She Sees Your Sneakers

Women might not take note of the hours you log working out, but they will notice if you wear your sneakers outside the gym.

"Your shoes send a message to women that you care about your appearance," says designer Michael Bastian. So ease back to the streets with cool and simple styles like these.

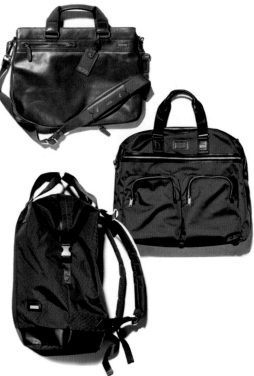

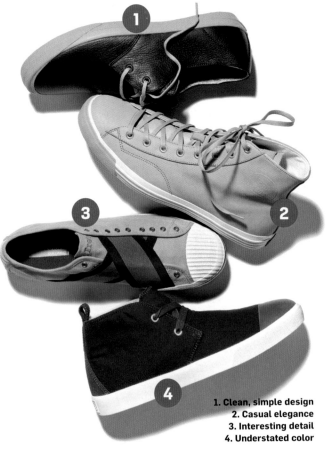

1. Clean, simple design
2. Casual elegance
3. Interesting detail
4. Understated color

The Wrong Bag Weighs You Down

A well-dressed professional carrying a shoddy bag is headed nowhere fast.

"It is important that the bag doesn't become an afterthought," says Phil Russo, vice president of design for Cole Haan. "If you invest in a quality piece, it will continue to look better over time." Let your bag reflect your ambition. Make that *bags*, because you need these.

Gym: You can carry this practical nylon bag as a tote or backpack. And it's smart enough to bring into the office.

Work: This is a modern take on the traditional leather briefcase. A zipper allows the bag to expand with your workload.

Weekend: The ballistic nylon can stand up to the wear and tear of travel. Extra pockets help keep you organized.

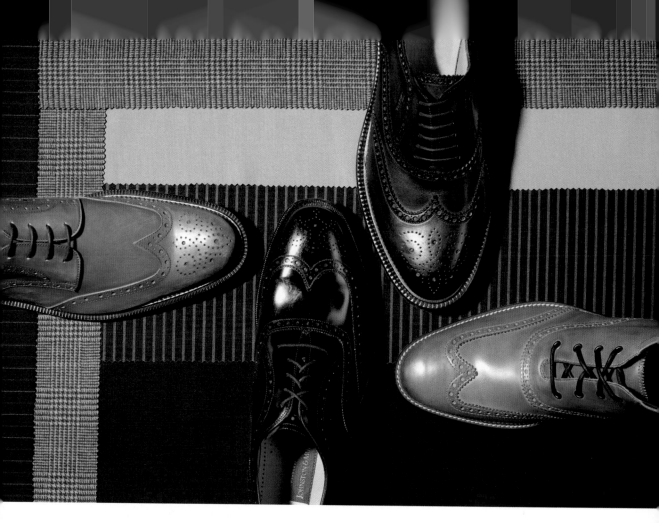

Always Pair with Care

You choose shoes to go with trousers every day. To pull it off in style, use this guide. The shoes on this page rest on fabric colors that work best.

Navy or tan trousers are your best bet to pair with medium-brown shoes. Use either of these shades to set off a shoe's unique pattern, texture, and burnishing.

Dark brown should be considered a neutral that goes best with navy, brown, tan, or gray.

Black shoes read as dressy; wear them when you want to add gravity to black or shades of gray. Wear black with navy for an evening event.

Gray shoes are an unexpected alternative and work best with black and gray. A sophisticated move: pairing them with a rich brown.

Socks: Match your socks to your pants, not your shoes, to lengthen the look of your legs. The other way creates the illusion of boots. And this isn't 1967.

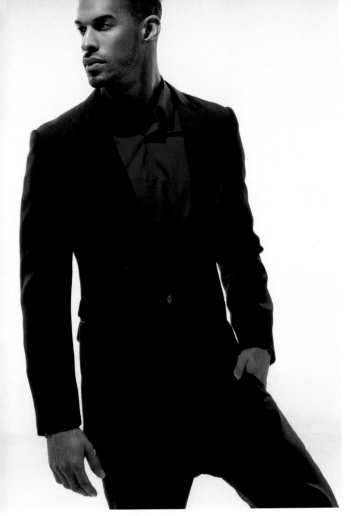

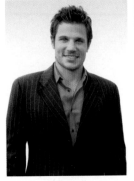
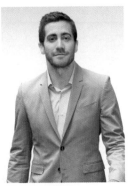
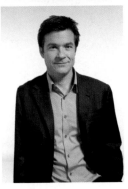
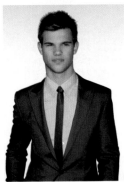

The Blues Speak Volumes

Every man owns at least one blue dress shirt. Buy some more; different shades carry different shades of meaning. Darker blues tend toward the corporate; lighter feels more fashion-forward and youthful. Do you see yourself here?

Buttons: The bottom button on your suit jacket or sport coat always stays undone. Period.

Banker blue: You're conservative. This popular shade is neither offensive nor risky. The upside is that just about any other color, from khaki to black, will be a match.

Powder blue: You have a casual, youthful attitude. You'll stand out in this subtle shade, which won't overpower pale skin but will also show off a tan. Ideal matches are navy, gray, and chocolate.

French blue: You're mainstream. This color was once risky, but now it's expected. Its mass appeal extends to matching: It goes with practically everything.

Steel blue: You're modern and cool. The gray tones give this color a contemporary feel. Wear it with neutrals and cooler hues, like gray or navy, to keep the look intact.

It's Okay to Ignore Your Father

Your dad's advice was not timeless. If he warned you never to mix navy and black, it's time to be your own man. Following conventional wisdom can make you look dated, says designer Michael Bastian.

"I'm a big believer in playing around a little with strong color," he says. For instance, black and brown and other dark neutrals make a sleek, modern statement when worn together, despite old-school edicts. "A confident, friendly man can pull anything off," he says.

Color Has Emotion

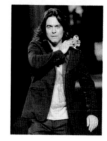

"Color is a vibration of light; it has an emotion, an intensity. You can enhance your life by adopting color in a therapeutic way. Take it step-by-step: Start with a pastel shirt and pair it with a traditional suit. Next, try new combinations of colors with shirts, pocket squares, or ties. When you're ready, dare to wear brighter colors, even for a jacket. Remember that black is the absence of light!"

—Kean Etro, menswear creative director, Etro

Color Rules Aren't Black and White

There are gray areas when it comes to restrictions on color combinations. Knowing a little color theory opens up endless possibilities.

USE NEUTRALS.
Red and tan work together because tan is neutral. So are black, brown, navy, and gray. Each of these goes with anything.

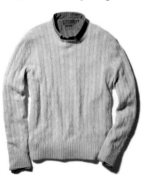

BLEND TEMPERATURES.
Orange is a warm color; blue is cool. This and other warm-cool combinations complement each other.

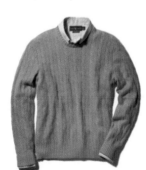

ENGAGE OPPOSITES.
Purple and green are easy on the eyes because they are directly across from each other on the color wheel.

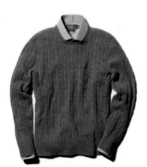

KEEP IT IN THE FAMILY.
A plum-lavender combination is monochromatic—that is, one hue paired with a related shade or tint.

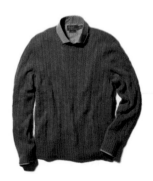

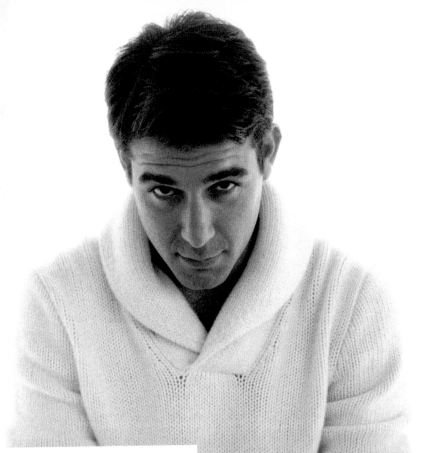

Denim Guide

Casual can be classic

James Wolk, who played the central character in Fox's series *Lone Star*, grew up in Michigan, where his father owned a high-fashion women's shoe store. He learned to appreciate quality accessories.

"The first thing I look at when I meet a woman is her shoes, because they say a lot about her," he says. "For a man, wear good shoes and you can get away with a lot."

In his real-world life, Wolk will dress up a plain pair of jeans and a T-shirt along with a good pair of suede MacAlister-style shoes from J.Crew. Another option: nice wingtips, which can dress up denim as well as they dress up trousers. Tip: Take them off before dangling your feet in water.

Your wardrobe doesn't have to be sloppy or garish to signal that you're off the clock. Wolk wears J.Crew T-shirts, Gap denim, and a flannel or crisp white shirt on his days off.

"There's something comfortable and calming about wearing classics, because they are so familiar," he says. Before you buy something new, ask yourself if it's something you can see yourself wearing in 5 years. If there's any hesitation, walk away and spare yourself present expenditure for future regret.

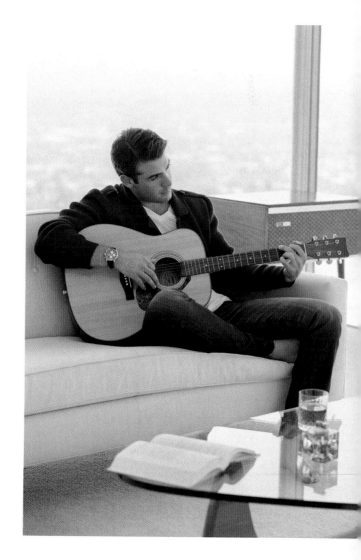

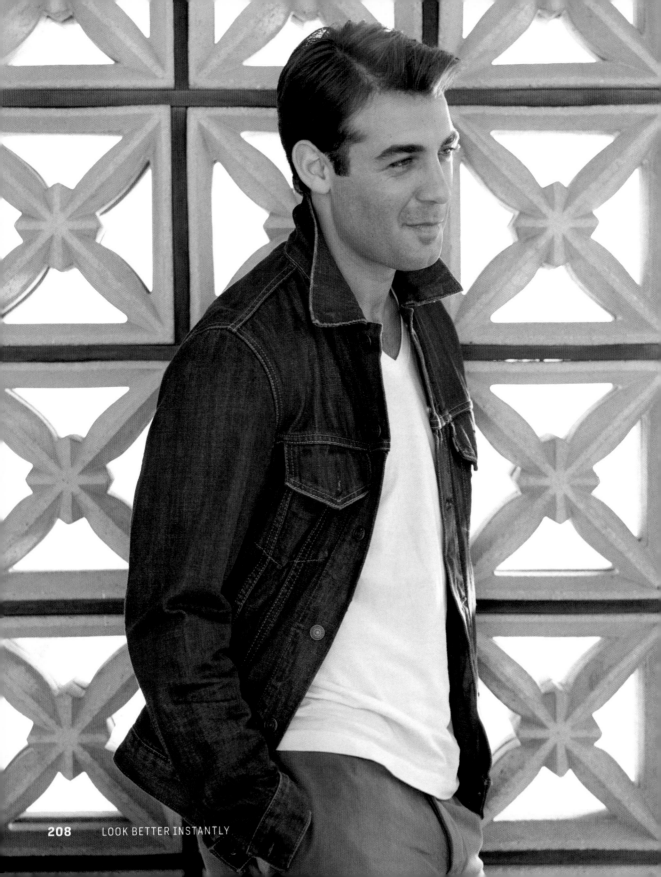

Playing a nice guy is hardly an actor's dream. But a nice guy with a dark side—now *that's* fun, says Wolk, who played a charismatic Texas con man in *Lone Star*. "I enjoy the adrenaline rush that he has from pulling off his cons," says the 25-year-old newcomer, who also stars in the comedy film *You Again*.

In *Lone Star*, Wolk played one man with two identities: schemer Robert Allen, who lives with his girlfriend in suburban Midland, and Bob Allen, who's married to an oil tycoon's daughter in Houston. Imagine *Catch Me If You Can* mixed with *Big Love* and *Dallas*, Wolk says.

"In my own life I carry myself pretty honestly," he says, "so it's fun to delve into this complex character, who's so comfortable with deceit yet experiences a lot of guilt and anxiety."

One thing about Robert/Bob is consistent: his sharp sense of style. "I wish I dressed in my daily life as well as this character dresses—he looks like a movie star out of the '40s or '50s," Wolk says.

In the big city, Bob Allen wears beautifully tailored business suits. "Even when he dresses as casually as Robert does, he's always very dapper, very manicured."

Off the set, Wolk favors a T-shirt or a button-front and jeans. When he dresses

You can't go wrong with a simple, classic pairing of a T-shirt, denim, and a relaxed jacket.

The Right Jeans for Your Body

New hybrid styles offer more chances for a perfect fit.

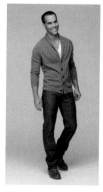 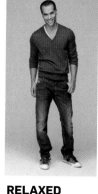 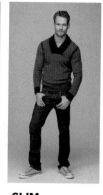

SLIM BOOT
Example: 597 Low Square Boot, by Levi's
The fit: Streamlined, with a lower rise. They fit like typical slim-cut jeans above the knee, and widen slightly to a subtle boot cut.
Best for: A lean build, but they can flatter a range of body types.
Length: The rear hem should be at least half an inch from the ground.
Perfect with: A blazer or sweater and cowboy boots.

RELAXED STRAIGHT
Example: Krooley, by Diesel
The fit: Normal rise and waist, tapering through the leg. The back pockets are set slightly lower.
Best for: The skinny guy who tends to wear jeans loose, as well as for the guy with athletic legs who wants a skinnier look.
Length: A little crinkling at the shoe tongue.
Perfect with: A dress shirt when the jeans are worn high on the waist.

SLIM STRAIGHT
Example: The Outsider, by Joe's Jeans
The fit: "It is our slimmest fit—not quite skinny, but an alternative to the skinny look," says Joe Dahan, the creative director and founder of Joe's Jeans.
Best for: Tall, lean men.
Length: Allow a slight break in the middle of your low-top shoes.
Perfect with: A T-shirt and blazer.

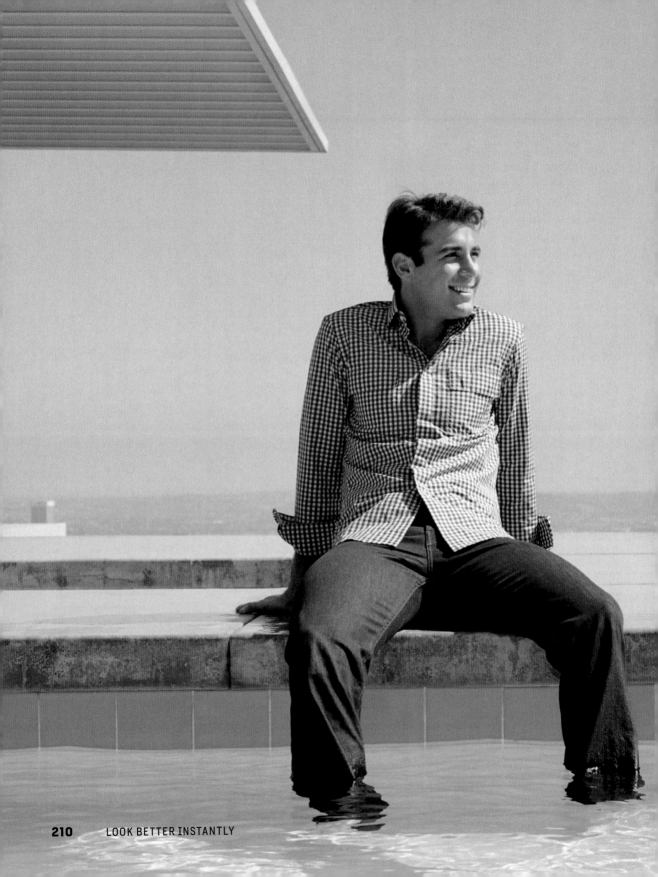

Nice wingtips can **dress up denim** as well as they dress up trousers. Tip: Take them off before dangling your feet in water.

up, he chooses fitted suits with sleek silhouettes that flatter but don't distract. "I love those vintage styles because the clothes were the frame for the man and the picture was the man," he says. "It allowed someone to ask, 'What are you made of? What are your stories?'"

Sounds like a line from a *Lone Star* script.

Here's how to steal Wolk's style.

SIMPLE IS FLEXIBLE.

No matter how the trend tides flow, Wolk stays with basic jeans. Their cleaner cuts offer more wardrobe options.

"They look just as good with a T-shirt as they do with a cool sport coat," he says. We like this season's dark denim styles from Gap, Lee, and Levi's.

NEUTRALS ARE BUILDING BLOCKS.

Patterns and colors can be confusing. But solid neutrals—like gray, white, black, and tan—always look clean and modern. Plus, they can easily be worn together.

"I consider them a foundation that helps me build and deconstruct," says Wolk. Add a layer for complexity when you hit the town, subtract one for simplicity when you hit the road.

BE COMFORTABLE.

Wolk was trained on a steady diet of classic films; striking figures like Steve McQueen and Paul Newman became his style icons. "Newman always looked put together and comfortable in his own skin," says Wolk. Whether it's Brando or Beckham who inspires you, learn from your icon's style.

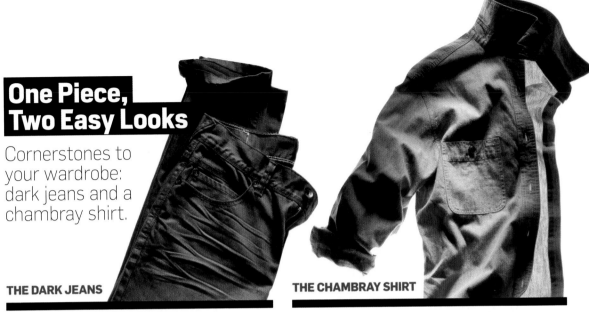

One Piece, Two Easy Looks

Cornerstones to your wardrobe: dark jeans and a chambray shirt.

THE DARK JEANS

KEEP IT CASUAL: Simplicity always works: A clean pair of dark jeans and a white T-shirt will never fail you. They can act as a classic canvas for a cool jacket (like the military-inspired one below) or a statement sweater. Add comfortable slip-on sneakers or a pair of boat shoes and you're ready to hit the town.

DRESS IT UP: Dark, fitted jeans with little or no back-pocket stitching can serve as a cooler alternative to casual cotton trousers. Try a cardigan instead of a blazer over a slim-collar dress shirt, and add a narrow tie for a sleek silhouette.

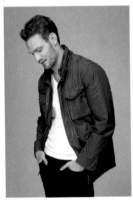

Where: Out after hours with buddies, when you still want to look good enough to run into an ex-girlfriend.

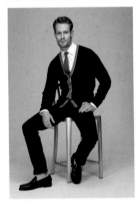

Where: On a first date, when you want to make a nice impression without looking like you're trying too hard.

THE CHAMBRAY SHIRT

KEEP IT CASUAL: A shirt made of chambray—the lightweight cotton originally popular among workmen (hence the phrase "blue collar")—should be part of your basic wardrobe. It says more than a plain tee or average button-front shirt does. Wear it with jeans, alone or paired with a chunky knit (especially a patterned one—see below) to strike a balance between rustic and refined. With sneakers or suede boots, you'll feel as comfortable as you look.

DRESS IT UP: Worn under a tailored jacket, it's a fresh alternative to a plain dress shirt. But know the limits: This is a relatively relaxed shirt. Make it more sophisticated with a wool or knit tie (not a classic silk). Try it with tailored separates or a two-button suit to inject some unexpected cool into a buttoned-up look. Since the shirt's vibe is contemporary, the suit's silhouette should be slim and modern, not traditional.

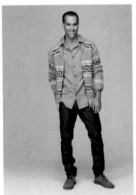

Where: A weekend brunch or backyard get-together.

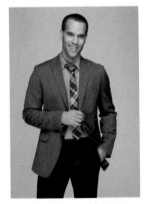

Where: A creative office on days you want to be taken a little more seriously. But don't wear it to an interview.

Make the Shoe Fit

Jeans are casual. But don't be casual about matching your footwear.

Pairing jeans with shoes is all about balance, says Los Angeles-based shoe designer George Esquivel. "You never want one overpowering the other," he says. A wide leg opening requires a wider shoe or boot; a slimmer cut calls for a narrower pair.

"It's important for jeans and shoes to fit the occasion," Esquivel says, "and to have one complement the other."

Slim and straight cuts are versatile and can be paired with several shoe styles, he says, from low-top sneakers, loafers, and desert boots to dressier shoes like bucks and wingtips. A straight cut can handle a more substantial shoe than a slim cut can. And watch the toe width when you're wearing slim-cut jeans: "You don't want to go too pointy or long because it will look funny," he says.

The biggest mistake Esquivel sees men make is wearing loafers with boot cuts. "Boot-cut jeans are meant for boots," he says. He recommends wearing your jeans while you're shoe shopping. And it never hurts to bring a woman along to the store with you. "You're literally looking down at your shoe," he says. You need another

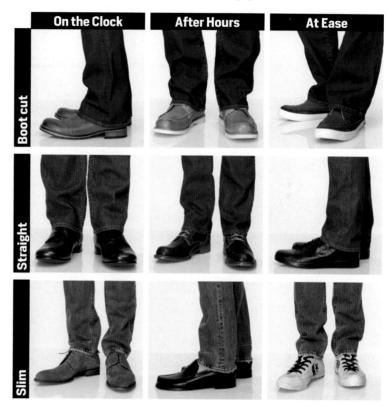

person to see it from everyone else's perspective.

As for length, "men forget that they can take jeans to the tailor," he says. You want just a slight break on your shoes so that enough of them will show. Plus, it looks

sloppy when you have a lot of wrinkles at the bottom.

Women look at these things, he warns. "They pay so much attention to detail that when a man pays attention to detail, it stands out in a good way."

Pairing jeans with shoes is about balance. Your jeans and shoes should complement each other and the occasion.

PROVE IT

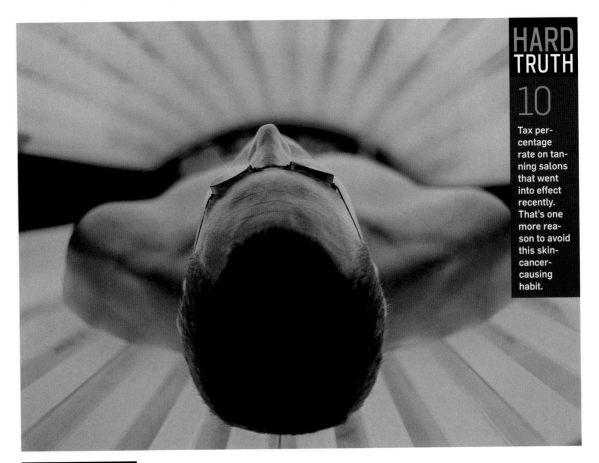

DON'T BAKE

Can you believe people pay to raise their risk of skin cancer? The really crazy thing? You might be one of them. Using a tanning bed is among the most dangerous activities of winter or any other season, reports a review by the World Health Organization's International Agency for Research on Cancer. The beds are so harmful, the IARC placed them in the highest cancer-risk category: "carcinogenic to humans." So if you think the fake 'n' bake is safe, wise up. UV rays from tanning beds are just as damaging to DNA as the ones at the beach.

EAT FOR YOUR SMILE

Not enough healthy fats in your diet may lead to too few teeth in your mouth. Harvard researchers found that consuming DHA (a type of omega-3 fatty acid) can lower your risk of developing periodontitis, a common gum disease, by 20 percent. The scientists believe DHA may discourage the growth of bacteria that attack gum tissue, and may also reduce inflammation-related tissue loss. To reap the benefit, eat 3 ounces a week of canned albacore (white) tuna, the amount used in the study.

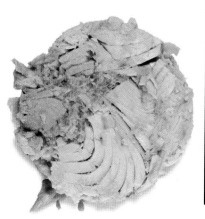

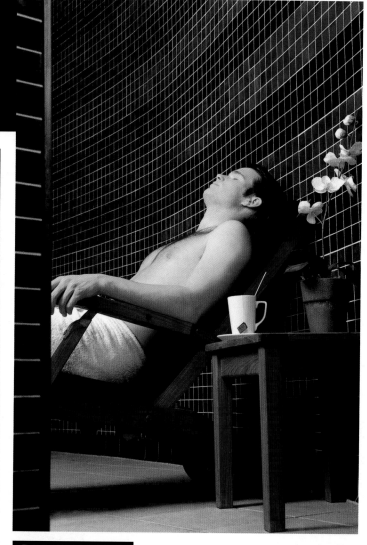

CALM DOWN

Feeling stressed? Channel Peyton Manning. Women prefer calm men, and can sense a man's calm just by looking at his face. Researchers measured levels of testosterone and cortisol, a stress hormone, in college-age men, and took their pictures. They then had women rate the photos for attractiveness, masculinity, and health. The women favored the men with low cortisol levels, says study author Fhionna Moore, PhD.

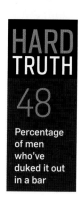

HARD TRUTH

48

Percentage of men who've duked it out in a bar

PROVE IT

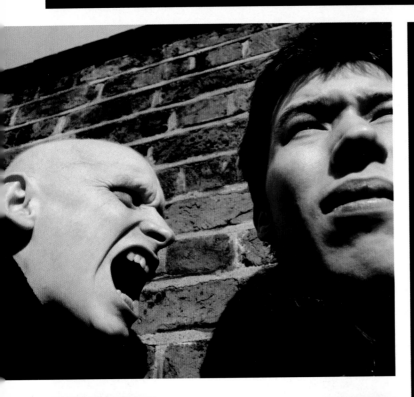

MAKE 'EM LAUGH

So three French guys walk into a bar . . . seriously: The men went on to prove that making your buddies laugh can catch her eye. In the study, three men went to sidewalk bars in France and sat near a woman who was alone. One of the trio told jokes, the other two laughed, and then one of them asked the lady for her digits. While they took turns being the joke teller, the guy hitting on the woman was the same each time. After 54 women, his success rate was 43 percent when he was the jokester, but only 15 percent when he was one of the guys laughing.

CHILL OUT

Tough guys don't wow women. A study in the *Journal of Experimental Social Psychology* shows that women find a man more appealing if he walks away from a jerk instead of responding aggressively. When researchers presented people with scenarios of men being harassed or insulted by other men, the men figured the women would find an aggressive response attractive. Instead, results showed, women prefer that guys detach themselves from trouble.

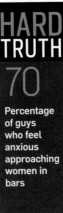

HARD TRUTH

70

Percentage of guys who feel anxious approaching women in bars

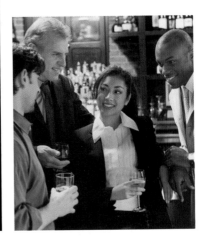

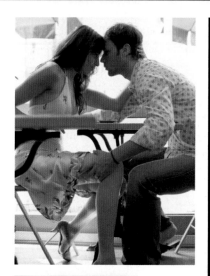

SEDUCE HER WITH ONE LOOK

You have her attention; now don't lose focus. Sideways glances during a conversation can be misinterpreted as the cold shoulder, say Purdue scientists who used videos to gauge the effects of eye contact. Looking away can make a woman think you hold her in low esteem, study author James Wirth, PhD, explains.

"The 'right' amount of gaze means matching hers," he says. If you glance away, choose a spot beyond her—not to the side— and quickly resume your focus.

CLIP AT YOUR RISK

Poor grooming is more than just ugly; it's dangerous. Careful with those clippers. Trimming your toenails the wrong way can expose you to MRSA, a potentially deadly form of antibiotic-resistant staph bacteria. Over the past 2 years, members of the American College of Foot and Ankle Surgeons have seen an alarming increase in cases of MRSA contracted as a result of ingrown toenails.

"When the nail grows into the skin, it causes a cut, which can then become infected," says spokesman Karl Collins, DPM. Trim your nails straight across; cutting on a curve increases the chances of the nail biting back. If you already have an ingrown nail, bandage it and see your doctor or a podiatrist.

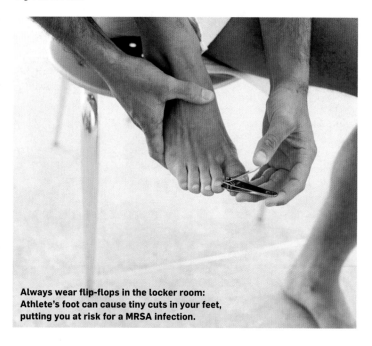

Always wear flip-flops in the locker room: Athlete's foot can cause tiny cuts in your feet, putting you at risk for a MRSA infection.

YOU ASKED

Q: **Should I worry about chemicals in grooming products sabotaging my swimmers?**

A: We're guessing you heard about the analysis of 35,000 grooming products by the Environmental Working Group, a nonprofit research organization. It found that 37 percent of those products contained chemicals, such as phthalates and parabens, that have the potential to wreak havoc on a man's hormones. Sure, that sounds scary, but for an actual health threat to exist, the chemicals not only have to be present in significant concentrations, but also need to be able to enter your bloodstream. These remain two big question marks.

"In rat studies, phthalates in higher doses than those found in grooming products have been shown to reduce testosterone during fetal development. Parabens, also in higher doses, have been shown to decrease sperm

SOAP: AUBREY ORGANICS

Ground almonds and clay help generate the friction needed to clean your skin, while shea butter moisturizes it. $5, **aubreyorganics.com**

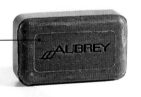

SHAVE CREAM: BURT'S BEES

Coconut oil provides lubrication in this paraben-and phthalate-free cream. $8, **burtsbees.com**

ANTIPERSPIRANT: CERTAIN DRI

It's not organic, but this roll-on is made with only three ingredients, none of them toxic. $6, **dsehealthcare.com**

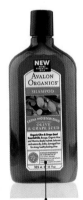

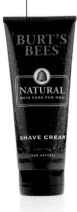

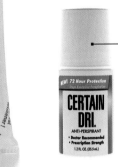

SHAMPOO: AVALON ORGANICS

It's free of phthalates and synthetic preservatives. Grape-seed oil and olive oil help clean and moisturize your hair. $9, **avalonorganics.com**

TOOTHPASTE: PERIOPASTE

Made with organic herbs and without sodium lauryl sulfate, a chemical that can give you canker sores. $8, **docharrison.com**

production in rats," says Kenneth Korach, PhD, principal investigator and chief at the Laboratory of Reproductive & Developmental Toxicology. "But we need more research to determine if grooming products can cause hormonal effects in humans." Still, if you want to play it safe with your sperm, go with the products at left—they'll clean you up without the chemical coating.

Organic grooming products are gentle on the planet as well as your body.

Q: How do I select a good dress watch?

A: Think timeless. "Less really is more with dress watches," says Ruediger Albers of American Wempe, a Manhattan-based watch seller. "You want a subtle face in black or white, with few subdials or apertures. Remember, you could still be wearing it in 50 years." Use these tips to choose your new arm candy.

The strap: Nothing is more elegant than a leather strap in black, brown, or navy. Crocodile adds flair.

The movement: There's something reassuringly retro about a watch that utilizes a handcrafted mechanism to keep time. But mechanical movements are expensive—quality ones start at $1,000—so if you don't have the dough, go with a quartz movement.

The size: Choose a face with a diameter of 37 to 42 millimeters so it doesn't look too

gaudy. And avoid big numbers or symbols; they look childish.

The face: Look for sapphire crystal, one of the strongest and most scratch-resistant face materials. Choose any metal you like, but keep in mind the rings you wear: Select a gold watch if you wear a gold wedding band.

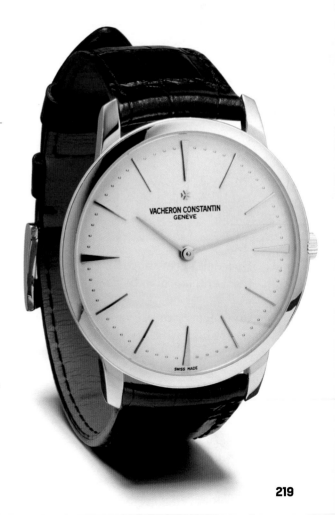

YOU ASKED

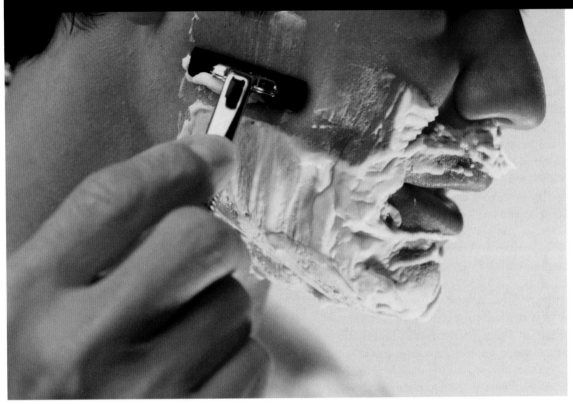

Q: **How can I prevent recurring razor burn and ingrown hairs?**

A: First, understand why your beard is burrowing back into your face. "If you cut too close to the follicle, the hair recedes beneath the surface," says Omeed Memar, MD, an assistant professor of dermatology at Northwestern University.

To achieve the right shaving height for your sensitive mug, use a basic dual-blade razor. The first blade will catch the hair and the second will cut it, giving you a shave that's close but not too close. (Buff your stubble with a toothbrush and warm water to dislodge any existing ingrown hairs.) As for razor burn, try lathering up with a shampoo, such as Aquaphor Baby Gentle Wash & Shampoo, that doesn't contain sodium lauryl sulfate. It's gentler than shaving cream and works just as well, Dr. Memar says. Then simply shave in the direction of your beard growth. When you're finished, slap on a lightweight, alcohol-free aftershave, like Topix Replenix Green Tea Serum.

Q: I've tried all kinds of face cleansers, but I still get pimples. What am I doing wrong?

A: Variety might spice up your life, but it can also screw up your skin. "The most common problem is inconsistency," says Adnan Nasir, MD, the *Men's Health* dermatology advisor and an assistant professor of dermatology at the University of North Carolina at Chapel Hill. "When you stop and start a regimen, you seesaw between improving and worsening your condition, which means you never allow your skin to clear."

He recommends sticking to the following strategy for at least 8 to 10 weeks—the amount of time it takes to replace old, infected, and inflamed skin cells with new, healthy ones. Wash once a day with an oil-free cleanser containing 2 percent salicylic acid, such as Neutrogena Oil-Free Acne wash, then spot-treat pimples with a 5 percent benzoyl peroxide product. The acid will unclog your pores, and the peroxide will kill bacteria and reduce redness. Sensitive skin? Use a mild pore-clearing cleanser, such as Cetaphil Gentle Skin Cleanser.

At the same time, watch what you put in your face: Dr. Nasir says that research suggests that just one serving of dairy may be enough to contribute to skin breakouts, and a study from the *Journal of the American Academy of Dermatology* cites a diet high in refined carbohydrates as another possible culprit. Aim for 25 grams of carbohydrates a day and trade cow's milk for a nondairy alternative, such as almond milk.

If, despite your best efforts, you get a zit, here's what Dr. Nasir advises: Spot-treat it with 10 percent benzoyl peroxide—the active ingredient in some Clearasil creams and ProActiv—and then put on a "dot" Band-Aid overnight. This combo allows the medicine to penetrate better and ensures that it doesn't smear off. Remove the Band-Aid during the day.

Q: What's the fastest, simplest way to soothe my face after shaving if I have no balm?

A: Robbing an ice cube on your skin for 15 seconds immediately after shaving decreases blood flow and causes the muscles that control your hair follicles to contract, says Kenneth Beer, MD, a dermatologist in West Palm Beach and the owner of ScientificSkin. com. "This will decrease redness and help your pores return to normal size, reducing irritation."

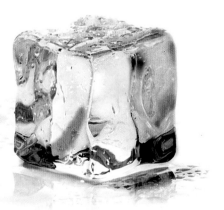

YOU ASKED

Q: My skin gets so dry that it cracks. What can I do to moisturize better?

A: After your shower, reach for the moisturizer before you grab a towel. When the outer layer of your skin is wet, it swells and expands the gaps between the cells; in doing so, it lets in more moisturizer to hydrate your hide, says Dr. Nasir.

Q: I'm considering veneers for my teeth. What can I expect?

A: Serious face time with your dentist. The process of putting porcelain on your teeth requires three visits, beginning with an initial consultation to determine how many veneers you need. If you want to remodel your entire mouth, go with eight to 10 on top and 10 on the bottom, since those are the teeth people see when you grin, says Mark Wolff, DDS, PhD, chairman of the Department of Cariology and Comprehensive Care at New York University's College of Dentistry.

On your second visit, your dentist will load you up with a local anesthetic and prep each tooth, sanding away about half a millimeter of enamel. Then the doc will take an imprint of your mouth and send it to a lab that makes the veneers. In the meantime, you'll be fitted with temporary veneers.

When the custom set is ready, you'll come back to have your new smile cemented in place. If money's tight, go with resin veneers; they cost about $750 a tooth (versus $2,000 for porcelain). But porcelain looks much more real, and it lasts longer—up to 15 years—so it's generally considered the best option. When you're ready to begin, ask for a recommendation from a friend or family member who has veneers (work that Facebook network!) or go to aacd.com and click on "Find a Cosmetic Dentist." Choose an "accredited member or fellow" (not just a "member") who specializes in veneers and performs two to four procedures a month.

Q: I'm 24, and my hair's starting to thin. Is there any danger in starting Propecia now?

A: Not only is popping Propecia a proven way to maintain your mane, but one of its side effects could someday save your life. Data from the Prostate Cancer Prevention Trial showed that men who swallowed a daily 5-milligram dose of finasteride (Propecia's active ingredient) for 7 years were 25 percent less likely to develop prostate cancer than those who didn't take the medication. A 2007 study in *Lancet Oncology* found that a dose of 1 milligram—the same amount used to treat hair loss—was equally effective at lowering PSA, a marker for prostate cancer.

"Finasteride blocks the conversion of testosterone to DHT, a hormone that activates cells in the prostate that can lead to cancer," says Robert Bernstein, MD, a clinical professor of dermatology at Columbia University.

Granted, your 24-year-old prostate may not need protecting yet, but if you start taking Propecia now, you'll probably still be on it as you hit your 40s, when your gland could benefit.

So what's the catch? Every drug has its drawbacks, and with Propecia it's that roughly 2 percent of men experience a dip in sexual desire. If you end up among the unlucky few, simply stop taking the med; your mojo will return. (And try treating your thinning thatch with Rogaine, also known as topical minoxidil.) There is one other hitch to Propecia: the price. Ask your doctor for generic 5-milligram finasteride tablets, says Dr. Bernstein, which you can then cut into quarters to approximate Propecia's dose.

Q: Can I make my Rogaine work better?

A: Ask your doctor to doctor it. A Korean study showed that spiking Rogaine with Retin-A, a vitamin A derivative, made the hair potion 25 percent more effective. (It's believed that Retin-A improves absorption of minoxidil, the active ingredient in Rogaine.) Most pharmacies that do compounding—custom medication mixing—will be able to fill a prescription for a blend of Retin-A and Rogaine.

But don't expect the combo to recarpet your scalp. "Rogaine is more effective at helping you hold on to your hair than at stimulating new growth," says Nelson Lee Novick, MD, a clinical professor of dermatology at Mount

Sinai School of Medicine, in New York City. So talk to your dermatologist about finasteride as well. This is the active ingredient in Propecia, a prescription oral medication that's proven to increase chances of hair growth. To save about $30 a month, ask for a prescription for Proscar, which has 5 milligrams of finasteride (versus Propecia's 1 mg). Then quarter it with a pill cutter for your daily dose. And don't stop taking Rogaine.

"Some men see a synergistic effect when they use both Rogaine and finasteride," says Dr. Novick.

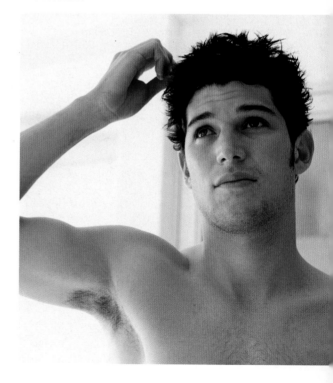

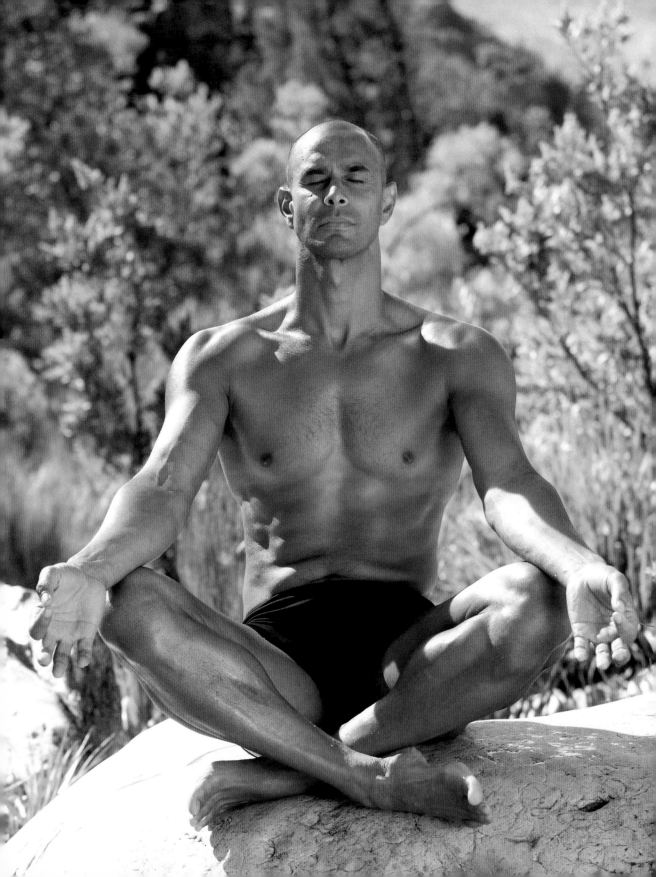

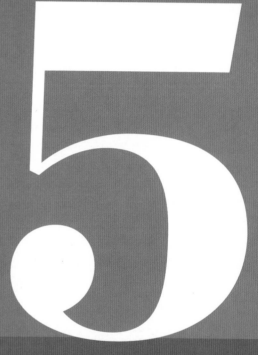

5

Live Longer, Live Better

Twitches, Glitches, Spasms, and . . . Blood

One moment these bodily pranks have you convinced you're a dead man.
The next, they've disappeared.
How seriously should you take your random health hiccups?

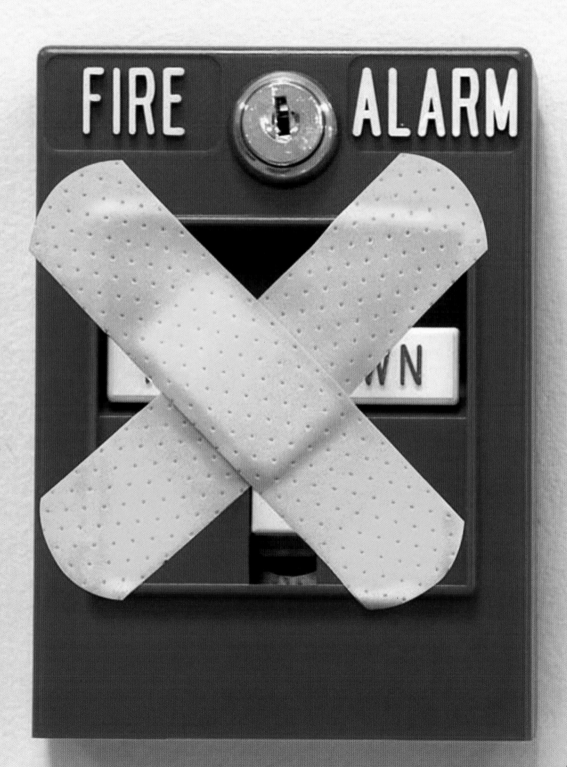

Occasionally your body shoots you the equivalent of a check-engine light—a weird spasm, say, or a sudden, piercing chest pain. Your brain races. Do you hustle to the doctor? Or just ignore it?

Doug Leawood of Kansas City defaulted straight to the doomsday scenario. His check-engine light: He saw red. In the toilet.

"I was scared," says Leawood, a 41-year-old insurance rep who was in great shape. "My mind went immediately to colon cancer. I thought I was a goner."

To Leawood's immense relief, blood didn't reappear in the following days, but he was sufficiently spooked to book an appointment right away with his doctor. Before he knew it, he found himself lying on his side in an outpatient surgical facility, counting backward from 10 as a gastroenterologist readied a scope that would snoop around his colon. Leawood checked out fine. No cancer, no worries—just an anal fissure, or small tear up his kazoo. But like the driver of the car that screamed "total engine meltdown," Leawood hasn't fully regained confidence in his machinery. Not that any of us have such confidence, given the strange and fleeting pains, spasms, gurgles, and clicks that surprise us at random moments. Are these signs of dangerous underlying conditions, or just harmless blips from a steady state?

With help from frontline doctors who've seen it all before, you can sort out which quirks you should take seriously—and which ones you can ignore.

PENETRATING CHEST PAIN

Worst fear: Heart attack
Likely culprit: Muscle spasm or stitch

"This is every man's nightmare," says Reid Blackwelder, MD, a professor of family medicine at East Tennessee State University. "But if the pain goes away relatively quickly, it's probably not a big worry."

Sudden, intense chest pain by itself can simply be a muscle spasm or even a stitch. It might also be pre-cordial catch syndrome—a very intense, sharp pain, typically in your left chest, that might feel like a heart attack to its unsuspecting victims. It's harmless, has no known cause, and can last for just a few seconds or up to several minutes. It's more common among children and teens but does occur occasionally in young men.

But combine intense chest pain with shortness of breath, nausea, dizziness, and/or sweating and you might indeed be facing a heart attack.

"As a general rule, when pain of any kind persists, you need to pay attention," Dr. Blackwelder says. Call 911, and chew two 81-milligram aspirin tablets to thin your blood and ease its flow to your heart.

TWITCHING EYELID

Worst fear: ALS, a.k.a. Lou Gehrig's disease
Likely culprit: Eyelid spasm

"I see this all the time," says Charles Cutler, MD, an internist in Norristown, Pennsylvania, and chairman of the American College of Physicians board of governors. Patients frequently think a twitching eyelid is an early symptom of

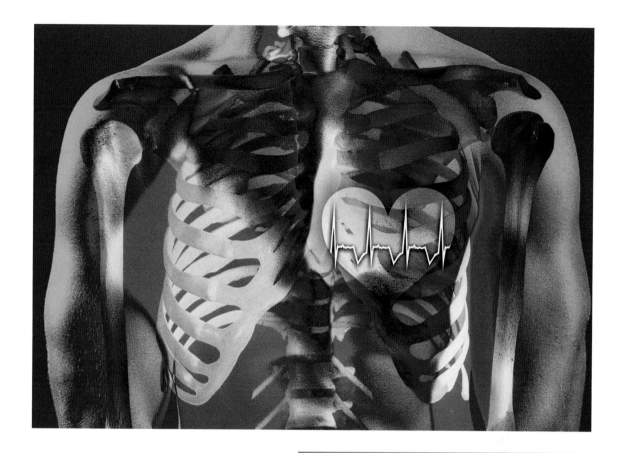

something horrible, he says—like ALS, a progressive, degenerative disease that affects nerve cells in the brain and the spinal cord. "But while it's uncontrollable and certainly annoying, the twitching is generally benign," Dr. Cutler says.

The medical term for this is blepharospasm. It's simply the result of uncoordinated muscle contractions in your eyelid. These spasms tend to come out of nowhere and occur every few seconds for a minute or two; episodes can continue for up to several weeks. Doctors aren't sure of the cause, although stress, fatigue, and caffeine may be culprits.

Talking Straight with Your Doc

Trying to describe symptoms to your physician can be excruciating, but you need to meet the doctor halfway. Cough up some details using our expert tips.

Spill your guts. Report everything unusual—sleep loss, mild aches. You may think it's not important, but it may be.

Open your mind. Follow the doctor's line of questioning closely. Don't become bogged down with what you found online, and be prepared for questions that seem unconnected to your problem.

Focus on the fix. Make clear what you want—for example, for your back to stop hurting at night. This is the clearest route to solving the problem, and it relays the key message.

Speak up. Describing how symptoms affect your life helps the doctor grasp their full impact, says Jaya Rao, MD, a health-care communications researcher at the University of North Carolina.

BUCKLING KNEE

Worst fear: Major joint damage
Likely culprit: Weak quads

A knee can buckle so swiftly you'll be looking for the sniper who shot you. But the pop or crunch you hear is due to a "reflex inhibition" of your quadriceps.

"It's a protective reflex—the same one that occurs when you step on a tack," says Sherwin Ho, MD, director of sports medicine fellowships at the University of Chicago Medical Center. "Your quad is looking to protect a painful knee by keeping weight off it."

The wobbliness is most likely a sign that the shock-absorbing cartilage under your kneecap has worn down, which is a condition that can lead to patellofemoral pain syndrome, says Dr. Ho. The fix: stronger quads, which take stress off your knee by acting as shock absorbers.

To build your quads, start with short-arc extensions, says physical therapist Jason Amrich, CSCS, director of the Boulder Center for Sports Medicine in Colorado. Lie on a mat with a rolled-up towel under the thigh of your injured knee. Straighten your leg, hold for 5 seconds, and lower. Do 10 reps, twice a day.

To reduce patellofemoral pain, work your gluteus medius—a hip muscle that helps move your thigh—with clamshell exercises. Lie on your side with your back against a wall, hips stacked, and hips and knees bent 45 degrees. Keeping your heels together, raise your top knee toward the ceiling, opening and closing your legs like a clamshell. Do 15 to 20 reps and switch legs. Complete 2 or 3 sets every other day.

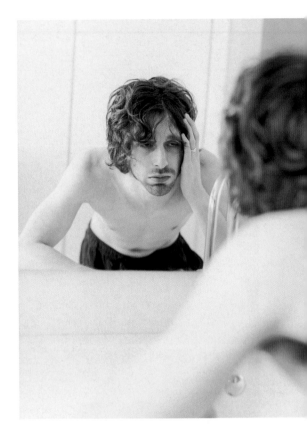

SEVERE HEADACHE

Worst fear: Brain tumor
Likely culprit: Tension or cluster headache

"Everyone thinks they have a brain tumor whenever they get a sudden, intense headache," says Dr. Blackwelder. "Despite the many brain tumors we see on TV, they really aren't all that common."

What's far more likely, he says, is that it's simply a severe headache—a migraine, a tension headache, or a cluster headache.

Migraines produce severe, throbbing pain, often on one side of your head. They're also frequently accompanied by nausea and sensitivity to light. Another clue: People who suffer from migraines tend to first experience them before they reach their 20s. So if you're over 40 and have never had a migraine, you probably have a tension or cluster headache. A tension headache produces dull pressure or tightness across the forehead, while a cluster headache includes sudden, severe pain, typically on one side of the face, usually surrounding the eye.

Brain tumor symptoms often vary with the tumor's size, location, and growth rate, but morning headaches tend to make doctors nervous. If you repeatedly wake up with headaches, see your physician to rule out a tumor. Do the same if you have a headache that worsens with sneezing, coughing, or any exertion, all of which increase the pressure within your head.

UNDERARM PAIN

Worst fear: Lymphoma
Likely culprit: Muscle spasm

Sharp underarm pain that comes and goes is probably the result of a muscle spasm or pleurisy, a medieval-sounding term for inflammation of the tissue that lines the chest cavity and covers the lungs. Pleurisy is usually caused by an infection, and betrays itself when the armpit pain is sharp and most pronounced when you take a deep breath. Massage and slow stretching can relax spasms, while nonsteroidal anti-inflammatory drugs can limit pain.

If the pain in your underarm is dull and you detect a small, tender knot in the area while feeling around, then your lymph nodes may be swollen. This happens routinely when you're battling an infection. Swelling could also be a sign of lymphoma, though the chance of that is very, very small, says David Ellington, MD, medical director of the Rockbridge Area Free Clinic in Lexington, Virginia. Have your doctor check out any knots, bumps, or persistent pain.

BLOOD IN THE TOILET

Worst fear: Colon cancer
Likely culprit: Hemorrhoids or anal fissure

If you spot bright red blood swirling in the bowl or on the toilet paper, you're probably dealing with hemorrhoids or an anal fissure, especially if the area is painful or tender. An anal fissure, which sounds worse than it is, is just a small cut in the lining of the anal canal. A fissure can develop when you pass a hard or large stool, and it typically heals by itself. (Deeper, chronic fissures may need surgical repair.)

Dark-colored blood mixed with your stool, on the other hand, might indicate a source farther up the gastrointestinal

Is that severe headache a brain tumor? Probably not.

tract, says Dr. Ellington. If any bleeding appears without pain during bowel movements, then you may have a colon polyp or perhaps an internal hemorrhoid. The occasional tarry or black stool (digested blood is black) indicates bleeding in the upper GI tract, perhaps due to a peptic ulcer. Call your doctor, who may schedule a colonoscopy to find the source and rule out colon cancer.

Male Hormones

Yes, men have hormones too. They help you beat stress, stay fit, and have better sex. Are yours slacking?

You might remember hormones from your sex-crazed teen years. Or your partner's most recent crying jag. But if you're sitting there smugly thinking that you're immune from hormonal chaos just because you're (a) no longer a teenager and (b) male, think again. In fact, if you knew all the ways hormones could mess up your life, you'd probably start crying like a little girl.

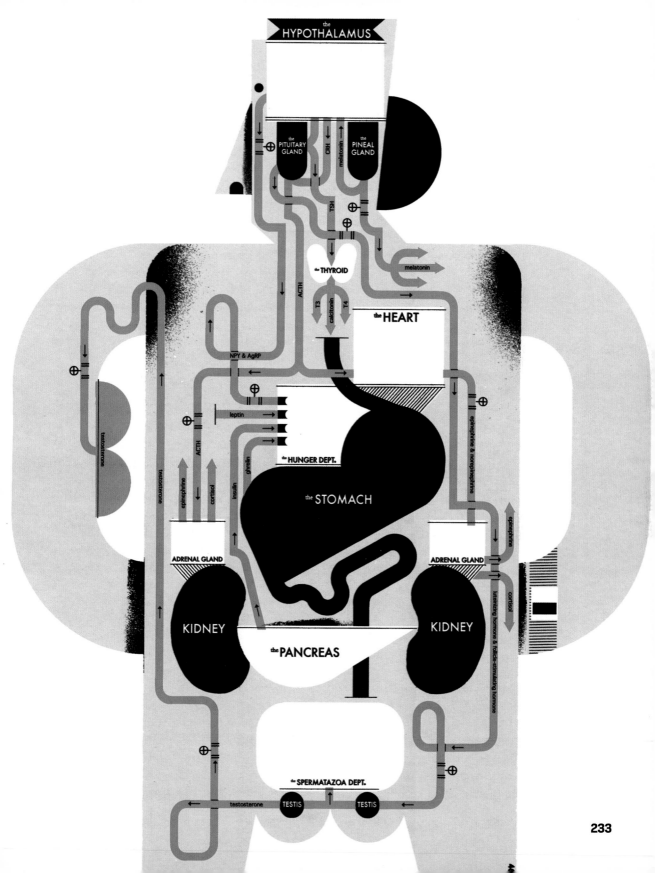

233

Off-kilter hormone distribution can make you store too much fat, hamper your ability to fight stress, and cause you to eat when you're full. It can lead to metabolic syndrome and diabetes and can adversely affect your sleep and sex life.

That's a lot that can go wrong. This is due to the vast reach of your endocrine system, which commands body activity utilizing powerful hormones.

"It's like your body's internal Internet," says pharmacologist John McLachlan, PhD, director of the Center for Bioenvironmental Research at Tulane University. "Your hypothalamus and pituitary glands are the control centers, like servers sending out messages going back and

Your hormones are part of a finely tuned system. That fine-tuning makes them vulnerable as it relies on complex feedback.

forth among your organs. Your pancreas, adrenal glands, thyroid, and testes are all part of this finely tuned system."

That fine-tuning increases the system's vulnerability, as it relies on complex feedback to regulate itself.

"If that feedback is distorted, it can disrupt the process," says Vivian Fonseca, MD, chief of endocrinology at Tulane University's Health Sciences Center.

Use our guide to ensure your hormones are doing their job.

STRESS HORMONES
Cortisol and Epinephrine

Whether you're fending off an angry rottweiler or an angry client, your body's response to stress is the same: Your hypothalamus floods your blood with hormones to frighten you into action.

"Cortisol and epinephrine are your body's alarm-system hormones," says Dr. Fonseca. They make your heart beat faster and dilate your bronchial tubes so they can feed oxygen to your brain and keep you alert. They also release fat and glucose into your bloodstream to provide emergency energy.

ARE YOUR HORMONES IN TUNE?

Too much stress can keep your cortisol levels consistently elevated, which disrupts your metabolic system. This, in turn, signals your cells to store as much fat as possible. Worse, the fat tends to accumulate in your belly as visceral fat, which resides behind your abdominal muscles and has more cortisol receptors than other fat does.

To defend yourself against stress-hormone disruption, make a habit of exercising for an hour a day, 3 days a week. Doing so helps regulate your cortisol levels, say researchers at Ohio State University. Also try to eat organic foods as much as possible in order to steer clear of the common pesticide atrazine. This chemical has been shown to affect hormonal balances in amphibians, reptiles, birds, and mammals. A National Health and Environmental Effects Research Laboratory study showed that atrazine produced extreme increases in stress-hormone levels in rats. In fact, the stress reaction was similar to that seen when the animals were restrained against their will, the study noted.

WEIGHT HORMONES
Leptin, Ghrelin, CCK, Insulin

You have an army of hormones telling you when to eat and when to put the fork down. The hormone ghrelin begins the cycle when your stomach is empty by prompting neurons in your hypothalamus to make you feel hungry. Then when you start eating, your stomach stretches and you secrete cholecystokinin (CCK), an appetite suppressant.

Hormones now begin working overtime to help you back away from the table. Your intestines produce peptide YY, which tells your brain you've had enough to eat, and your pancreas sends out insulin. This signals that you're metabolizing a meal and that you shouldn't consume any more. Leptin, a hormone produced by fat cells, also tells your hypothalamus that you're full by prompting the secretion of alpha-MSH, another appetite-suppressing hormone.

All this helps your body maintain a balance between hunger and satiation. Why so many hormones in the game?

"Energy regulation is necessary for survival, so we have many redundant pathways in case any fail," says Robert Lustig, MD, an endocrinologist at the University of California at San Francisco. "But we were never supposed to have so much food so readily available, and certainly not this much sugar."

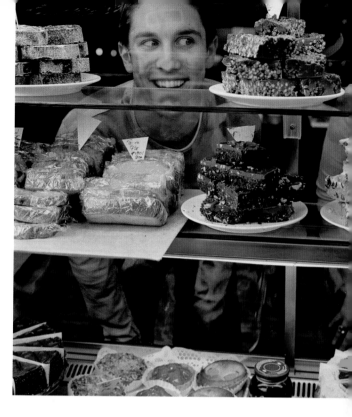

ARE YOUR HORMONES IN TUNE?

Hungry? Full? You may not be able to trust your gut. When you put on extra weight, you start secreting excess leptin.

"And if you secrete a lot of leptin on a chronic basis, it should tell your brain, 'Look, you're putting on weight; you need to cut back,' " says Dr. Fonseca. But disruptions in leptin (mostly from too much sugar) instead tell your brain to send out hunger signals, even if you've just eaten. This can lead to fatty liver disease and insulin resistance. "When your insulin goes up, it blocks leptin signaling, which means your brain thinks you're starving," Dr. Lustig says. This, of course, sets up a wicked feedback cycle as you pack on the pounds.

Beyond losing weight, your best defense against leptin disruption is to reduce your sugar intake. Americans consume an average of 22 teaspoons of sugar a day;

the American Heart Association recommends that men eat no more than 9. And it's not just high-fructose corn syrup that you need to avoid; table sugar and fruit juice can be as bad as soda. In fact, 100 percent fruit juice has 1.8 grams of fructose per ounce, while soda has 1.7 grams per ounce, Dr. Lustig notes.

SEX HORMONES
Testosterone, LH, FSH

That rock-hard erection you're so proud of? Thank your hormones—specifically testosterone, the key ingredient for normal sexual health in men. Its production is prompted by something called luteinizing hormone (LH), while the follicle-stimulating hormone (FSH) helps produce the actual sperm. When you're aroused, your adrenal glands pump out epinephrine and norepinephrine, raising your heart rate and moving blood into your muscles, brain, and penis. Then the hormone dopamine increases your sexual appetite and communicates with the hypothalamus to orchestrate your erections.

ARE YOUR HORMONES IN TUNE?
Elevated estrogen levels can eclipse your testosterone, zapping sex drive. Yes, men have estrogen too.

"In fact, the most widely spread hormone receptor in the body is the estrogen receptor," says Dr. McLachlan. When a man is exposed to estrogenic chemicals—such as bisphenol A (BPA), the endocrine disruptor found in plastics and food-can linings—he can experience erectile dysfunction and weight gain.

Your best defense against an estrogen invasion is to lose weight and build muscle.

"Fat converts your testosterone to estrogen," says Jack Mydlo, MD, chairman of the Department of Urology at Temple University School of Medicine. Dropping pounds will improve your testosterone-to-estrogen ratio, which improves your sex drive as well as your erections. And when you're actively building muscle, you become more sensitive to insulin, which means you can push more glucose into the muscle, says Dr. Fonseca. This produces more fat-burning, libido-boosting energy.

ENERGY HORMONE
Thyroxine

Your thyroid gland controls your metabolism, which is your body's mechanism for turning calories into energy. It's yet another chain of command: Your hypothalamus detects fatigue and then your pituitary gland signals your thyroid to secrete thyroxine. This hormone enters almost every cell in your body.

"It boosts sugar burning and oxygen intake in cells," says Dr. McLachlan. "This raises your body temperature and increases your heart rate."

ARE YOUR HORMONES IN TUNE?
When this system is out of whack, the result can be muscle breakdown, weakness, fatigue, and weight gain. While most thyroxine disruptions are genetic, there is growing evidence that some environmental compounds can block thyroxine, says Dr. McLachlan. A 2009 study suggests that BPA can displace thyroxin from its

receptor and block it. Brominated flame retardants (BFRs) and polychlorinated biphenyls (PCBs) also both interfere with your thyroid. (BFRs are found in clothes, furniture, and electronics; PCBs, which are no longer in use in the United States, can still be found in the environment, particularly in farmed salmon.)

"If you're exposed to these, you could end up with a form of hypothyroidism—an underproduction of thyroxine that causes low energy and weight gain," says Dr. McLachlan. On the other end of the spectrum, hyperthyroidism, or overproduction of thyroxine, can cause anxiety, increased heart rate, weight loss, an enlarged thyroid, and swelling behind the eyes. Your doctor will be able to identify thyroid problems by prescribing a thyroid-stimulating hormone (TSH) blood test; fixes for both may include surgery or dietary changes, as well as lifelong daily doses of prescription drugs.

SLEEP HORMONE
Melatonin

When the sun goes down, your pineal gland switches on like clockwork to secrete melatonin, a hormone that helps you fall asleep and regulates your circadian rhythm. It lowers your core body temperature, which if too high promotes wakefulness. Production of melatonin peaks in the middle of the night, and the process can be disrupted by even very low levels of artificial light.

ARE YOUR HORMONES IN TUNE?
Mounting evidence suggests that exposure to light at night—whether you're asleep or awake—might play a crucial role in cancer, diabetes, and obesity. The World Health Organization classified "circadian disruption" as probably carcinogenic, and light at night is considered by some to be an endocrine disruptor that may affect melatonin, cortisol, ghrelin, leptin, and testosterone.

"Most people think, and the drug companies want you to think, that waking up at night is bad for you," says Richard Stevens, PhD, a cancer epidemiologist at the University of Connecticut Health

People think waking up at night is bad for you. It's actually exposure to light that's bad.

Center. But that's not the case, he says. It's exposure to light at night that's the problem. "If you wake up at night, as most of us do, that is a period of quiet wakefulness—stay in bed, in the dark, and enjoy it," Dr. Stevens suggests.

You don't have to be asleep to have good melatonin rhythm, but you do need to be in the dark. Buy heavy curtains, cover your alarm clock, and turn off gadgets.

"Make it dark enough that you can't see your hand," Stevens says. "If you go to the bathroom and turn on that bright light, you'll lower melatonin almost immediately," says Stevens. "I actually have a red night-light in my bathroom, because red light has less effect on melatonin than white or blue light," he says.

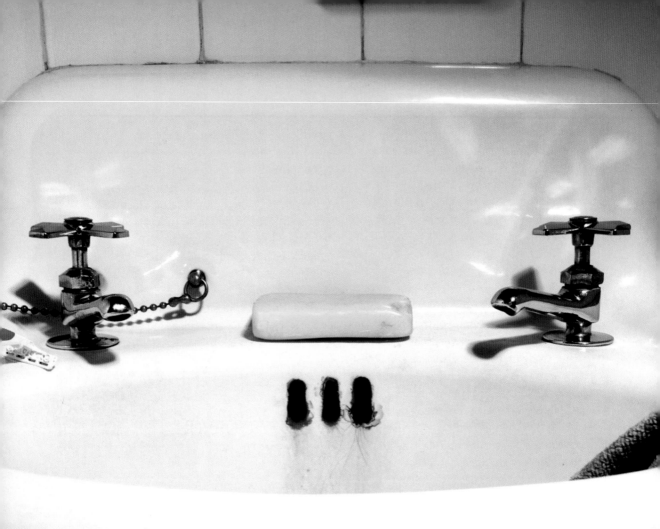

Dirty Talk

Your girlfriend is right: Your house is filthy.
Use our guide to eliminate germs before they eliminate you.

The next time you cut up chicken for dinner, do it on a clean surface. We recommend your toilet seat.

"It has the least amount of bacteria of all the spots in your home," says Charles Gerba, PhD, a professor of environmental microbiology at the University of Arizona. In fact, there are 200 times more fecal coliforms—otherwise known as feces bacteria—on the average cutting board than on the typical commode.

Blame the fact that most people just rinse their cutting boards instead of washing them thoroughly—and that all the little grooves made by knives provide perfect homes for bacteria. (Run your cutting board through the dishwasher after each use—or, if it's wooden, sanitize it with a few drops of bleach mixed with water.)

Want to know what else is scary? The filth on your washcloth. And your water bottle. Even your remote control. You probably don't want to fess up to how often you clean these items, but there's a good chance that at least one of these has made you sick. In a recent multicountry study by the public-education group Hygiene Council, a whopping 28 percent of households were found to be heavily contaminated with bacteria, which can live on dry surfaces for days, or even months. In that time, they can migrate from, say, bathroom to hand to cutting board to mouth.

"It's something to be reckoned with," says Philip Tierno Jr., PhD, a microbiologist and immunologist at New York University Langone Medical Center and the author of *The Secret Life of Germs*. "In fact, 50 to 80 percent of foodborne illnesses are contracted in the home, not in restaurants." There are no health inspectors watching you make the food.

But before you start spraying bleach on everything in your house, relax: Simply being consistent about cleaning key items—some of which you may have never even thought about cleaning—can keep a lid on viruses and bacteria. Read on to discover some frequently neglected targets, along with smart antimicrobial strategies to make all of them safe.

Towels

THEY ABSORB MORE THAN JUST WATER

Whenever you use a washcloth, hand towel, or bath towel, skin cells slough off your body and stick to the fabric. Those cells serve as food for bacteria, Dr. Tierno says. Plus, bacteria thrive in the damp, densely woven material, which has lots of nooks and crannies for them to hide in. As you reuse towels, these bacteria can transfer back to you and cause skin infections.

"If you have any kind of wound, you may be infecting yourself with whatever is on the towel," says Elizabeth Scott, PhD, codirector of the Simmons College Center for Hygiene & Health.

Your cleanup: Dr. Scott suggests washing your bath towel at least weekly if you're the only person using it, and using fresh towels daily if you share. Anything that gets soaked—like a washcloth—should be washed after every use. And don't forget about guest towels; wash them every time you have visitors. Who knows where those people have been?

Office Coffee Mug

YOUR HANDY DESKTOP CESSPOOL

Reusing your coffee mug is great for the environment but may not be so great for your health.

"Colonies of germs are living in your favorite cup," Dr. Gerba says. Twenty percent of office mugs carry fecal bacteria, and 90 percent are covered in other germs, according to Dr. Gerba's research. That's because in an office, most people tend to clean their cups with bacteria-laden sponges or scrub brushes instead of in a dishwasher. Those bacteria transfer to the mug and can live there for 3 days, Gerba says.

> **SERIOUSLY: Employees Must Wash Hands Before Returning to Work**
>
> This classic directive just isn't enough of a reminder for some folks. If you suspect your coworkers aren't washing their hands after using the bathroom, try hanging a sign that says, "Is the person next to you washing with soap?"
>
> In a recent study in the *American Journal of Public Health*, researchers found that those exact words most effectively sent people to the sink.

Your cleanup: You're not going to down that scalding cup of coffee as soon as it's poured, but don't nurse the cup for longer than an hour or so, Dr. Gerba suggests. Bring your mug home daily to be washed in the dishwasher, and make sure it goes through the dry cycle, which uses the hottest temperatures and zaps every last germ. At the very least, wash it with hot water, soap, and a paper towel. If it sits unwashed on your desk after being used, germs will start reproducing immediately, and bacterial colonies grow even when the cup contains nothing more than a coffee ring.

Sheets

YOU NEVER REALLY SLEEP ALONE

When you're rolling around between the sheets, you're basically rolling around in your own filth. Studies have found feces, salmonella, and *E. coli* on bed linens—even ones fresh out of a washer, Dr. Gerba says. His research shows that sheets can contain 0.1 gram of feces, salmonella, and *E. coli* after just one night's rest. That means they'd collectively contain about 10 billion microbes.

Your cleanup: Wash your sheets once a week, and make sure the water is hot. According to Dr. Gerba, only 5 percent of Americans use high temperatures when they wash their linens, and germs can live through a cold or even a warm wash. And the dryer may not be much of a backup: Although *E. coli* is usually zapped in the drying cycle, salmonella and mycobacteria, which can cause pulmonary diseases, can survive, says Dr. Gerba. Your best bet is to kill them off with hot water in the wash cycle. Then rest easy.

The Bugs Stop Here

Fueled by flu fears, hand sanitizer sales spiked 71 percent last year. But to be really clean, you can't buy just any bottle.

Not every bathroom sink has antibacterial soap, so it helps to be prepared. When used properly, hand sanitizers rid your hands (and you) of illness-causing bacteria and viruses—even the flu. Follow these tips to find the strongest kind and use it to its fullest potential.

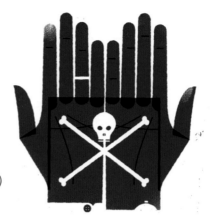

CHECK THE ALCOHOL CONTENT

Most hand sanitizers use alcohol to kill germs, but make sure you buy one with at least 60 percent alcohol; it won't be as effective with less, warns the CDC. Major brands offer that amount—Germ-X has 63 percent and Purell has 65 percent—but some budget brands may contain less. However, don't assume that super-concentrated is better. A recent *American Journal of Infection Control (AJIC)* study found that sanitizer with 95 percent alcohol doesn't have enough moisture to work properly.

SOAK YOUR HANDS

If you can rub your hands dry in 15 seconds, you didn't use enough sanitizer. In a University of North Carolina study, a silver-dollar-size dollop—7 grams—killed germs more than twice as effectively as 3 grams did. That amount will take 30 seconds or more to rub dry.

LOOK FOR MOISTURIZER

Alcohol can dry your skin, and excessive sanitizer use can make your hands uncomfortable, rough, or even cracked—especially in winter. If you're prone to skin dryness, help yourself out by buying a bottle of sanitizer that's infused with a moisturizer. Aloe vera is one of the most common additives; it moistens your hands and has been shown to boost the sanitizer's microbe-fighting power, according to another *AJIC* study. Purell with aloe is one good choice.

USE WIPES AND GEL

Gels are often thought to be better than wipes, but that may not be the case. A recent *AJIC* study found that when gels and wipes have the same amount of alcohol, wipes kill almost 50 percent more of certain types of bacteria than gels do. Buy gel for when you're on the go, but keep a box of wipes around the office. We like Sani-Hands wipes.

Water Bottle

BACTERIA TO GO

What better way to save cash and keep trash out of landfills than to drink from reusable plastic water bottles? Just don't let the bottles become bacterial bombs. Researchers at the University of Calgary found significant levels of coliform bacteria in 9 percent of water bottles used by elementary school students—suggesting that when thirsty youngsters open the bottles with dirty hands, they can dump a host of fecal matter into the water. When they empty the bottle, the damp, warm, closed space becomes a perfect breeding ground for bacteria.

Your cleanup: Because water bottles tend to have narrow necks, they can't undergo a thorough cleaning in the dishwasher. If you

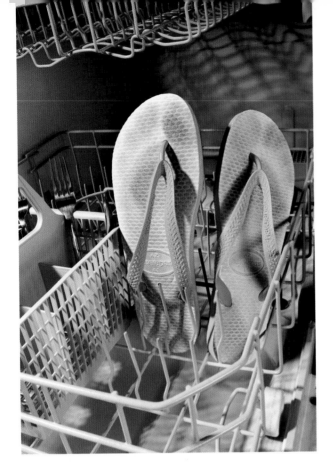

for bacteria such as MRSA, which causes skin infections," Dr. Gerba says. Since bacteria like MRSA can live for at least a day, reaching into your bag while you have a cut on your skin could lead to a potentially lethal infection.

Your cleanup: After you remove your gear, sanitize the inside of the bag with a disinfectant wipe like the ones made by Clorox. You can stash packets in one of the side pockets so they stay handy but separated from the clothes.

"That should cut back on the bacteria significantly," Dr. Gerba says. "But if the bag is machine washable, you should also toss it into the machine every week." (Throw in your shower flip-flops as well, he says; they can become equally filthy.)

Carpet

WALL-TO-WALL GERMS

Dr. Tierno's research indicates that your carpet probably contains about 200,000 bacteria per square inch, making it 4,000 times dirtier than your toilet seat.

"Rugs are botanical and zoological parks," says Dr. Tierno, who says hundreds of thousands of different types of species live there. These invasions occur because the average person sheds about 1.5 million skin cells every hour; these cells hit the rug and serve as food for germs. Add in food particles, pollen, and pet dander and you have a gratis buffet, he says. And because a vacuum cleaner's suction and rotating beater brush don't usually reach the bottom of the carpet, you're bound to have communities of *E. coli*, salmonella, staphylococcus, and other

must reuse your bottle, wash it with hot, soapy water and use a bottle brush like the Oxo Good Grips model ($5, oxo.com). Feel free to reuse the bottle, as long as you wash it after every use and air-dry both the bottle and cap completely, Dr. Gerba says.

Gym Bag

HAVE YOU EVER CLEANED IT?

Probably not, but you should. Now. Think about it: Even though spray bottles are usually placed around gyms to wipe down equipment, most patrons don't use them. When you toss your clothes into your gym bag, the sweat from who-knows-how-many people transfers to the bag.

"It becomes a terrific breeding ground

bacteria down there. Every time you walk on the carpet or roll around on it with your kids, you disrupt the bacteria, bringing some closer to the surface, Dr. Gerba says.

Your cleanup: Hire a company to do a deep steam cleaning at least once a year, and consider covering high-traffic areas with machine-washable area rugs.

Remote Control

170 CHANNELS OF HIGH-DEF FILTH

One day we'll change channels using our brain waves. When that day comes, we'll all be a lot healthier, because 50 percent of television remotes tested positive for rhinovirus, according to a University of Virginia study. The rhinovirus can live there for a few days, and other germs can survive for up to a few months, thanks to the many hideouts found amid the rubber buttons and various LEDs.

Ever have popcorn with your DVD movies? You're making matters worse, Dr. Tierno says. "If you eat something greasy, then cough in your hands and go back to the remote, you've deposited an organism with some oil, which offers the germs protection on a device that isn't cleaned very often to begin with."

Your cleanup: Sanitizers don't work well on remotes because you can't get the cleaner into the cracks. Dr. Tierno suggests using a plastic-sleeve protector that can be wiped clean daily with a disinfecting wipe or other type of sanitizer. When you're traveling, bring along a few zip-lock bags to slip onto the remotes in hotels.

HARD TRUTH

34

Percentage of men who don't wash their hands

Things That Aren't Gross

We live in a microbe-laden world. But there are things you don't need to be particularly obsessive about. Here are three of them.

1 YOUR HAIRBRUSH

The only reason you'd want to clean out the brush would be to remove gel or spray residue and unclog hair from the bristles, says Carolyn Jacob, MD, the director of Chicago Cosmetic Surgery and Dermatology. Infections from hairbrushes are rare, she says. So if those residues and hair knots don't bother you, leave them alone.

2 YOUR JEANS

There are no studied health risks associated with wearing most clothing items several times without washing them. (Your underwear, however, contains feces, and needs to be washed after each wearing, says Charles Gerba, PhD, a professor of environmental microbiology at the University of Arizona.)

3 YOUR BODY

Daily showering strips away necessary oils and some of the 150 good kinds of bacteria found on your skin, says New York University microbiologist Philip Tierno Jr., PhD. The bacteria guard against pathogens that can cause infections. The average person can shower every other day—or at least skip one shower a week, Dr. Tierno says.

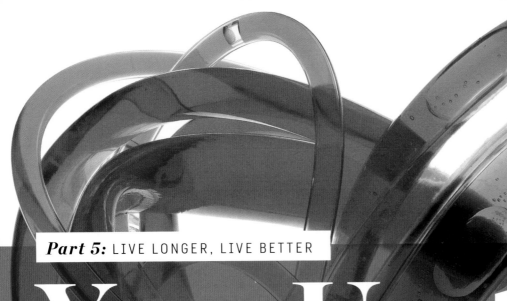

Your Unstop

If your doctor says you have elevated LDL cholesterol,
here's what you need to know: Only a portion of LDL is actually dangerous.
Before you swallow a pill, read what writer Paul Scott learned.

Here's the really tricky part about that dangerous portion of LDL: Standard blood tests do not measure it. Blockbuster pills do not target it. "Healthy eating" increases its numbers. So what on Earth do you do now?

pable Heart

Two laboratory machines have played a role in perhaps the greatest medical misadventure of our time: the indictment of a villain—LDL cholesterol—with the ultimate crime of the heart, coronary artery disease.

One machine delivered the early, misleading evidence of cholesterol's guilt, and another might have just nabbed the actual killer. And because the killer's likeliest and earliest targets are men, we'd all better pay attention to the new case being made against it.

The first machine, an early prototype of a device called an analytical ultracentrifuge, was crucial to the 1949 discovery of high-density lipoprotein (HDL) and low-density lipoprotein (LDL). These common blood fats would become cemented in people's minds by their angel/devil personas, "good" and "bad" cholesterol. But now the halo-and-pitchfork images seem a little simplistic. And hardly useful.

These cholesterol characterizations were spun out of a wall-size contraption that rotated plasma at 40,000 revolutions per minute from the late 1940s until the machine's retirement in 2004. When you consider its role in the powerful beliefs we hold about heart disease, the sprawling, rattling beast should be mounted under flattering light in the Smithsonian.

SIMPLER, NOT ALWAYS BETTER

For decades, a tidy narrative about the relationship between LDL cholesterol and heart disease has affected everything from the food we eat to the drugs we take to the test results we track and the worries we harbor. This oversimplified view of cholesterol—that all LDL is the same and that all LDL is bad—has enabled an accompanying oversimplified dietary belief: that all saturated-fat intake raises your risk of heart disease.

The LDL hypothesis has also encouraged many of us to swallow the most-prescribed class of drugs in recent history. Americans spent more than $14 billion on LDL-lowering medications in 2008. Whether that money came out of their own pockets—straight up, or through ever-escalating co-pays—or out of the hemorrhaging U.S. health insurance system known as Medicare, it's a huge expenditure. Twenty-four million Americans take statins, and the latest health directives suggest that those numbers should be higher. And why stop at grown-ups? Some pediatricians want to start feeding Lipitor (and the like) to kids.

As John Abramson, MD, wrote in his book *Overdosed America*, "Largely as a result of these guidelines, cholesterol control has become the main focus of preventive health care in the United States."

So it's more than a little disconcerting that the other machine in this story, a complex pile of gadgetry quietly clicking away on a countertop in Berkeley, California, is only the most recent breakthrough that has called the entire LDL cholesterol premise into question.

On a balmy Sunday last August, Ronald M. Krauss, MD, the director of the department of atherosclerosis research at Children's Hospital Oakland Research Institute, showed me into his workplace to demonstrate a novel new system for tabulating LDL. Using a particle-spitting process known as ion mobility analysis, Dr. Krauss and his colleagues have developed the first device capable of counting LDL and other lipoproteins down to their smallest subcomponents. (Several other ways of analyzing LDL subparticles exist, but they involve indirect methods.)

A New Jersey company, Quest Diagnostics, worked for 7 years with Dr. Krauss—who is helping to set the new cholesterol recommendations from the NIH's National Cholesterol Education Program—to develop a method of analyzing cholesterol. Borrowing the same processes used for testing air pollution and residue from explosives, the quarter-million-dollar prototype is very sophisticated technology.

"It determines the size of the particle based on physics," says Dr. Krauss with nerdy admiration, "on the speed at which it flies through the air."

In other words, this machine won't be coming to your community health clinic any time soon. But even if it's not ready for mass production, the information gleaned using technologies like ion mobility means that LDL cholesterol can no longer be identified as the single source of all heart trouble. Those pamphlets adorning your doctor's waiting room may portray LDL as a kind of lone gunman taking a bead on your heart, but they hide a basic fact of science: "Bad cholesterol" is

Small LDL, Big Risk

If you have a high risk of heart disease, it's time to measure the cholesterol that matters most. Not all LDL cholesterol is created equal. Some particles of this blood fat are large and buoyant and breeze easily through your circulatory system. But other particles are small and dense—and four times as likely to cause heart disease.

"In order for cholesterol to cause disease, it has to embed in the wall of the artery," says Paul Ziajka, MD, PhD, a clinical lipidologist with the Southeast Lipid Association. "And the smaller the particle, the easier it can do that."

That means even a low cholesterol reading may not be an all-clear if you have predominantly small, dense LDL particles known as pattern B. For a quick indication, have your doctor check your triglycerides using a standard blood test. If your reading is over 200, you're probably pattern B, says Dr. Ziajka, which means you should lower your LDL cholesterol target another 30 points. (Calculate your recommended baseline LDL at aristos.com/ldl-target.php.)

But even a healthy triglyceride number isn't a free pass exempting you from coronary artery disease. The blood tests described below measure not only the amount of LDL coursing through your veins, but also its average particle size. Have your doc refer you to an area lab offering advanced lipid-profile testing; the referral often means a cheaper rate.

LDL-S3 GGE Test

Proteins from your blood are spread across a gel palette. As the molecules move from one end to the other, the gel becomes progressively denser. Large particles of LDL cholesterol can't travel as far as the small, dense particles can, Dr. Ziajka says. After staining the gel, scientists determine the average size of your LDL cholesterol particles. (Berkeley HeartLab, bhlinc.com, about $15 with insurance)

The VAP Test

Your sample is mixed into a solution designed to separate lipoproteins by density. "The proteins in your blood have to find their equilibrium," says Dr. Ziajka. "Small, dense particles sink, and large, fluffy particles stay at the top." The liquid is stained and then analyzed to reveal 21 different lipoprotein subfractions, including dominant LDL size. (Atherotech, thevaptest.com, direct cost $40)

NMR Lipoprofile Test

Inside a magnetic field, radio waves charge the lipids in your blood. When the magnetic field is turned off, the protons give off energy, and that energy can be captured. Because energy emissions vary by particle size, this can be used to determine the type of LDL coursing through your veins. (LipoScience, lipoprofile.com, $100)

---

at best a poor shorthand for four major types of independently behaving LDL cholesterol, each one with its own implications for heart disease. We ignore the distinctions at our peril.

Some of these forms of LDL are relatively safe and some are dangerous, and treating them all as one and the same—

the way we do every time we pay our clinic for a three-part lipid panel that simplistically says "LDL: 125"—is telling us little about the LDL cholesterol that matters, all the while sending health costs through the roof. We might be medicating many people who have no clear need for medication, using drugs that don't target the right particles, and replacing foods that are benign with foods that are anything but.

So in the heart-disease world, we've been stalking the devil we know instead of the devils we don't know. But we need to get to know them if we hope to dodge the number-one killer of men.

LDL comes in four basic forms: a big, fluffy form known as large LDL, and three increasingly dense forms known as medium, small, and very small LDL. A diet high in saturated fat mainly boosts the numbers of large-LDL particles, while a low-fat diet high in carbohydrates propagates the smaller forms. The big, fluffy particles are largely benign, while the small, dense versions keep lipid-science researchers awake at night.

But here's the problem: The typical LDL test doesn't distinguish between large and small LDL particles; it can't even spot the difference. And people can have mostly large LDL or mostly small LDL in their overall LDL, depending upon a host of genetic, lifestyle, and environmental factors. Your own personal mix might make all the difference between living to a heart-healthy old age and becoming a Monday-morning casualty at your desk.

Dr. Krauss and collaborators from Harvard and Malmo, Sweden, have helped identify what influences the difference. Working with blood samples from 4,600 healthy Swedish men and women, they used ion mobility analysis to count 11 forms of cholesterol subparticles for each person, and then ran the data through a complex statistical sorting program. After looking for relationships correlating with the 8 percent of people who went on to develop cardiovascular disease, they found three scenarios that predicted it, from the most powerful predictor to the least:

1. High levels of smaller and medium LDL combined with low HDL (a dreaded diabetes-linked syndrome Dr. Krauss had previously called atherogenic lipoprotein phenotype, or pattern B)
2. Low HDL levels
3. High total LDL levels

According to Dr. Krauss, the three risk factors appear to represent three separate processes that put your cardiovascular health at risk. For men, the first two scenarios are more predictive of heart disease, but the third—high total LDL—was only marginally predictive of heart disease in men. Nowhere to be seen, of course, is the "total cholesterol" number doctors have been bashing us over the head with for decades. Turns out that number is not as useful a predictor for individuals.

"LDL cholesterol is used as a marker for heart-disease risk," Dr. Krauss explains. "It's not a perfect marker, and the particle story is part of the reason for that."

In other words, when you tease apart the subsets of LDL that are preferentially involved in heart disease, total LDL is a less reliable bio-marker. It's like the sniffles that could signal allergies, or the onset of swine flu, or nothing at all. This ambiguity works both ways. Just because you have less of the symptom (statin users take note) doesn't mean you'll have less of the disease. A drop in your total LDL cholesterol might mean nothing at all. A higher LDL cholesterol reading, for that

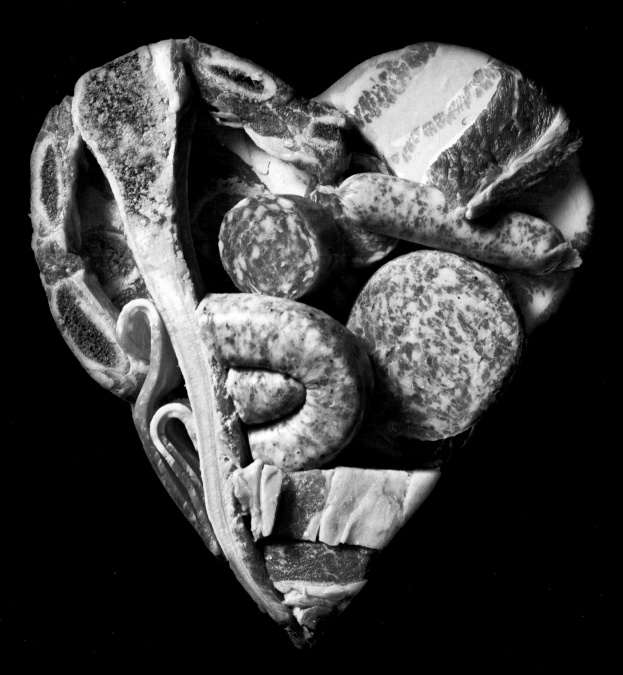

Americans spent $14 billion on cholesterol drugs in 2008.
Some doctors want to feed them to kids.

matter, could simply mean you are a healthy person who has learned how to build an amazing sauce out of wine, garlic, shallots, butter, and heavy cream.

We currently test for a number that tells us less about our health than we think it does, and then we busily (and expensively) medicate it downward. It would be more effective to test the numbers that do

We might be medicating many people who have no clear need for medication.

matter, of course, and then to learn how we can keep those meaningful numbers in check, whether we do it through different meals, more miles on the pedometer, or better-targeted medications.

ARE YOU REALLY WHAT YOU EAT?

Cholesterol is a natural substance your body produces for a variety of uses. It's carried through the body in three containers—LDL, HDL, and VLDL—that deliver it to cells along with triglycerides. The average man reasons that the cholesterol in his scrambled eggs must surely end up in his arteries somehow, and this makes him do things like order egg-white omelets for breakfast.

There is indeed a link between the cholesterol you eat and the cholesterol in your arteries. It's just not the "eat more, have more" worry that's been drummed into you for years. In fact, your body's production and uptake of cholesterol is highly regulated; eat a six-egg omelet and

your body simply produces less cholesterol because of the dietary onslaught.

"There is a very weak connection between the LDL cholesterol we measure and dietary cholesterol," Dr. Krauss says. "I spend a lot of time talking to reporters and trying to explain that dietary cholesterol is not the same as blood cholesterol." He adds that the 200 milligrams of cholesterol most people eat every day is nothing compared with the 800 milligrams their bodies produce. But you don't have to take his word for it.

"It is now acknowledged that the original studies purporting to show a linear relation between cholesterol intake and coronary heart disease may have contained fundamental study design flaws," wrote the author of a recent review in the *International Journal of Clinical Practice*.

So eggs are off the heart-disease hook. But what about saturated fat? One of the major types of saturated fat we eat—the stearic acid that makes up one-third of the saturated fat in beef—has little or no impact on blood cholesterol. And you may well imagine that pizza grease and butter are magically transported from your gut to your arteries, but that's like using sock puppets to explain the workings of a supercomputer. Other types of saturated fat do increase LDL, it turns out (sometimes HDL, too), and high LDL is modestly associated with heart disease, but the saturated fat on your plate never goes anywhere near your arteries. Saturated fat increases bad-cholesterol levels by interfering with receptors responsible for removing LDL from the blood. Whether or not that's a health concern is anyone's guess.

"If you substitute polyunsaturated [good] fat for saturated fat, you see a reduction in heart-disease risk," Dr. Krauss says, casting more doubt on four decades of diet advice. "The interpretation of that finding has been that saturated fat is bad. My view, based on the data I have seen, is that it means polyunsaturated fat is good; it doesn't necessarily say anything about saturated fats being bad. . . . Does that mean saturated fat is bad fat? Or just that saturated fat is not a good fat?"

Of course, that isn't the message we're all accustomed to hearing.

And for that you can blame the analytical ultracentrifuge—or, more specifically, the fact that so many heart-disease authorities weren't ready for what it discovered. The first one ever used in the United States arrived in Berkeley thanks to the efforts of John Gofman, PhD, MD, a physicist-turned-physician previously employed by the Manhattan Project. After the war, Dr. Gofman wanted to cure heart disease in the worst way, and he thought the answer might lie in the newly discovered particles known as lipoproteins, the fat-protein particles that encircled cholesterol and triglycerides to shepherd them through the bloodstream. He took plasma samples from people with and without heart disease and used his new machine to spin the samples like nobody's business. Because of the physical properties of the plasma, the fatty lipoprotein particles separated and floated, with the lightest ones making it to the top first. Thanks to his analytical ultracentrifuge, Dr. Gofman discovered three major classes of lipoproteins. He named the lightest

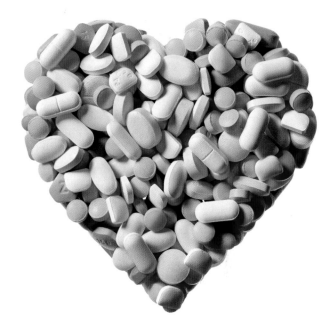

lipoproteins VLDL, for very-low-density lipoproteins (chicken-fat-type globules carrying triglycerides); the next most buoyant came to be known as LDL, and the heaviest were called HDL.

Then Dr. Gofman asked people about their health and diet. He learned that having high LDL or high triglycerides correlated with an increased risk of heart disease, high HDL correlated with a low risk of heart disease, and that the two profiles responded entirely differently to foods in the diet. (He also learned that cholesterol could be packaged either tightly clustered or loosely assembled within LDL; measuring it did little to reflect this risk.) Saturated fat raised LDL, while carbohydrates raised triglycerides, ultimately lowering HDL. (Dr. Gofman even recognized that LDL was made up of subtypes, although the meaning of the diversity was unclear at first.) It was groundbreaking work, but too advanced for the movement it ultimately spawned. With so few analytical ultracentrifuges available, researchers began using cheaper methods of counting lipoproteins, methods now offered during routine physicals. One form of cholesterol became "good," the other "bad."

"It sort of lost the details," says Dr. Krauss.

By the time Dr. Krauss arrived at Berkeley in 1976, the ideas of Dr. Gofman,

Targeting the Killer LDL

WITH SMALL CHANGES, YOU CAN HAVE FEWER SMALL PARTICLES.

"Small, dense particles of LDL are much more inflammatory than larger particles," says Paul Ziajka, MD, PhD, a clinical lipidologist with the Southeast Lipid Association. Here's how to snuff the little devils.

Crack an egg. Down an omelet every morning and you may lower your small-particle count, University of Connecticut researchers recently found. People who ate three whole eggs a day for 12 weeks dropped their small-LDL levels by an average of 18 percent.

Choose your meds wisely. A class of drugs known as fibrates, which includes Tricor, specifically targets small, dense LDL, says Dr. Ziajka. The effect is significant only when your triglycerides are also elevated, he says.

Pop some niacin. "Most drugs shift particle size after the cholesterol is made," Dr. Ziajka says. "Niacin causes the liver to produce larger particles." Try a no-flush variety (Dr. Ziajka recommends Slo-Niacin) starting with 500 milligrams a day and building to 2,000. There are side effects, so talk to your doctor first.

Lighten your load. Deflating your spare tire may reduce your small, dense LDL cholesterol, say scientists at Children's Hospital Oakland Research Institute. The majority of overweight men who were pattern B (mostly small LDL) switched to pattern A (mostly large LDL) after they lost an average of 19 pounds.

Have a glass. That nightly beer does more than relax you—it may also lower your small, dense LDL, a recent *Journal of Clinical Endocrinology & Metabolism* study found. Men who drank 7 to 13 alcoholic drinks a week had 20 percent fewer small-LDL particles than men who didn't drink at all.

who had left for greener pastures, began attracting support. A 1977 NIH study—an early set of papers from the now legendary Framingham Heart Study—confirmed that high HDL is associated with a reduced risk of heart disease. It also confirmed that LDL and "total cholesterol" tell us little about the risk of having a heart attack, language that heart-disease authorities would downplay years later. Given this finding, as Gary Taubes writes in *Good Calories, Bad Calories*, we would have been better off to start testing for HDL—or even triglycerides—and nothing else.

Dr. Krauss was working part-time in Dr. Gofman's old lab and flipping through some data cards when he noticed a correlation that would change everything. As he combed through a recently completed study of 80 men and 54 women in Modesto, California, Dr. Krauss noticed that the people with low HDL tended to have high LDL. But not just any LDL was elevated; only the smaller forms observable to Dr. Gofman's analytical ultracentrifuge.

"I started studying these readouts, and what popped out were some amazingly strong inverse correlations," he says, still amazed at his good fortune. "It was just sitting there in the data." Dr. Krauss had found that small, dense LDL particles were the evil twin of good cholesterol. HDL and small LDL tended to move at the same time, he discovered, but in opposite directions. If your smaller forms of LDL were high, your HDL was low; if your smaller forms of LDL were low, your HDL was high. Whether one was the cause and the other was the effect was unclear, but given the newly discovered importance of HDL, the importance of smaller forms of LDL was now real.

This created a practical problem. Lumping all forms of LDL cholesterol together, as labs currently do when they count it in your basic blood draw, tells us little about how much of that LDL is small and how much is large.

"Everyone doesn't necessarily have the same amount of very small LDL in their LDL," Dr. Krauss explains. Some people have mostly large LDL, a group Dr. Krauss would describe as "pattern A," while others have mostly small LDL (and usually, low HDL and high triglycerides), a group Dr. Krauss would label "pattern B." The second group has an increased risk of heart disease (a finding suggested again this year through the use of ion mobility). Large LDL, on the other hand—and large LDL is usually the majority of the LDL that shows up in a standard blood profile—is mostly benign.

The heart-disease community was not impressed.

"It took me 4 years to publish that paper," he says, recalling his early work on subparticles in the late 1970s. "That's beginning to tell you some of the obstacles I was going to face."

The cost of that resistance had become apparent by the mid-1980s and into the 1990s as Dr. Krauss began to test whether changes in diet could change a person's LDL profile from good to bad, or from pattern A to pattern B. Using data from the Framingham Heart Study—the longest-running study of its kind—health organizations had begun to roll out the message of "good" and "bad" cholesterol, a

message that in turn created the concept of good fats and bad fats. But during experiments, Dr. Krauss discovered that while a diet high in saturated fat from dairy products would indeed make your LDL levels rise, "saturated fat intake results in an increase of larger LDL rather than smaller LDL particles," as he wrote in an *American Journal of Clinical Nutrition* review he co-authored in 2006. A diet heavy in full-fat cheese and butter—but not overloaded in calories—triggered the relatively harmless health

Reducing saturated fat in a way that increases carbohydrates in a diet can shift a person's LDL profile from safe to dangerous. The stearic acid in beef has little or no impact on cholesterol levels.

profile described as pattern A. (Having demonstrated the benign consequences for cholesterol from consuming dairy fat, he is currently conducting studies to find out if the same holds true for diets high in saturated fat from beef.)

Not only is dairy fat unlikely to increase heart-disease risk, Dr. Krauss and others have learned, but reducing saturated fat in a way that increases carbohydrates in a diet can shift a person's LDL profile from safe to dangerous. That's pretty much what happens when-

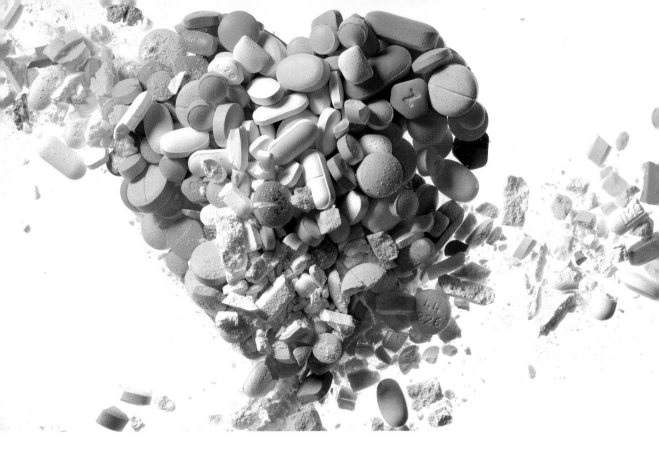

ever some well-meaning person with "high LDL" starts eating "low-fat" frozen dinners filled out with corn-derived additives, all the while engaging in the customary ravaging of a basket filled with dinner rolls.

"I like Ron Krauss and admire his work," says Dean Ornish, MD, a fellow Bay Area heart-disease researcher and surely the most visible proponent of the idea that a diet low in saturated fat and high in carbohydrates can help reduce the risk of heart disease. But Dr. Ornish says Dr. Krauss shifted his study participants from pattern A to pattern B by having them eat more of the processed carbohydrates.

"The carbohydrates they fed people were predominantly refined, like sugar and white flour," says Dr. Ornish. "That's not what I've been recommending."

Dr. Krauss concedes that it's possible that refined carbohydrates are the problem when it comes to small LDL, but adds that his study used both complex and simple carbohydrates "in a manner consistent with many people's dietary practices when they adopt a low-fat diet." Low-fat diets are old news, you say? Try telling that to the makers of, say, Baked Lays. It will take us years to shake off the damage done by broadly implicating fat in the diet. "Everybody I know in the field—everybody—recognized that a simple low-fat message was a mistake," says Dr. Krauss.

Dr. Krauss learned about the safety of saturated fat from dairy thanks to a grant from—guess who?—the dairy industry. He also receives royalties on patents for two of the five methods for measuring small forms of LDL, including ion mobility. These are no small details, of course, and to his credit, he readily places his conflicts of interest on the table when the talk turns to heavy cream or particle-measurement technology. You could raise an eyebrow at these potential biases, but if you did, you'd also have to rethink the guidelines we now follow about healthy LDL. Their authors, nearly to a person, have taken money from a drug industry that's made a lucrative mission out of LDL mythology. Then there is this: Dr. Krauss is not sure we should all race out to have our small LDL measured just yet.

"I have not been an advocate of widespread testing for small LDL to assess heart-attack risk," he says. "It would be hard to justify the added expense for many people." At this point, he sees a role for small-LDL testing primarily in the management of people with heart disease or people who have a high risk of developing it. More research needs to be conducted before national guidelines make tests routine, he says. Until then, we have to live with the knowledge that the tests most commonly offered tell us only part of the story. (If you fall into either of the categories above, or you want a more detailed test, see "Small LDL, Big Risk" on page 247.)

But what about statins? Dr. Krauss believes statins probably offer beneficial effects on heart-disease risk beyond those of lowering LDL (anti-inflammatory properties, for example). Interestingly, statins might help men who want to reduce their small-LDL levels. However, because they increase the removal of LDL from the blood (a process partial to larger LDL), "the benefit may be less than what you would expect from the drop in total LDL," he says.

So with small-LDL testing far from standard (your doctor can request an ion mobility analysis from Quest Diagnostics), the surest way you can reduce your numbers of the LDL that matters is to rely on time-tested advice. Eating fewer carbohydrates, losing weight, and engaging in more physical activity have all been shown to reduce small LDL. Weight loss, in fact, has been demonstrated to reverse the dreaded pattern B all by itself. In other words, worry less about eggs or butter and their effect on LDL, and focus more on eating fewer processed foods and staying in motion.

"I am very much an advocate of starting with lifestyle first," Dr. Krauss says.

Standing over his ion-spitting device quietly tabulating microscopic blood particles as the weekend wears on, Dr. Krauss invokes his admiration for Dr. Gofman, who died of heart failure at the age of 88. Dr. Gofman spent the second half of his career sounding the alarm about the dangers of low-level ionizing radiation, the type emitted from CT scans. (He was years ahead of his time on that subject, too.)

"Like the analytical ultracentrifuge, this process of ion mobility is based on first principles of physics," says Dr. Krauss. "So it's my attempt to leave a legacy, I hope, having been around to put Dr. Gofman's ultracentrifuge out to pasture."

It's in a warehouse, actually. Next door to a carpet store.

How Long Do You Last?

Not since Viagra has a prescription medication held so much potential to affect the sex lives of American men. Here's why that could hurt you.

Matt knows how to close the deal. He can meet a woman, charm her, land her in bed . . . and that's when the worrying begins. More often than not, he reaches orgasm too soon. He desperately wants his body to be cooler and calmer, to handle the great gift he's been rewarded with. When it doesn't, he feels inadequate, defective.

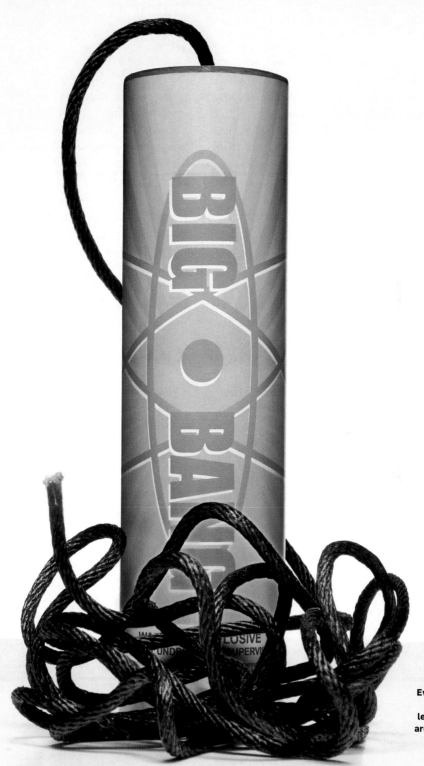

Every man's fuse
is a different
length. But there
are ways to make
yours longer.

"I can't control it," the 23-year-old Iowan says, "and I can't figure out why."

Science has a name for Matt's problem, one that sounds both sterile and judgmental: premature ejaculation, or PE. As a study in the *Archives of Sexual Behavior* notes, PE is the most common male sexual

"There's some cultural expectation that the longer you last, the better you are."

dysfunction. According to estimates, somewhere between 20 percent and 30 percent of men experience it, with many men doing almost anything to last longer in the sack. Those we spoke with said they've downed beers, undergone hypnosis, and even tied elastic bands around their penises.

It's easy to see why Big Pharma is betting they'd also pop a pill.

In 2009 in Europe, Johnson & Johnson began selling the first prescription drug designed specifically for treating PE. It's called Priligy, and clinical trials reveal that it can triple the time to ejaculation for men who normally last just a minute or two. Right now it's available in a handful of countries, including Germany, Spain, and Italy. Matt, however, is out of luck. Priligy isn't for sale in the United States. In 2005, the US Food and Drug Administration rejected Johnson & Johnson's application for approval, although a company officer says it has a raft of new research and plans to renew discussions with the FDA.

If the FDA eventually does approve Priligy, it will be a watershed moment for a condition that received little attention from researchers until a decade ago. Doctors will have a proven solution for men who've been robbed of sexual satisfaction. As Priligy advertising infiltrates the media and PE becomes acknowledged as common and treatable, the stigma surrounding it will fade. A conversation will begin, and suffering men will become emboldened with the knowledge that they're not alone.

But a much-heralded, mass-marketed release of a PE drug could also have an entirely different, more dangerous effect. Some researchers believe that a Priligy advertising blitz could bend men's expectations by stressing stamina as their sole measure of sexual prowess, sowing self-doubt and fears of PE in the minds and beds of perfectly normal guys.

In other words, they worry that the treatment could cause the condition.

Doctors still don't fully understand PE, nor can they pinpoint what leads to it or who has it. Some say it can be the result of psychological problems. Others liken ejaculation to sneezing after a sniff of pepper; everyone eventually lets out an achoo! but some people can hold theirs in longer. In fact, some experts believe that many men—and perhaps even most men—who say they suffer from PE have completely normal levels of sexual stamina.

Case in point: The average guy lasts about 6 minutes during sex. Matt says he sometimes lasts 5, but usually goes 15.

The problem is that the "P" in PE may often be a matter of perspective: Some men believe they're supposed to last longer, says Marcel Waldinger, MD, PhD, a neuropsychiatrist at Haga Hospital Leyenburg, in the Netherlands, and one of the world's leading PE researchers.

"The majority of men who complain of PE just aren't satisfied with the way they have sex," he says. "I call these men premature-like ejaculators. They may have a psychological, cultural, or relationship problem, and we should not treat them with medication at first. We should talk with them."

Last year, Dr. Waldinger provided timers to about 500 couples in five different countries, and he asked them to time themselves having sex. Self-timing is typical in PE research; such glorified stopwatches might not be the sexiest items brought into bed, but they sure beat a guy in a lab coat peeking out of the closet.

After the men had sex on the clock for a month, Dr. Waldinger asked them if they were dissatisfied with their time to ejaculation. Almost 40 percent said yes. Then he asked if they'd be willing to take medication to make themselves last longer; 23 percent said they would. The men who wanted drugs lasted an average of 4.9 minutes. The average time for all 474 men in the study? Six minutes.

"There's nothing medically wrong with most men, but so many think they have PE," says Dr. Waldinger. "It's wonderful for the pharmaceutical companies, but it's not really a medical issue."

That's why many experts say premature ejaculation needs a strict, universally accepted definition. The only diagnostic criteria doctors have to go by were pub-

lished in 2008 by the *International Society for Sexual Medicine*: A man with lifelong PE cannot last longer than 1 minute, and his time to ejaculation is harming his relationships.

Even though the 1-minute threshold would address what Dr. Waldinger says are the distorted perceptions of men like Matt, some doctors argue that this definition takes the discussion in the wrong direction. In their minds, PE should never be diagnosed with a watch.

"It's not so much the length of time that matters," says Derek Polonsky, MD, a

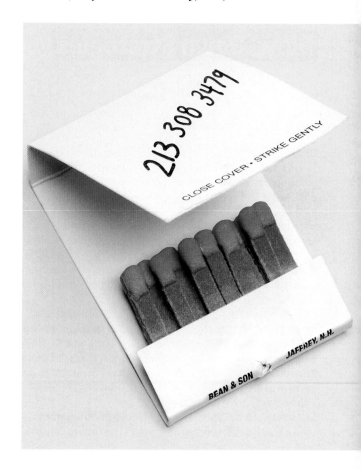

psychiatrist in private practice in Brook-line, Massachusetts, "but the satisfaction for men and their partners."

Urologist Michael Werner, MD, agrees. He believes a man can have PE whether he lasts 1 minute or 5. When he opened his first practice in Purchase, New York, 15 years ago, about 5 percent of his patients complained of PE. Today, that number is about 30 percent. For Dr. Werner, the matter is simple: "If you spend the whole time during sex thinking about not ejaculating, that's PE, and that's not the way sex is sup-posed to be."

It seems natural that a man would want to last longer during sex. Why wouldn't we be hardwired to prolong something so pleasurable? But in reality, men's sexual desires are malleable, influenced by external factors that scientists are only beginning to understand.

"There's some cultural expectation that the longer you last, the better you are," says Gale Golden, LICSW, a clinical associate professor of psychiatry at the

Slow-Down Strategies

Men often resort to home remedies to defeat PE. Here's what works and what doesn't, according to *Men's Sexual Health* coauthor Barry W. McCarthy, PhD.

Distraction.
Sex is part body, part brain. So in the heat of passion, some men think about baseball stats; others think about roadkill. "It works because you're less sexually present," psychologist Dr. McCarthy says. But beware: If you picture something disgusting or morbid, you'll train yourself to think that way during sex—and that in itself can lead to erection problems, he says. Go with the sports.

Stop and squeeze.
In a *Men's Health* survey, 98 percent of women said they'd be happy to help train their partner to last longer. So ask your honey to lend a hand: Relax your pelvic muscles as she manually stimulates you. When you're about to reach the point of no return, ask her to stop and, if necessary, squeeze the head of your penis. Rest until the urge passes, and then resume. You're teaching your body restraint, says Dr. McCarthy; you can use a similar strategy during intercourse by changing positions or slowing down.

Pre-sex orgasm.
It's the most obvious move: Go it alone first and you'll last longer in round two. But there's a downside, says Dr. McCarthy: Second orgasms are less intense.

Numbing agents.
The lube in Trojan's Extended Pleasure and Durex's Performax condoms contains benzocaine, a topical anesthetic that reduces sensation in your penis so you can last longer. The catch: Once your penis is slightly numbed, you must keep the condom on. (Men who suffer from PE often take it off.) Why? The residual benzocaine can also numb her vagina.

Timed imbibing.
Drink too much and you won't be able to get it up. But some alcohol before sex may depress your central nervous system and delay ejaculation. Don't rely on it, though: You could become sexually dependent on alcohol, and then develop erectile dysfunction.

University of Vermont and the author of *In the Grip of Desire*. And yet different cultures have different expectations, as shown by the results of a 2002 survey from the pharmaceutical firm Alza (owned by Johnson & Johnson). In the survey, American men said they should last about 14 minutes, but British blokes thought 10 was plenty, and German guys figured 7 was enough.

Another and perhaps even more important factor is how men think their partners want to be pleased in the bedroom—that is, the means to the orgasmic end.

"They believe that if they last longer, they'll be better able to bring a woman to orgasm," Golden says. But for women, sex is far more complicated than that. Most can't reach orgasm through intercourse alone, so to be a truly great lover, a man needs to know what else turns her on. Foreplay is huge, clitoral stimulation is important, and, not surprisingly, women report more orgasms when a vibrator is in the mix. In fact, women are far less likely than men to care (or perhaps even notice) how long intercourse lasts. Of couples surveyed in a 2003 study published in the *Archives of Sexual Behavior*, 24 percent of men claimed they had a PE problem—but only 10 percent of their partners agreed. The rest were unbothered.

The difference was more dramatic when *Men's Health* surveyed couples who typically have intercourse for about 6 minutes. Asked if that time was satisfying, only 34 percent of the men said yes—but 82 percent of the women said their sex lives were perfectly fine. That may not be a scientific sampling, but it does reflect what PE experts like Stanley Althof, PhD, hear when they talk with clients.

"Everything can become so focused on how quickly the man ejaculates rather than on being loving and sensual," says Dr. Althof, a psychologist in private practice in West Palm Beach, Florida. He says it doesn't matter if a man lasts a minute or far longer: If the man believes there's trouble, he needs to talk with his partner about it and learn what she wants. That's the first step in making sex more satisfying.

Dr. Althof's prescription for communication before chemicals sounds sensible, if not exactly in his own best fiscal interests: He serves as an advisor to pharmaceutical companies, including Johnson & Johnson.

THERE'S A PILL FOR THAT

If a man wants a pill to increase his staying power, he doesn't have to wait for Priligy. For the past 10 years, physicians have been prescribing certain types of antidepressants for the off-label treatment of premature ejaculation. Prozac and Paxil, both selective serotonin reuptake inhibitors (SSRIs), are two of the most popular choices. This isn't because PE is making men depressed (although it probably is, in many cases); it's because delayed ejaculation can be one of the side effects of SSRI use.

Both Prozac and Paxil (and Priligy) boost levels of serotonin, a neurotransmitter that affects such basic body functions as appetite, sleep, and sexual desire. When there isn't enough serotonin in a small area of your brain stem known as the (get ready now) nucleus paragigantocellularis, your time to ejaculation speeds up, says Dr. Waldinger. In one study review, Prozac was shown to increase men's time three-fold. Paxil increased their time eightfold, although that drug comes with a higher risk of side effects, such as drowsiness and nausea.

"You have to deal with the impact PE has had on your relationship."

So if Prozac and Paxil work on PE, why do we need Priligy? Because Priligy seems to be better tolerated than the other two—and, because of its faster absorption into the bloodstream, it works more quickly than they do. You can take it an hour or two before sex instead of having to pop it regularly; plus, the effects wear off a few hours later.

More notably, if Johnson & Johnson resubmits Priligy for FDA approval and receives it, the company would be the first manufacturer allowed to market a drug for the treatment of PE. Its advertisements could then set the tone for how future PE drugs are advertised, and researchers who work on PE drug trials say it's only a matter of time before Priligy has company. (Dr. Althof says he's been helping other pharmaceutical companies develop PE drugs, and although he can't provide details, he notes that none are as far along in the process as Johnson & Johnson is.)

So what would a Priligy campaign look like, and what kind of men would it target—those who struggle to last a minute, or those who already last an average amount of time? It's impossible to say. There are no examples to go by, because prescription drugs can't be advertised to consumers in the countries where Priligy is now sold. But Johnson & Johnson may be dropping some clues. It has already sponsored at least two studies that document the emotional toll PE takes on a man. And at its June conference for investors and analysts, a company presenter stressed that PE creates "difficulty in a man's ability to manage his relationships, and directly impacts self-esteem."

That focus on self-esteem might sound familiar. When Viagra went on sale in 1998, its first public face was a 75-year-old Bob Dole. And although it's doubtful anybody wanted to think much about the former senator's sex life, choosing him as a spokesman made a lot of sense: Viagra was being targeted to older men because they're the ones most likely to be stricken with erectile dysfunction.

But 4 years later, in 2002, Dole's gig was taken by Rafael Palmeiro, then a 38-year-old slugger for the Texas Rangers. "Let's just say it works for me," he said in commercials, delivering a coy, swaggering line that matched a shift in ad strategy: Instead of focusing on the lack of an erection, ads targeted the quality of an erection. Men were convinced, and the fastest-growing segment of users that year became men between 18 and 45—an age range in which erectile dysfunction is rare, according to a study in the *International Journal of Impotence Research*.

Some experts worry that Johnson &

Johnson will follow the same game plan.

"There are tons of men out there who think they should be doing better and who will buy into a PE campaign," says Joel Lexchin, MD, a professor of health policy at the York University School of Health Policy & Management, in Toronto, who has studied the Viagra campaign. "It could implicitly or explicitly define what PE means so that any man could identify with the condition."

And if that happens, he says, even more men will have exaggerated expectations of how long sex should last. The mirage of those 45-minute romps in porn would seem even more attainable.

But that's not to say that drugs for PE are inherently bad. Stephen Lefrak, MD, a professor of medicine who teaches medical ethics at the Washington University School of Medicine in St. Louis, argues that from an ethical standpoint, SSRIs (and Priligy by extension) offer a perfectly legitimate treatment for PE.

"I don't see a problem, provided that the patient knows the upsides and downsides to taking a drug," he says. "If someone's unhappy in life, we give them SSRIs to treat depression anyway, no? To me, that's part of medicine. We treat chronic pain, even when it's hard to determine its exact cause."

Johnson & Johnson says it understands the complexities of PE and knows that not every man with time-sensitive desires actually has a medical problem or should be treated. That's as much as the company will say, though. "It would be premature—no pun intended—to discuss how we might or might not approach a conversation with a consumer for a product that is not yet approved," says company spokesman Greg Panico.

Dr. Althof, the Johnson & Johnson consultant, says doctors should be responsible for determining which patients need a PE drug and which ones don't. But he doesn't believe a drug will ever be a complete solution, which is why, when he recommends SSRIs, he also encourages his patients to go through counseling.

"It's too simplistic to think that people who have a lifelong problem can take a tablet and make everything better," he says. "You have to deal with the impact PE has had on your relationship."

Matt hasn't yet taken any drugs to extend his time. He does regularly use condoms with an anesthetic cream that slightly numbs his penis, but they don't give him the kind of control he craves. And so he continues to worry and to flounder, and he's come to see this problem as a measure of his manhood: He can entice a woman to bed, sure, but that's no success on its own.

"I want to last until she orgasms," he says.

It's that simple. He figures 25 to 35 minutes should be long enough.

Your Life: On the Line

As scientists test whether cell phones cause tumors, they're receiving lots of static from the telecom industry. Here's what you need to know before you point a loaded phone at your head.

Lloyd Morgan, an old man with a hole in his head, had no business discovering the fatal flaw. After all, this was a $30 million effort to answer the question of whether cell phones can give you brain cancer.

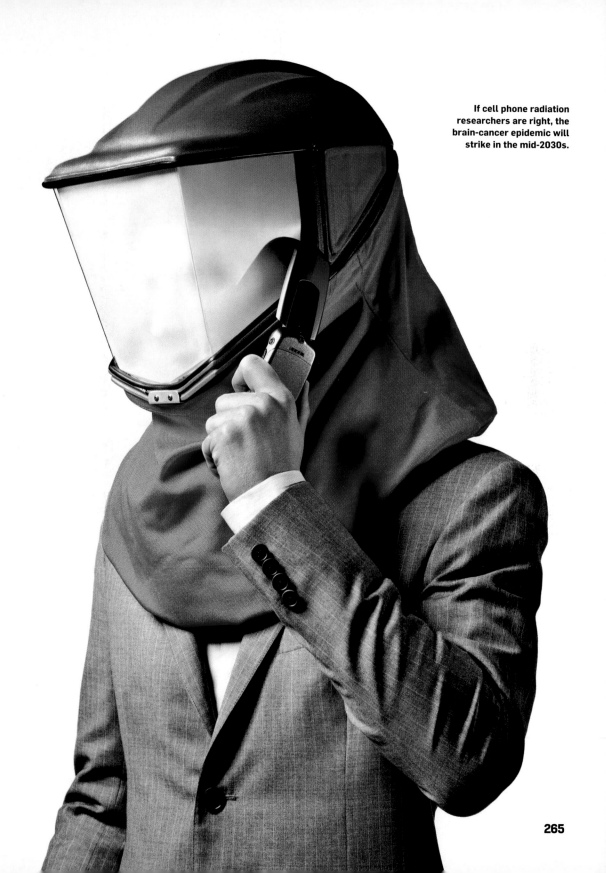

If cell phone radiation researchers are right, the brain-cancer epidemic will strike in the mid-2030s.

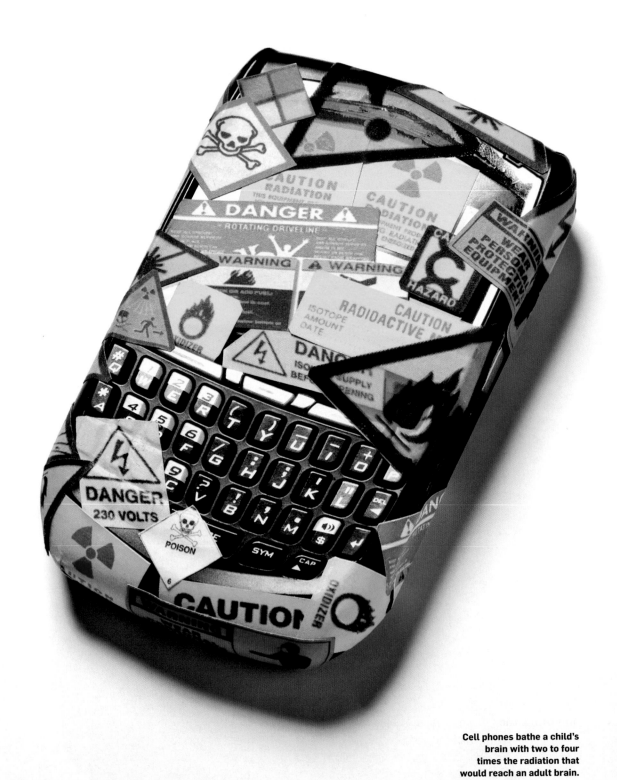

Cell phones bathe a child's brain with two to four times the radiation that would reach an adult brain.

Morgan, 68, is a survivor of brain cancer. Based in Berkeley, California, this retired electronics engineer and self-trained epidemiologist has made it his mission to spread the message that cell phone radiation is carcinogenic. He does this more or less as a wireless communications vigilante, however. The American Cancer Society, the National Cancer Institute, the U.S. Food and Drug Administration, and the World Health Organization all regard the radio waves emitted from cell phones as safe. But another growing body of experts believes cell-phone use can promote tumors, and momentum has been shifting to their side. A researcher in Sweden, for instance, recently reported that people who started using cell phones before the age of 20—including 80 percent of the readers of this magazine—have four to five times the odds of developing one type of brain tumor. An unpublished (and therefore not peer-reviewed) analysis by researchers at the University of Pittsburgh Cancer Institute shows an increase in brain tumors among Americans in the under-30 age group.

And according to new research, studies showing that cell phones are safe tend to be (a) less rigorously designed and (b) funded by the cell phone industry, while studies showing that cell phones carry risks are (a) produced with better science and (b) have no financial conflicts of interest.

And if the slow spread of distress within the halls of government means anything, the topic no longer causes eye rolling among lawmakers. The National Institutes of Health (NIH), for example, has recently authorized a $25 million study to analyze rats that have been bathed in cell phone radiation for a period of 2 years. Both houses of Congress have held hearings on the issue. And in Maine, legislation might soon require warning labels on cell phones sold in that state.

The cell phone industry has responded with studies, mind you—ones that exonerate the technology, including a new study showing that tumor rates are steady in Scandinavia, where cell phones were adopted early. But if you dig deep, those findings aren't as reassuring as you might

A growing body of experts believe that cell phone use can promote tumors.

hope. For one thing, they tend to limit their good news to people who've been using cell phones for less than 10 years.

And then there's the trouble unleashed by Morgan, an unfunded retiree armed only with personal suspicions and plenty of time to read the fine print. Thanks to his pursuit of answers, we now know the biggest cell-phone study of all produced a biologically impossible conclusion: It determined that not only do cell phones not give you cancer, but they protect you from it. Another recent study claims that they ward off Alzheimer's. It makes some people question whether the defenders' cases are riddled with wrong numbers.

The laws of physics dictate that it should be impossible for cell phones to cause cancer, let alone act as tumor-busting force fields or magical memory sharpeners. While radiation from x-rays and CT scans is strong enough to knock electrons from molecules and damage the double helix, radio waves from cell phones are too weak to subvert your operating code in this way.

"It's the equivalent of holding a flashlight up to your head," my friend Steve, a high school physics teacher, explained to me with a shake of his head over dinner. His analogy has not been lost on the defenders of the technology. "Radio waves,

Researchers report that people who start using cell phones before age 20 have greater odds of developing brain tumors.

or radiofrequency (RF) energy, is a range of the electromagnetic spectrum that includes AM and FM broadcast radio, television, and many other devices and technologies, including cordless phones, baby monitors, radar, and microwave ovens," says Linda Erdreich, PhD. Erdreich is a spokeswoman for Exponent, the consulting company chosen by the cellphone industry to represent its position before the U.S. Senate.

In selecting Exponent to argue its case, the Wireless Association has hired the scientific equivalent of Mr. Burns from *The Simpsons*. In its 43-year history, Exponent has defended nearly everything that is bad in American industry: buildings that fail. Amusement-park rides that

exceed G-forces inflicted on astronauts. Soda machines in schools, rocket-fuel chemicals in groundwater, chromium in the workplace. Atrazine, asbestos, even the *Exxon Valdez*.

"Visible light is also part of the electromagnetic spectrum," Dr. Erdreich continues, propping up my friend's flashlight defense of cell phones. "But it's at a higher frequency and shorter wavelength than RF."

But Dr. Erdreich might be on shaky ground at the troubled intersection between biology and physics. The BioInitiative Report, a research project authored by an international team of scientists, sought to gather all the evidence against RF radiation in one place. Released in 2007, the report cites experiments showing that radio waves can in fact damage human cells, though they do it through indirect means. The damage doesn't happen in every instance, but studies have documented RF radiation causing cells to produce molecules known as "heat-shock proteins," a sign that the cells sense environmental stress. Animal studies confirm that exposure to RF radiation can also cause leaks in the blood-brain barrier, which could allow carcinogens into the brain.

Other studies included in the BioInitiative Report show that radio waves can break both strands of the double helix.

"A double-strand break is a big problem," says Henry Lai, PhD, of the Department of Bioengineering at the University of Washington. "The cell loses the information on how to repair DNA."

David O. Carpenter, MD, director of the Institute for Health and the Environment

How Much Radiation Are You Absorbing?

The Federal Communications Commission limits the output of U.S. cell phones to 1.6 watts/kilogram of radiofrequency energy per gram of tissue. But outputs vary depending on a phone's design and function, so you can shop for lower numbers. Other strategies: Hold your phone farther from your ear, use a headset, and avoid calling when your phone shows only one or two bars: Straining for a signal boosts the radio-frequency output. Another solution: Talk less.

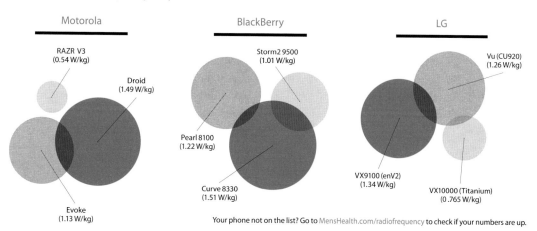

Motorola

RAZR V3
(0.54 W/kg)

Droid
(1.49 W/kg)

Evoke
(1.13 W/kg)

BlackBerry

Storm2 9500
(1.01 W/kg)

Pearl 8100
(1.22 W/kg)

Curve 8330
(1.51 W/kg)

LG

Vu (CU920)
(1.26 W/kg)

VX9100 (enV2)
(1.34 W/kg)

VX10000 (Titanium)
(0.765 W/kg)

Your phone not on the list? Go to MensHealth.com/radiofrequency to check if your numbers are up.

at the University at Albany and an expert on radio waves, believes it causes some genes to become more active and other genes to become less active. "This may be how cell phones cause cancer," he says. Finally, another theory suggests that radio waves might damage DNA by creating free-radical activity: RF radiation could trigger a chemical process known as a Fenton reaction, a chain of events in which radio waves meet molecular iron in cells, turning hydrogen peroxide into hydroxyl, which is, in the words of Dr. Lai, "a very potent and toxic free radical."

The explosive debate over cell-phone safety comes down to finding out whether the brains of people who use them grow meningioma, glioma, acoustic neuroma, or parotid gland tumors more readily than those of people who ring up their friends over corded landlines. (Cordless phones emit the same type of radiation that cell phones emit, although at lower levels.) In an attempt to settle the issue, the International Agency for Research on Cancer commissioned an epidemiological study in 1998 big enough for cell-phone critics to choke on. The 13-nation Interphone project asked more than 6,000 patients with brain tumors about their cell-phone use, and compared their answers with those of a matched group with no brain cancer.

So what did they find? When the paper was published, the study found no overall increase in the risk of brain tumors in regular cell phone users. However, the researchers noted that they have virtually no information on cell phone usage beyond

15 years. Press accounts have asserted that the coauthors were bitterly divided over what the study found. Most of the patients studied used their cell phones for less than 10 years. That matters, because brain tumors could take decades to develop, and widespread cell-phone use in the United States began only in the mid-1990s.

"It took 40 years for brain tumors to show up after Hiroshima," says Devra Davis, PhD, MPH, founding director of the Center for Environmental Oncology at

The Interphone researchers are bitterly divided on the study's results.

the University of Pittsburgh Cancer Institute (UPCI). "How can you expect to see effects from cell phones in 10?"

Studies that look at cell-phone use for more than 10 years are less comforting. According to a 2002 study of more than 1,400 brain-tumor patients by Swedish cancer epidemiologist Lennart Hardell, MD, PhD, as well as a review by Dr. Hardell of data from other researchers' studies, regular use of a cell phone for longer than 10 years increases your risk of some types of brain tumors.

And that's just the bad news for adults.

A former cell-phone-industry researcher from the University of Utah, Om Gandhi, ScD, has discovered that children's brains absorb far more RF radiation than adult brains do. Having routinely subjected adult-size dummy heads to RF waves, in 1996 Gandhi created models of the smaller, thinner skulls of children ages 5 and 10. In what would mark the beginning of the end of his financial relationship with the cell-phone industry (its decision, not his), Dr. Gandhi reported in the journal *IEEE Transactions on Microwave Theory and Techniques* that the cell-phone radiation that hits an adult brain with 72 milliwatts per kilogram of brain tissue (mW/kg) of wireless radiation, for instance, zaps a 10-year-old's brain with 160 mW/kg. Worse, it invades a 5-year-old brain with nearly 240 mW/kg.

Gandhi's research was replicated by the French cell-phone industry, and France has joined several other nations in issuing advisories limiting the use of cell phones by children.

"We have children running around with these cell phones up to their ears and sleeping with them under their pillows," says Andrea Boland, a lawmaker from Maine who introduced the first piece of legislation in this country to require warning labels on cell phones.

Lest readers over the age of 10 take comfort, the window of increased vulnerability to cell-phone radiation might not be limited to kids' *Dora the Explorer* years. According to Ronald Herberman, MD, former head of UPCI, it takes decades for the brain to lay down the electrical insulation (known as myelin) that presumably shields the nerves, for the most part, from radio waves. Dr. Herberman thinks our increased vulnerability to RF radiation could extend well into our 20s.

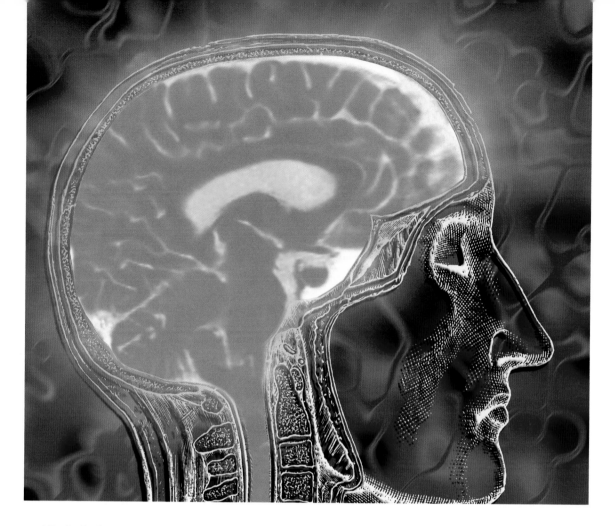

All of which might explain the latest bad news out of Sweden. According to data published by Dr. Hardell in the *International Journal of Oncology* in July 2009, brain-tumor patients who went wireless as teenagers had four to five times the risk of developing an astrocytoma, a type of brain tumor. If this data is correct, you can forget about having a leisurely decade to wean yourself off your mobile-phone habit. These patients had used their cell phones for only a 1-year minimum.

Brain cancer is rare, affecting just 27 in every 100,000 U.S. men. It's also an illness of middle age, with 56 being the median age of diagnosis. But the signifi-

cance of Dr. Hardell's latest finding, if it's true, is pretty stunning. With 277 million cell phone accounts in the United States alone, a quintupling of brain-cancer risk has the potential to translate into hundreds of thousands of preventable cancers.

The critics of cell phone radiation compare our position today—at the dawn of wireless communication—to that of our grandparents upon the widespread introduction of tobacco and asbestos into the environment in the past century. It took decades for these carcinogens to leave a mark on official health statistics, but the body counts grew exponentially: few cancers in the beginning, then a sharp slope upward. If this scenario's cost in human suffering doesn't bother you, consider its financial repercussions: It can cost $200,000 to treat a brain tumor.

Lloyd Morgan's path to cell phone evangelism was personal. In 1995, when he was 53 and working in Silicon Valley, he suffered a grand mal seizure. Doctors removed a softball-size meningioma from his left frontal lobe, and told him he might have raised his risk of brain cancer from having been around electromagnetic radiation on the job. (He'd also raised his

Are cell phones the equivalent of asbestos and tobacco?

risk by having full dental x-rays as a child and by using a ham radio as a teenager.) Today there is a dimple in his scalp, and MRIs show a hole in the space where his tumor was removed.

Morgan immersed himself in brain-cancer research, and his self-education eventually led to his discovery, 2 years ago, of a baffling characteristic buried deep within Interphone statistical tables. Not only do cell phones not cause cancer, argued some of the project's dozens of authors, but according to their results, the brain-cancer risk associated with cell phones routinely produces an "odds ratio" of less than one. That means, incredibly, that Interphone has quietly found that cell phones protect you from cancer.

"They never say it that way," says Morgan. "They always just say, 'We found no increased risk of cancer.' " One Inter-

phone study even found that using cell phones keeps brain tumors smaller. "Either holding a radio transmitter up to your head protects you from developing a brain tumor," Morgan says, "or the studies have major design flaws."

If RF radiation does cause brain tumors, we'll see a precipitous rise in cancer by the mid-2030s. If rates stay where they are, on the other hand, gadflies like Morgan will have undermined the case for environmental causes of cancer. Morgan believes it's a risk worth taking. "I worry, and I pray that I'm wrong," he says.

When he broke ranks in 2008 to testify before Congress about his concerns, the UPCI's Ronald Herberman, MD, became the most prominent member of the American cancer research community to describe long-term use of cell phones as a potential carcinogen. In September of that year, Dr. Herberman appeared before a sparsely attended subcommittee meeting—it was the week the banking crisis came to a head—to argue that while more research was needed, enough data was available for him to warn his staff to begin using headsets and speakerphones and to keep their cell phones away from their children. He based his recommendation on the work of Dr. Gandhi and Dr. Hardell.

After studying 1,400 brain-tumor patients and an equal number of healthy people, Dr. Hardell found not only a doubling of brain-tumor risk after 10 years of heavy wirelessness, but also a specific risk on the side of the head patients remembered using their phones on. (Critics say that recollections by

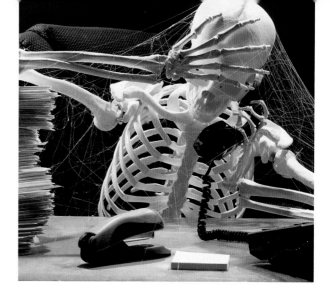

brain-tumor patients would be colored by where the tumor grew.) In 2003, Dr. Hardell looked at the same data and found that the risk from using cell phones rose with a patient's total hours of use. Two years later he sorted the people in his study by address and discovered that rural cell-phone users—whose phones must emit much more power to reach towers than urban phones do—faced a higher risk of tumors.

For Dr. Herberman, it was the idea of RF radiation saturating the heads of children that most troubled him. "Of all the studies I had read linking an increased risk with cell-phone use," he says, "none had been done with kids."

Now retired from the UPCI, Dr. Herberman remains in the minority on the issue. "A number of my colleagues in the cancer community wonder whether I did the right thing," he says, "whether there was enough evidence to sound an alarm. But most of them didn't take the trouble to assess the published results. Whenever they ask me why I spoke up, I ask them if they've read the research, and what I usually get is, 'No, I hadn't seen much about that.' "

Dr. Herberman and Dr. Davis are now waiting for the publication of the troubling findings presented by Davis in 2009 in Davos, Switzerland. After parsing the NIH database of brain-tumor incidence in the United States, Dr. Davis discovered an "increasing incidence of brain tumors in the United States in people under age 30," she wrote in an e-mail. "The reasons for this trend could include changing patterns of use of cell phones, diagnostic radiation, or even aspartame." Dr. Davis, who moved on from Pitt's Cancer Institute to found the Environmental Health Trust, thinks it's lousy that her findings remain mired in review while the authors of a recent article in the *Journal of the National Cancer Institute* made headlines for suggesting that there had been no increase in brain tumors in Scandinavia between 1998 and 2003, a period still early in the use of cell phones.

When you come down to it, though, we might simply be arguing about headsets. That's right: Whatever the outcome of these clashes between RF wonks, no one has proposed a ban on cell phones. "In general," says Dr. Carpenter, "merely pulling the phone 6 inches away will dramatically reduce your exposure."

This entire seemingly apocalyptic argument, in other words, is over whether the cell phone industry should warn us to wear our headsets, keep the things away from our kids, and use the speaker feature. That seems like an easy enough suggestion. But it's like suggesting to an NRA member that he put a lock on his gun. Not over my dead cell phone battery, the industry shouts back.

PROVE IT

TAKE YOUR TIME

When it comes to knowing the best time to pop a pill, your body may be even smarter than your pharmacist. Use this daily dosing guide based on *The Body Clock Guide to Better Health*, by Michael Smolensky, PhD, to maximize your meds' effectiveness. Of course, talk with your doctor before making any changes to your medication schedule.

Take in the Morning

Decongestants: Some compounds that clear up congestion may also keep you awake at night. Pop decongestants in the morning to take advantage of their adrenaline-like effects.

Proton-pump inhibitors: Treat heartburn in the a.m. Scientists in Canada determined that taking a PPI in the morning is a better way to suppress acid production for 24 hours than taking it at night is.

Antidepressants: Depression can be caused by low levels of the brain chemical serotonin. Some antidepressants, such as Paxil, work by keeping levels steady. But take them early, because they can sabotage sleep.

Take in the Evening

Antihistamines: Nasal allergies worsen overnight, so many of these medications work better when they're taken at bedtime. Plus, one side effect of some antihistamines is drowsiness.

Aspirin: People taking low-dose aspirin before bed had a 5.2-point drop in systolic BP and a 2.4-point drop in diastolic BP; those taking it in the morning had no change, reports a study in *Hypertension*.

Cough suppressants: While you sleep, you experience a drop in anti-inflammatory hormones, leaving cold symptoms unchecked. Take a suppressant at night to halt your hacking.

BLOW OFF THE FLU

The seasonal flu actually has a very long "season"—from fall until well into March. So if you still haven't been vaccinated, what are you waiting for? Just make sure you opt for the shot, not the spray. University of Michigan researchers found that adults given the injectable vaccine were 50 percent less likely to contract the flu than those who received the nasal-spray version. (More research is needed to explain why the spray is so much less effective in adults.) Can't stand needles? Before the jab, press your thumb on the injection site for 10 seconds. Hong Kong scientists showed that this trick significantly reduced the pain of being pricked.

Here's another stay-well trick: A humidifier can help keep your home influenza-free, say Oregon State University researchers. They found that increasing the moisture level in the air causes 80 percent of the flu virus to die within an hour, compared with a 30 percent drop in a dry environment.

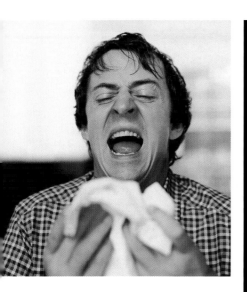

One theory holds that a boost in humidity may deactivate flu molecules while they're airborne, possibly by altering their size or shape. Set your humidifier to 50 percent, and be sure to empty, dry, and refill it every day—otherwise you'll be wheezin' for different reasons: mold and bacteria.

SURVIVE THE 9-TO-5

Your office is like a playground: You have to know how to handle the bullies. Rule 1: Don't run. Swedish researchers found that men who often retreat from obnoxious bosses and coworkers are five times more likely to have a heart attack than those who stand up for themselves.

"Coping with the situation internally may cause a temporary spike in blood pressure, which could trigger an attack," says study author Constanze Leineweber, PhD. So the next time you're a target, stay put and respond calmly. (Of course, tread lightly if it's your boss.)

HAVE A HAPPY HEART

Death is depressing. So it's fitting that one of the best meds for the blues may also repel the Reaper. Taking an SSRI antidepressant, like Paxil or Zoloft, could save you from a heart attack. Researchers at Loyola University tested 50 people and discovered that those swallowing SSRIs showed a decrease in blood-clot formation. That's important, because clots are often the cause of a heart attack. This doesn't mean everyone at risk of heart disease should pop Prozac, but taking an SSRI may be smart for people with depression. Talk to your doctor.

DON'T BE A SITTING DUCK

We have some bad news, and you should stand up for it: Sitting all day could hurt your heart, according to a recent study in *Medicine & Science in Sports & Exercise*. Men who sat for most of every day were 35 percent more likely to die of heart disease than those who were often on their feet.

"Your legs are a large part of your total muscle," says study author Peter Katzmarzyk, PhD. "When they're inactive, you don't break down fats in your blood as well." Your Rx: Walk for a few minutes every hour.

PROVE IT

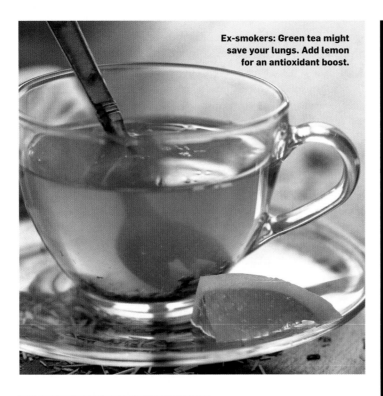

Ex-smokers: Green tea might save your lungs. Add lemon for an antioxidant boost.

HAVE A SPOT OF TEA

Drinking green tea may undo damage from years of smoking, according to researchers in Taiwan. In the study, current and former smokers who never sipped the stuff were 12 times more likely to develop lung cancer than those who quaffed at least a cup a day.

"Antioxidants in green tea may trigger the production of compounds that stop the spread of many cancers, including lung cancer," says study author I-Hsin Lin, PhD(c). If you don't feel like brewing a cup, try Honest Tea Organic Honey Green Tea. It's low in calories and loaded with antioxidants.

WATCH YOUR WEIGHT

Eighty ounces. That could be the difference between beating prostate cancer and watching it return with a vengeance. In a new Johns Hopkins study, researchers found that men who gained 5 or more pounds prior to or up to a year after prostate surgery were nearly twice as likely to battle cancer again than those who maintained their weight.

"Obesity and weight gain are associated with inflammation, which might influence prostate-cancer recurrence," says study author Corinne Joshu, PhD.

While we're on the topic of prostate cancer, know this: The PSA test isn't perfect. In fact, only one out of four men with high PSA levels actually have prostate cancer, which means the rest undergo unnecessary biopsies. That's why a new study in the *Archives of Internal Medicine* is so alarming: Only 20 percent of men who take a PSA test are told the pros and cons of the screening before-hand. Unfortunately, one reason physicians stay mum about the shortcomings of PSA comes down to CYA.

"Doctors fear they'll be sued if they don't order the test and the patient later finds he has cancer," says study author Richard Hoffman, MD. If your doctor doesn't review the pluses and minuses of a PSA test with you—including its diagnostic downsides—find a new doc.

WASH UP

Think only shopping carts are crawling with germs? Loma Linda University and University of Arizona scientists recently found that nearly half of the reusable grocery bags they sampled contained fecal bacteria, including *E. coli*. One path to contamination: You put fresh fruits and vegetables in your bag, and germs on the produce slough off and stay behind. Or maybe you buy a package of raw meat and some juices leak out. Either way, the danger is the same: food

poisoning from groceries that sat in the tainted tote.

"The cross-contamination risk is similar to the risk you have with cutting boards," says study author Charles Gerba, PhD. Protect yourself by using cotton bags that you can wash after every shopping trip.

GET YOUR Zs

What a nightmare: Too little sleep may raise your risk of type 2 diabetes, say scientists in the Netherlands. People who slept 4 hours a night saw their insulin sensitivity (ability to process blood sugar) fall 25 percent, compared with those who slept 8½ hours. Rough night? Top your cereal with cinnamon. It might lower blood sugar.

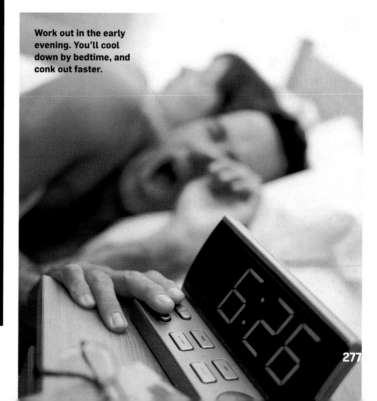

Work out in the early evening. You'll cool down by bedtime, and conk out faster.

YOU ASKED

Q: What's the best plant to put in my office?

A: You need a mind-body tag team: a fragrant shrub to stimulate your brain, and a leafy plant to scrub your office air (which can be five times more polluted than the air outside). Finding the right foliage for you depends on a number of factors, however, including the amount of sunlight in the room and the color of your thumb. Clear your head (and the air) with this guide from James Dillard, MD, an integrative medicine physician in New York City, and Bill Wolverton, PhD, the author of *Plants: Why You Can't Live Without Them.*

1 ARECA PALM
Dypsis lutescens
Benefit: Cleans the air
Light: Direct
Attention: Moderate
Thanks to its huge fronds (which can reach 6 feet in height and feature 60 leaflets), this palm is especially effective at filtering airborne particles.

2 PEPPERMINT
Mentha x piperita
Benefit: Stimulates your brain
Light: Direct
Attention: Easy
Sniffing mint can increase your alertness and enhance your memory, according to a study in the *International Journal of Neuroscience.*
Bonus: It can also help suppress your appetite.

3 ENGLISH IVY
Hedera helix
Benefit: Cleans the air
Light: Indirect
Attention: Easy
Tests at the University of Georgia show that English ivy is particularly efficient at absorbing volatile organic compounds, airborne pollutants spewed by office machinery that cause headaches and nausea.

4 LEMON BALM
Melissa officinalis
Benefit: Stimulates your brain
Light: Indirect
Attention: Easy
Researchers at Ohio State University found that the scent of lemon improved people's moods and raised their levels of norepinephrine, a brain chemical linked to mood and behavior.

5 GOLDEN POTHOS
Epipremnum aureum
Benefit: Cleans the air
Light: Indirect
Attention: Easy
This hardy vine reduces indoor ozone, Penn State researchers found. Exposure to even low ozone levels can cause chest pain and throat irritation.

6 GARDENIA
Gardenia augusta
Benefit: Stimulates your brain
Light: Direct
Attention: Moderate
It's like a long-acting antidepressant. A gardenia can live for 25 years, and every time you smell its flowers, your emotional outlook improves, according to research from Rutgers.

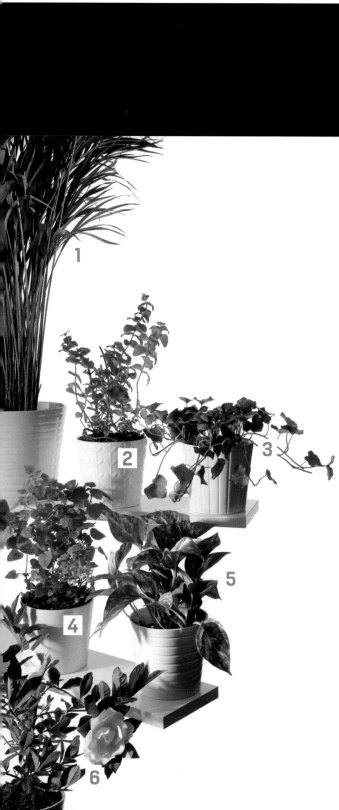

Q: Just how many germs are people leaving behind when they double-dip at a party?

A: It comes down to the consistency of the condiment. When Clemson University researchers tested various dips that had been contaminated by double dunkers, they found significant amounts of bacteria in all their samples—but salsa contained seven times more bugs than other dips. Salsa's watery texture makes it easier for it to drip off the half-eaten chip and back into the communal bowl, while thicker mixtures stay put, says study author Paul Dawson, PhD.

So if you're not sure whether your fellow partygoers are minding their manners about microbes, steer clear of the red, runny stuff. While unlikely, H1N1—among other illnesses—can be passed from person to person through dip.

"Microbially speaking, double dipping is the equivalent of swapping spit," says Dr. Dawson.

Q: My gums bleed when I floss. Does that mean I should worry about my heart health?

A: It depends on why you're spitting blood. "If you floss only occasionally, then your gums will likely bleed because they're inflamed from excess plaque," says periodontist Sally Cram, DDS, an advisor for the American Dental Association. "Rev up your regimen: Brush for 2 minutes twice a day, and floss every day."

If your gums still run red after a week of diligent care, see your dentist. You probably have either gingivitis (a mild gum infection) or periodontitis (an infection that has spread below your gums into the bone and tissue). If it's periodontitis, inflammatory chemicals and bacteria may be flowing from your gums into your bloodstream, where they can contribute to the buildup of arterial plaque.

But the good news is that periodontitis is reversible. Your dentist should do an initial deep cleaning (though surgery may be necessary) and have you return every 3 months to make sure the infection is under control. To help reduce bacteria, use a mouthwash containing the essential oils thymol, menthol, and eucalyptol, such as Listerine.

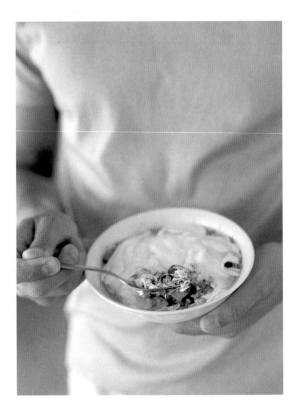

Q: Should I have my CRP tested to gauge my risk for heart disease?

A: It depends on what else is in your cardiac crystal ball. "The C-reactive protein (CRP) test provides an additional coordinate to triangulate your risk of heart disease," says John Elefteriades, MD, chief of cardiac surgery at the Yale University School of Medicine. "It's useful for men who have normal cholesterol levels but are borderline for other reasons." Here's why: Elevated CRP levels in your body reflect inflammation, which can cause arterial plaques to rupture, triggering a heart attack—even if you don't have high cholesterol. Dr. Elefteriades says it's worthwhile to have your CRP tested if you have two or more of these risk factors for heart disease: family history, obesity, smoking, or prehypertension (systolic blood pressure 120 to 139 mm Hg, diastolic 80 to 89 mm Hg).

Q: Will consuming foods or drinks that contain probiotics help my digestive system?

A: "Probiotic beverages can provide relief from gassiness equivalent to the benefits from yogurt with or without added cultures. However, some relatively expensive products claim to have 'higher' concentrations of 'good' flora and are promoted for gastrointestinal health. The data behind these claims is not scientifically rigorous and does not support the added cost," says Mark Welton, MD, chief of colorectal surgery at Stanford University School of Medicine and the author of numerous research articles on colorectal cancer and other gastroenterological diseases.

Q: Should I avoid meat containing nitrates if I'm concerned about colon cancer?

A: "The research isn't clear about whether avoiding nitrates can lower your risk of colon cancer," says Dr. Welton. "However, a high-fiber diet plus daily exercise speeds food through your system, which is good for your colon. If you have a family history of colon cancer, go for a colonoscopy at 40, or 10 years before the age your relative was diagnosed with cancer, whichever comes first."

Q: What's the best natural sleep enhancer?

A: Valerian. Your ticket to dreamland is a tincture (alcohol solution) made from the roots of this perennial. Studies show that valerian not only reduces the time required to fall asleep, but also limits nighttime awakenings. "It acts like a natural Valium, reducing anxiety," says W. Christopher Winter, MD, director of the Sleep Medicine Center of Martha Jefferson Hospital in Charlottesville, Virginia, and *Men's Health*'s sleep-medicine advisor. For best results, mix 1 teaspoon of valerian tincture with a glass of water, and drink the mixture an hour before bed. We like HerbPharm's organic valerian extract (herb-pharm.com).

Q: Is there any way to remember more of my dreams?

A: "The key is to wake up near or during a rapid eye movement (REM) sleep cycle, which is when you dream," says W. Christopher Winter, MD, the medical director of the Sleep Medicine Center of Martha Jefferson Hospital, in Charlottesville, Virginia. Set your alarm to go off a few minutes earlier. You may catch the tail end of the longest REM phase of the night. Writing down your dreams can also help.

Q: Is it a bad sign that my urine stinks in the morning?

A: "Your first morning urine is concentrated with urea, salts, and organic compounds. Just drink more water to dilute it. If you have additional symptoms, such as fever, burning while urinating, or pain above your pelvis or near your kidneys, you could have an infection. You should see your doctor," says Larry Lipshultz, MD, a professor of urology at Baylor College of Medicine.

Q: Why do paper cuts hurt so much?

A: Location: The real estate on your fingertips has about 100 free nerve endings per square millimeter; your palms have only 4 to 5. "And the paper's edge slices a relatively deep gash for such a sensitive area," says Elaine Gilmore, MD, PhD, an assistant professor of dermatology at the University of Rochester Medical Center. Next time, start by washing the cut with warm water and a mild soap, and let it dry. Then press firmly on your white-collar wound.

"Constant pressure overwhelms the nerve endings—like jamming a call center—which prevents them from sending the pain signal," says Dr. Gilmore. After a minute or two, apply a liquid bandage, such as Band-Aid Single-Step. By going the liquid route, you're actually sealing the wound, which prevents the infiltration of more pain-inducing irritants and speeds healing.

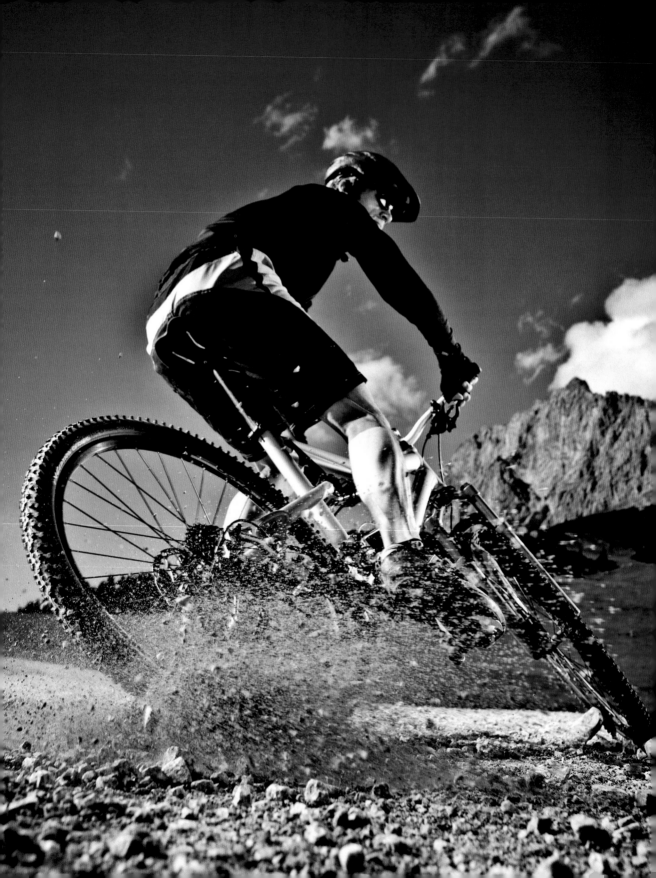

6

Improve Your Game

MVP Training

Elite trainer Todd Durkin, author of *The IMPACT! Body Plan*, shows writer Mike Zimmerman how even you can go from average Joe to pro

"Li'l quarterback, li'l quarterback," taunts the man right in my face, **"number 56 is coming to get you!"** My feet, already dancing in and out of the squares of rope ladder laid on the floor, move faster. The man is Todd Durkin, CSCS, trainer of some of the biggest names in pro sports. Number 56 is linebacker Shawne Merriman of the San Diego Chargers (he's since become number 56 for the Buffalo Bills), who is indeed coming to get me. He's behind me in this agility drill and closing in fast. It's like tap-dancing in hell, I think, wondering how anyone that big can move his

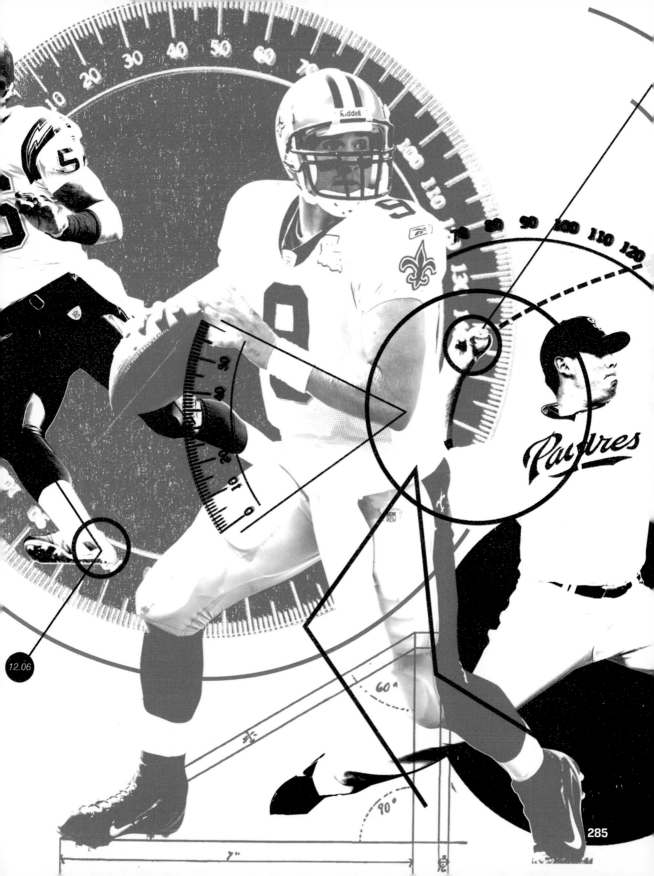

feet that quickly. If you're wondering why a scary MVP like Merriman is training next to a NVP like me, it's because we're more alike than different. All the clients at Durkin's gym, Fitness Quest 10 in San Diego, do the same workouts, and they often train next to each other.

"I train average Joes the same way I train the pros," Durkin says. "Why separate them? They're searching for the same thing. I've got grandmothers and housewives here who look unassuming, but they can outwork, outperform, and outlast you."

It's true. I've met them. I put in some serious sweat equity with Durkin as a coauthor on his new book, *The IMPACT! Body Plan*, a 10-week fitness, nutrition, and mental toughness program. I hung out at his gym, did his workouts, and felt that tasty pain. I also watched and sweated with several of his star athletes: Merriman, Saints quarterback Drew Brees, Packers QB Aaron Rodgers, Jets running back LaDainian Tomlinson, and many others.

The benefits of Durkin's workouts came fast. I dropped 12 pounds in the first month. That crunchy pain in my left knee? Gone. Those chronic lower-back problems? History. When I climb a flight of steps, I feel a subtle plyometric bounce in my legs. Durkin calls this "springy strength," when your feet behave like flexible steel bands. I'll never go back to 5-mile jogs and 3 sets of 10 on the bench. Not when I'm having this much fun.

Yes, the workouts are fun, even when

Fitness on the Go

A lack of time or equipment shouldn't make you miss your next workout. You can still challenge your whole body and blast away your belly in as little as 10 minutes. Kick your metabolism into a higher gear with this express regimen from Durkin.

Perform this 5-exercise workout as a circuit. Complete one exercise after another, resting as little as possible. After you've finished the circuit, rest 90 seconds and then repeat.

Squat jumps (10 reps): Place your fingers on the back of your head and pull your elbows back so they're in line with your body. Dip your knees and lower your body until your thighs are parallel to the floor.

Explosively jump as high as you can. When you land, squat and jump again.

Pushups (as many as possible): Assume the classic pushup position, with your hands slightly beyond shoulder width apart and your body in a straight line. Lower your body until your chest nearly touches the floor. Pause, and push yourself back to the starting position as quickly as possible.

Lunge jumps (20 reps per leg): Stand in a staggered stance, your left foot in the front. Lower your body until your right knee nearly touches the floor. Jump and switch the position of your feet so your left leg ends up behind you. Alternate back and forth with each rep.

Pushups (as many as possible): See instructions at left.

Skater hops (20 reps per leg): Stand on your left foot with your left knee slightly bent and your right foot slightly off the floor. Lower your body toward the floor, then bound to your right by jumping off your left leg. Land on your right foot and bring your left foot behind your right as you reach toward the outside of your right foot with your left hand. Reverse the movement back toward the left, landing on your left foot.

you're beating the heck out of yourself. They change constantly. And eventually you realize you're changing as well.

"Conditioning drives success in every area of your life," Durkin says. "You want to change a relationship? Start with your conditioning. Change your energy? Start with your conditioning. Change your financial status? Start with your conditioning. Everything comes back to that."

Change your workouts, change your life. Is it really that easy? Well, no, there's nothing easy about Durkin's body-blasting workouts. Before you even start, you'll have to change your mind about what a workout is supposed to be, and what you need to do in the gym to make it work for you. Below are five examples of training principles I learned from Durkin. They were game changers for me, and I'm confident they'll work for you, too.

START FAST, LIFT MORE

The way most men warm up—5 minutes on a treadmill to start, a set of bench presses using an empty barbell to finish, with perhaps a couple sets of crunches or some stretches in between—is worse than useless. It actually fails you in two crucial ways: First, it doesn't warm your body up properly, so you become more susceptible to injuries. And it doesn't prepare your body for the kind of effort you need to put in if you want your workouts to pay off.

"A proper warmup makes you sweat," Durkin says. "It fires up your entire neuromuscular system. A warm muscle generates more energy and force."

Durkin uses a dynamic warmup consisting of 15 exercises that challenge mobility, coordination, and conditioning. All you need is 20 to 25 feet of floor space. The exercises typically include jumping jacks, pogo hops, high-knee skips, Frankenstein walks (with each step, raise one straight leg as high as you can and try to touch your toe with the opposite hand), and walking lunges with core rotation (twist to the side of your forward leg). He also uses inchworms: Bend forward to put your hands on the floor, and walk your hands out until you're in an extended pushup position. Now walk your toes up toward your hands until your legs are straight and your butt pikes up in the air. Start the next rep by walking your hands forward again. After you've covered about 20 feet moving forward, perform the exercise in reverse, ending up where you started.

Once you're used to it, a dynamic warmup takes 7 to 10 minutes.

SWEAT MORE IN LESS TIME

A fast warmup prepares you for a fast workout. And by fast, I mean *fast*. For me, the tempo was the hardest part of the program to handle, although it does come with a nice perk: When you're working this hard and taking little if any rest between sets and exercises, you don't need to do traditional cardio. Brees says his heart rate stays between 160 and 190 beats per minute in an average session.

"My program is all about efficiency. I don't want you spending 2 hours in the gym," says Durkin. "You should be focused and immersed in the activity," not standing around discussing your social plans for the evening. The workout is so efficient that you'll accomplish in 45 minutes what would ordinarily take more than an hour.

To keep you moving, Durkin uses giant sets—three or more exercises performed consecutively, with no rest in between. The key to a successful giant set is the setup. You need to progress from one exercise to the next without stopping to adjust or move a piece of equipment. If

Want to make a change? Conditioning drives success in every area of your life.

you're using a barbell, for example, you want to make sure you can do all three exercises with the same weight. So you might choose the high pull (an explosive upright row in which the bar starts on the floor), bent-over row, and shoulder press. You do all your reps of one exercise, then the next, and then the last. Set the bar down, rest 90 seconds, and repeat.

"This is an extremely time-efficient way to combine multiple movements and rev up your metabolism," Durkin says. Sometimes he'll conduct fitness classes that consist of nothing but giant sets, with participants rotating through four or five stations of three exercises each.

TRICK YOUR BODY INTO BIG GAINS

You know how to move forward in a linear direction. When you're trying to go from one place to another, it's called walking. If you're exercising, it's called cardio. Either way, it's

forward movement at a steady speed, which isn't enough to make big changes.

"All exercise is good, but if you don't change direction and speed, you're not challenging your body enough," Durkin says. "It could lead to overuse injuries and muscle imbalances."

That's why his workouts are designed for real-world movements, which means performing multidirectional exercises. In addition to doing traditional lunges in a forward direction, you'll do them backward, side to side, and diagonally as well.

Try these changeups to your routine: For each "push" exercise (pushup, shoulder press, or bench press), do an equal number of "pull" moves (row or pullup). If you do steady-state cardio, add intervals. If you run sprints, do hill sprints. If you do hill sprints, try reverse hill sprints, running up a hill backward. The point is to always surprise your body.

One of the hardest multidirectional exercises for me to master—and I still look stupid doing it—is the reverse lunge with a reachover. That is, as you step backward, you twist your torso and reach up and back with both hands. (Always twist toward the side of your forward leg.) The plain-vanilla lunge is a terrific lower-body exercise that targets your quads and glutes. But when you add the twist and reach, it lengthens your hip flexors. These muscles, near the top of your front thighs, are almost always tight because of all the sitting you do at work.

I hated this exercise the first time I tried it, which prompted this observation from Durkin: "If you hate doing something, it means you need it."

DARE TO HAVE FUN

Durkin is always looking for new exercises and tools to add to his workouts—anything that challenges muscles in new ways and teaches the brain to expect the unexpected. He was one of the first adopters of the Bosu balance ball (the half Swiss ball with the plastic base) and the TRX suspension trainer (nylon straps with handles and stirrups that allow you to suspend your hands or feet above the floor). He also loves Superbands and Sport Cords, which may not look like they'll help much—until you use them properly. That's when you notice a bunch of muscles you never knew you had.

"Again, it's about constantly changing things up, keeping your workouts fun, and challenging your muscles," he says.

Try the death crawl: Assume a pushup position as you grip a pair of dumbbells. Do two pushups, two plank rows with your right hand, and two rows with your left. (To perform a row, maintain the pushup position, but bring one elbow up close to your torso as you balance on the dumbbell in your opposite hand.) Now do a walking plank, moving forward several feet by lifting the dumbbells and your feet and taking tiny steps. (You should remain in the up position of the pushup.) Repeat the sequence twice, then do it three times moving backward.

SHATTER YOUR LIMITS

This last one leaves you collapsed in a puddle of yourself—in a good way.

"I love to design my workouts with some grand finale, so you can leave everything behind and empty the tank," Durkin says.

The final drill is brutal, requiring all the mental toughness you can muster. Durkin's goal is to give his athletes an edge. Tomlinson told me that he walks onto the field feeling untouchable after an off-season with Durkin. For the rest of us, there's value in pushing beyond our personal boundaries to achieve something we didn't think we could.

Here's one of Durkin's favorites.

At the end of your workout, do six squat jumps and six lunge jumps (three with each leg, in an alternating fashion). Then, without rest, do seven squat jumps and seven lunge jumps. (Remember which leg did more reps, and start with the opposite leg on the next set.) Keep going until you can't finish a set (or can no longer feel your legs). Durkin says a final set of 10 is good, "but 15 is MVP-worthy. No one said it was easy being great!"

Fuel Your Workouts

What you eat is just as important as how hard you work in the gym.

TD's Preworkout Shake

8 to 12	ounces water
2	scoops protein powder (your favorite flavor)
1	banana
6	ice cubes

Combine all ingredients in a blender. Blend for 30 seconds.

Makes 1 shake

Per serving: 325 calories, 35 g protein, 39 g carbohydrates, 3 g fat, 2 g saturated fat, 3 g fiber, 96 mg sodium

How You Roll

Choose the right equipment when you hit the road—or the trails

Credit Lance Armstrong's decision to stop chasing skirt and hop back on the saddle: Bicycling participation in America picked up with his return a few years back. Mountain biking has seen the greatest boost, with a solid 10 percent, according to a recent Outdoor Foundation survey. Part of the sport's thrill is sleek new road and trail equipment. (That and Lycra, of course.) These rides will make you feel as spirited as you did the day you ditched your training wheels.

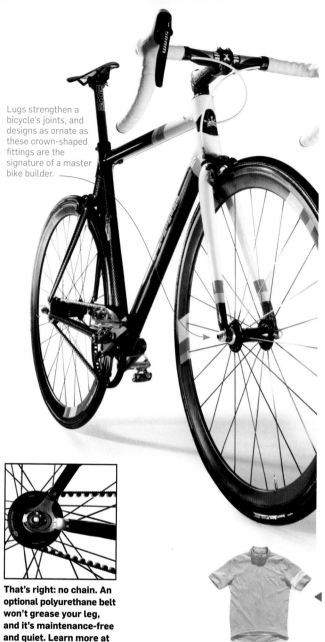

Lugs strengthen a bicycle's joints, and designs as ornate as these crown-shaped fittings are the signature of a master bike builder.

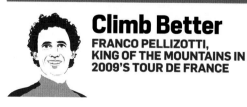

That's right: no chain. An optional polyurethane belt won't grease your leg, and it's maintenance-free and quiet. Learn more at carbondrivesystems.com.

Going Up
Corvid by Independent Fabrication

Few activities challenge your body like riding a bike uphill fast, which requires cardio fitness, core strength, and mental toughness. Well, the Corvid is here to help: Custom-built by exacting craftsmen, its featherweight carbon-fiber frame weighs just 2 pounds. Prepare to climb as effortlessly as a Sherpa at sea level. Order turnaround is a quick 6 to 8 weeks. From **$5,500** (frame and fork), *ifbikes.com*

Budget alternative
Felt Z5: Ride a race-worthy carbon-fiber frame fitted with high-performance Shimano 105 components for better shifting and braking. **$2,000**, *feltbicycles.com*

Instant upgrade
Easton EC90: SL Clincher Carbon fiber wheels help road bikes climb faster, and these hoops stand up to braking almost as well as aluminum ones do. **$1,800**, *eastonbike.com*

Best accessory
Rapha Lightweight jersey: Perfect for a long ride on a spring day, this full-zip top blends soft merino wool with polyester to help you look sharp, even if you're sucking wind. **$175**, *rapha.com*

Climb Better
FRANCO PELLIZOTTI, KING OF THE MOUNTAINS IN 2009'S TOUR DE FRANCE

"To climb fast, you have to stay relaxed. Try to do most of your climb while seated; this requires 5 percent less energy than standing. Keep your cadence at 70 revolutions per minute or higher. If you're feeling tired or the hill turns steeper, shift to a harder gear and stand up for 5 to 30 seconds. Then shift to an easier gear and sit back down."

Riding Around

Crosby by Swobo

Here's a versatile bike: Its wide forks can accommodate fat tires or skinny ones, for dirt or asphalt. Commuters can opt for disc brakes, additional gears, and fenders. It's also an affordable ride for cyclocross, an off-road event of puddles, tight corners, high-speed dismounts, and bunny hops. Participation has more than doubled in 5 years. (For a peek at why, search YouTube for "An hour in hell.") **$1,000**, *swobo.com*

Budget alternative

Linus Roadster Classic: Inspired by French and Italian cinema from the '50s and '60s, this single-speed bike's upright riding position lets you cruise the streets in style. **$390**, *linusbike.com*

Instant upgrade

Hold Fast Foot Retention System: Slide into these fabric foot straps for easier pedaling, or just stomp on them if you're in a hurry. **$55**, *holdfastordie.com*

Best accessory

Cordarounds Bike to Work Pants: Roll up the cuffs and pull out the rear pockets of these office-ready pants—their linings are highly reflective for commuting. **$90**, *cordarounds.com*

With a few turns of a screw, the SRAM Torpedo hub switches from fixed-gear to freewheel.

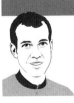

Defy Gravity

JEREMY POWERS, #1 RANKED CYCLOCROSS RIDER OF 2009

"In cyclocross, bunny-hopping the course's 16-inch-high obstacles saves time. Stand on your pedals, grip the handlebar's top section, and pull back. Try to lift your rear tire, or let it tap the barrier. Start 'slow and low' . . . and wear a helmet."

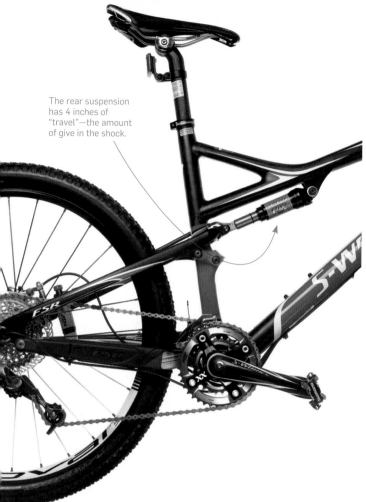

The rear suspension has 4 inches of "travel"—the amount of give in the shock.

The quick-stopping front disc brake will buck you over the bars if you're not careful.

S-Works Epic Carbon Disc by Specialized

The Epic might look brawny, but it has brains to match. Its revolutionary suspension system constantly senses the terrain and your pedaling and adjusts for a smoother, more precise ride. It's the only full-suspension mountain bike to win the Cross Country World Championship. Epic line from **$2,800**; **$8,800** as shown, *specialized.com*

Budget alternative
Kona Dawg: With 5 inches of travel and ace handling, this dual-suspension bike can handle a variety of backcountry terrain. **$1,600**, *konaworld.com*

Instant upgrade
Crank Brothers Joplin 4R: A handlebar remote adjusts the height of the hydraulic seat post. You'll never dismount again. **$285**, *crankbrothers.com*

◄ Best accessory
Take the *Bern Brentwood multisport helmet* on bike trails in summer; in winter, add a liner and take it snowboarding. **$80**, *bernunlimited.com*

Improve Your Cornering

DAVE WIENS, THE MOUNTAIN BIKER WHO BEAT FLOYD LANDIS AND LANCE ARMSTRONG

"Many riders tend to watch the front wheel. Instead, watch the trail ahead. When entering corners, scan the trail for the best possible traction for your front tire—rock, solid earth, or even tree roots. Use that surface to make as much of your turn as you can. The rear tire may wash out, but it'll always follow your lead."

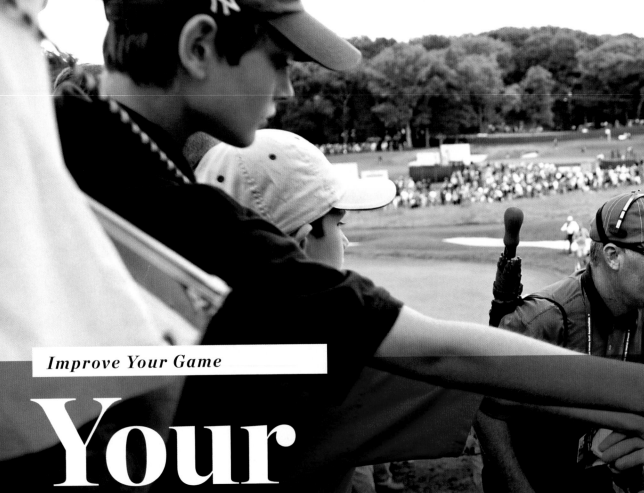

Your Drive, Refocused

Golfer Ricky Barnes went from near-washout to near-champ. His secret?
A change in attitude can change everything.

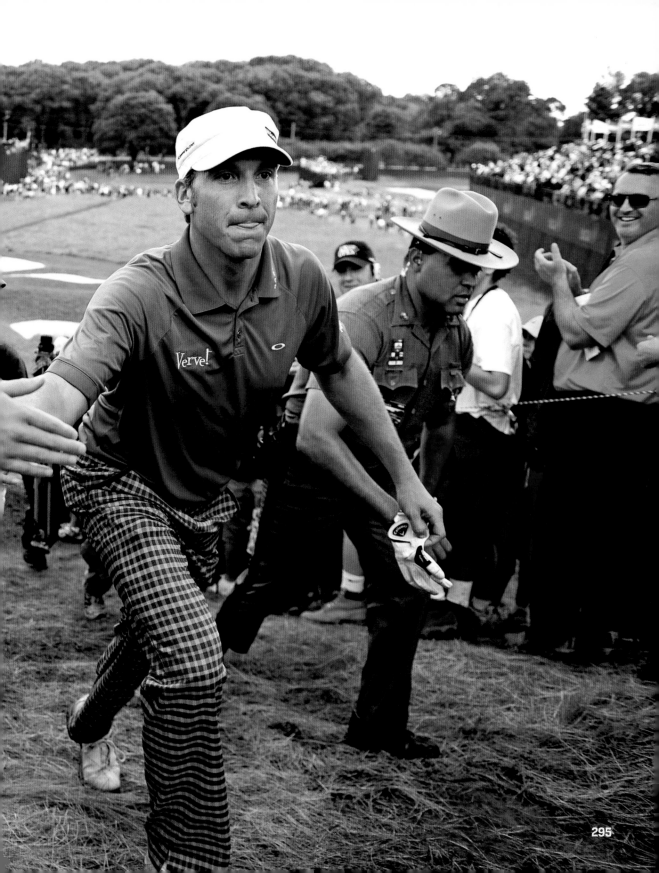

Ricky Barnes once assaulted a tree. He'd missed a few shots in a professional golf tournament, lost his cool, and just cocked his club back and let the tree have it. He had a few choice words for the people around him, too. The organizers fined him for the spectacle, but whatever.

"I've been fined a few times," he says. That was in 2004, at the beginning of a 5-year career stall-out, and Barnes is bad at hiding frustration. Two years earlier, as a junior in college, life had been different. He'd won the U.S. Amateur, earning a spot in the 2003 Masters. As amateur champion, he was paired with the reigning Masters champ, one Tiger Woods. Barnes promptly shot a 3-under-par 69, seven strokes better than Woods. For that glorious weekend, at least, Barnes was the Next Big Thing, an aggressive young man with serious game. The cameras loved him. Fans cheered him. He was exciting.

That's when the trouble began.

"The Masters made me feel as if things would always come easy," he says. "I thought I was better than 90 percent of the guys—that I should almost be handed my PGA Tour card, or that it would just come to me." So he stopped working as hard. Stopped practicing as much. Why bother, when he was so secure?

Shortsighted, egotistical, lazy—and understandable. You've probably done it yourself. You set a goal, reach it, and forget what led you to victory. You start thinking that the secret weapon is you—just you, a complete package, as potent as a neat scotch—and not all the hard work you did before everyone started watching. And because the gleam of success takes time to fade, nobody questions your swagger. Which only makes you swagger more.

Barnes did a lot of that. He shouted and fist-pumped his way through tournaments. He even flexed for the crowd. Of course, this was the Nationwide Tour, pro golf's equivalent of Triple-A baseball. Fans recognized him, though—as that guy from the Masters.

"People were always coming up, offering me deals. In the back of my mind, the last thing I was thinking about was, 'Heck, I'm not even on the PGA Tour.' They almost made me feel like I was."

Then they all disappeared. It was just Barnes and the tree. *Whap.*

He searched for fixes, but they didn't come easy. Then, 3 years ago, Barnes decided to find someone who could tell him, with fresh eyes, what he was doing wrong. So he hired a new coach, who gave it to him straight. And Barnes listened. He remembered that success was earned, not owed.

His game improved. He gained his PGA Tour card. And that summer he was back on national TV, leading the U.S. Open after three rounds over the punishing Bethpage Black course, on Long Island. In the final round, he bogeyed five of his first nine holes and finished second by two strokes. Translation: He pocketed more than half a million dollars. The course's trees lived to breeze another day. And most

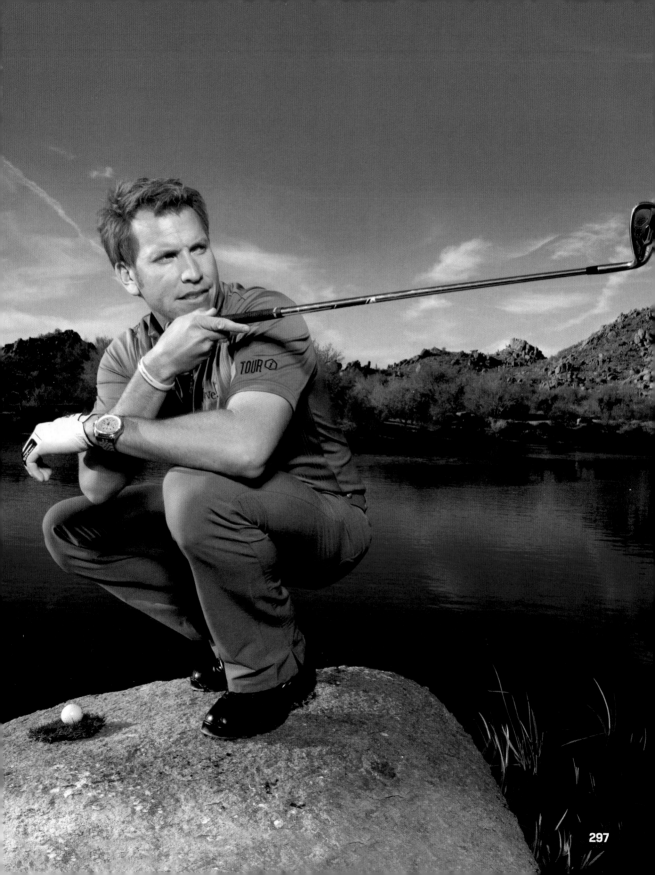

important, he qualified for the Masters.

Barnes is on a hot streak, but now he knows what brought him there, and what he'll have to keep doing if he wants to come back.

For Barnes, it's hard to forget the past. Sounds of "Hey, Ricky, I saw your mom this morning" echo in his memory.

High school's rough as it is, but try adding this indignity: You're a pudgy, 225-pound freshman, and every morning some smart-ass kid tells you he's gawking at your mom. That was Barnes's life. He'd ballooned on years of big meals and bigger desserts, but his parents were fitness buffs. His dad, Bruce, was a punter for the New England Patriots, and his mom ran 6 miles every morning—which in their part of Stockton, California, meant most kids saw her on their way to school. When they'd mention it, Barnes would be reminded of how out of shape he was.

Which, as it turns out, isn't such a bad thing. Needling is helpful. Try it yourself if you need a push: Sign up for a service like the one at textreminders.net and send yourself prompts to hit the gym. Or set a workout schedule with a friend so you can rely on each other for motivation.

By age 16, Barnes was following his parents' lead. He started eating smaller portions and discovered that they left him satisfied. He began a cardio routine in the gym and switched it up every so often so his body wouldn't plateau. By graduation he'd lost 65 pounds.

"Then fitness just became a part of my life," he says.

Need proof that you're stronger than any obstacle? Think back to the last time you felt trapped, and remember that you found a way out. When his career was in the can, Barnes thought about how he'd beat back his weight.

"It helped knowing that I could overcome tough times," he says. Then, step by step, just like before, he figured out what was wrong.

First up: his golf game. Barnes's new coach went through every part of it, to identify flaws and refocus on the fundamentals—because in any job, it's often the little things, the ones nobody praises you for, that matter most. The two men worked their way through the bag, driver to wedge to putter.

"You have to understand yourself—your mentality and your actions. He taught me where my misses were and why I was missing," Barnes says. Only then, once you see the origins of your screwups, are you able to fix them.

Next: Barnes didn't act like other golfers. Some of those guys are dreadfully boring. Fist pumps are about the closest they show to signs of life. Barnes, meanwhile, thought his showiness was part of what made him a success. Attention drove him.

When you're different from the older men around you, you might think you're better—less bound by tradition, fresher with ideas. Says Barnes, "You have to sit back and say, 'Okay, why is he doing what he's doing? I feel like I'm bigger, stronger, more athletic, and more talented, and I'm still not beating him.' "

The answer, he now knows, is that temperament is as important as anything else. Golf, like most endeavors, is about patience and focus. As Barnes watched veterans play, he realized that they never had to stop and refocus. They were always on, even if they always seemed off. That's why they stayed so calm.

It might make for slow television, but why should they care? Like every smart worker, golfers know how to separate the glamour from what matters. They're paid to win, not to entertain. Barnes still shows some emotion; it's part of who he is. "But now when I'm at the ball," he says, "I'm ready to go."

Today, Barnes is standing outside Grayhawk Golf Club, in Scottsdale, Arizona, about to play in a small tournament. With his invite to big tournaments secured, he doesn't really need to be here. But he met with his coach 2 days earlier and they spent hours working on some basics. "So I'm going to go out and compete today," he says. "There's the time to assess your game and your problems, and there's the time to take the test and put it to use."

And if he blows a shot, he'll react differently than he once did. He used to rush to the ball, eager to make up for his mistake. "But I was carrying frustration over— the next shot, the next two shots, the next hole. *How do you miss that shot, Ricky? You question yourself.*"

Then you hit the wall. Or the tree.

So he'll walk more slowly to the ball, consciously pacing his footsteps, buying a few extra minutes to cool down, to reflect, to be like the successful golfers he once looked down on but now looks up to.

And he'll earn whatever comes next.

Work the Angles

Renowned golf instructor Marius Filmalter shows you how to save strokes—with geometry!

MEASURE YOUR ESCAPE

The shot: Out of trouble, under or over a tree limb
The trick: To navigate the branch, step on the clubface of your iron with the shaft pointing in the direction you want the ball to go. The angle of the shaft is a rough gauge of the path of a well-hit shot, says Filmalter. If the path runs smack into a branch, club up or down.

PLAY MORE BREAK

The shot: A putt with a big sweeping break
The trick: To hit the apex point of your putting line, start the ball outside that point. People tend to underread the break, Filmalter says. A putt rarely falls if it skirts the low side of the hole. On the high side, it just might.

TAKE THE RIGHT ANGLE

The shot: Any full swing, from tee or fairway
The trick: Your leading arm stays relatively straight throughout the swing, but your dominant arm should form a 90-degree angle at the top of your backswing, says Filmalter. "You'll create width and generate maximum clubhead speed at impact," he says.

CHIP SMART

The shot: A chip from just off the green
The trick: On a chip from a shaggy lie, the temptation may be to scoop the ball up. Instead, tip the butt end of your wedge toward your leading hip and strike downward, says Filmalter. "You'll deloft the club and create a more controlled chip," he says.

Your Scientifically Enhanced, Can't-Lose Golf Bag

Golf-gear technology changes so quickly you need a physics professor to explain the updates. We found one: Raymond Penner, MSc, a professor of physics and engineering at Vancouver Island University, who happens to study golf. Follow his tips to upgrade your game.

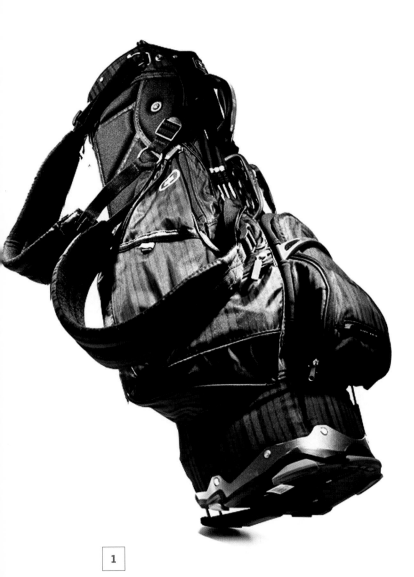

1

Strap Up
Golfers who carry a double-strap bag feel less tired and have lower heart rates than those who carry a single-strap bag, a 2008 *Journal of Strength and Conditioning Research* study notes. Try the Ogio Grom **1** ($220).

Buy MOI
Clubheads with high "moment of inertia" twist less on off-center hits, reducing hook and slice. Nike's Method putter **2** ($250) provides faster forward roll for better accuracy; the Callaway Big Bertha Diablo Hybrid **3** ($140) helps with distance and accuracy in any turf condition.

Go Groovy
The grooves on wedges help maximize ball spin, especially when grass is in the way. (The more spin, the quicker a ball stops.) The TaylorMade TP wedge with xFT **4** ($130) can be refreshed with replaceable faces ($40 each) to give you the teeth of a new club anytime you need it.

Pick a Size
Changing your driver's weight or size may require you to change the timing of your swing, Penner says. So pick a club and learn it. Cleveland's Launcher DST **5** ($300) weighs 25 grams less than the market average, the company says, and is designed to produce a more balanced swing.

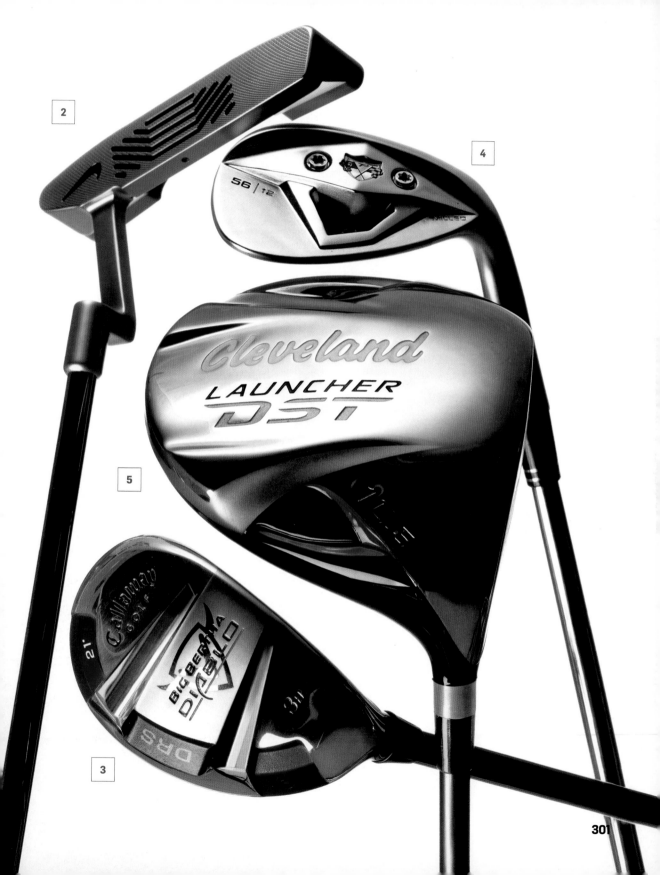

The Revolutionary New Science of Speed

Exercise visionary David Weck developed a theory about
how "spiraling" your arms could make you run faster.
Then Tyson Gay tested that idea and beat Usain Bolt in the 100-meter dash.
Suddenly, people began to take notice. Maybe you should, too.

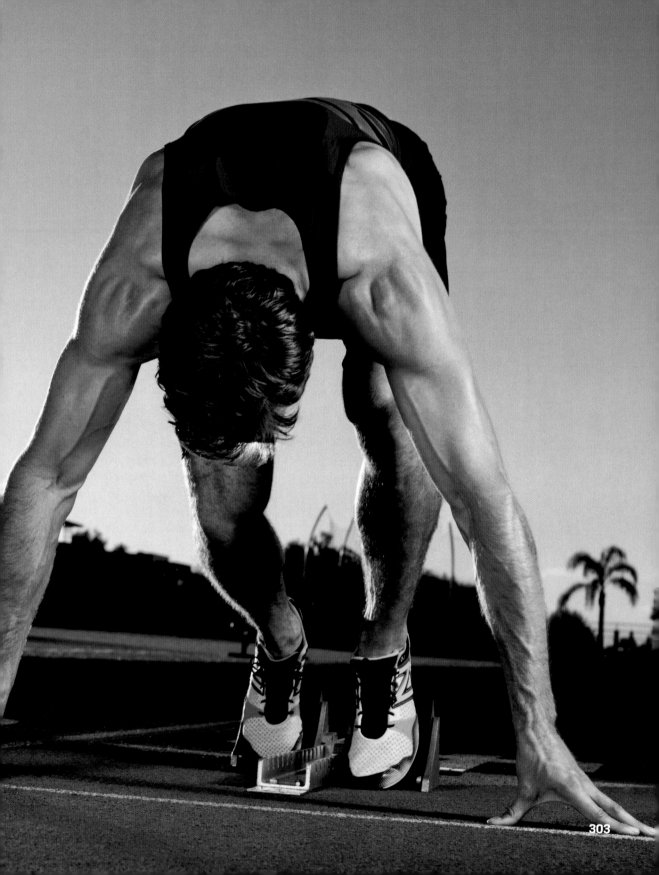

If you study the clip, you can almost freeze-frame the moment in the summer of 2010 when Tyson Gay realized he was about to dust Usain Bolt. Bolt is the fastest man on Earth, a 6′5″ Jamaican who shattered records in the Beijing Olympics and who has owned the 100 and 200 meters ever since. Gay is the fastest American 100-meter runner ever, but he's also a superstar who toils in the shadow of the most awe-inspiring sprinter of all time. They say everyone can be beaten, however, and Bolt's moment arrived just past the 5-second mark during the DN Galan race in Stockholm, when video found his face corkscrewing in frustration while Gay stared ahead wide-eyed with wonder.

Holy shit, he seems to be thinking, *I'm pulling away from Superman.*

But photos of Gay's win captured something else as well—a fleeting quirk of arm movement that could signal a new way of thinking about sprinting, anatomy, balance, and the spillover value of training both sides of the body equally. Side views show Gay's forward hand rotating slightly outward at the wrist, his fingers curling slightly toward the base of the thumb. Exercise geeks call it supinating. His back arm is doing precisely the opposite, though to a lesser extent. It is pronating—rotating slightly inward at the wrist, with the palm facing the rear in a whipping action. His arms are basically making spiral movements.

And here begins a tale of something either very novel or very nutty. You see, winding and unwinding a spring with each swing of your arms is not exactly the norm in track.

"Most sprinters are taught to move their hands from hips to lips, hips to lips, with a simple tomahawk action," says David Weck, the San Diego–based balance-training evangelist who taught Gay how to spiral his arm swings.

Weck believes that spiraling unleashes a little-understood benefit to controlling muscular tension in the fascia. The fascia is the network of tissue that envelops your muscles and organs—and seems to connect them all together as well. Fascia is also key to balance—like muscles and joints, it houses position sensors that tell your brain where your body is in space. Weck believes movements that spiral muscles and fascia might promote greater running efficiency and help keep your body aligned with its gravitational center.

Gay didn't need all this conjecture. He says he found the spiraling idea interesting, which was enough for him to give it a try.

"I'm always looking for new ideas," he says. "I liked the whip action and flip of the wrist; I liked that when I saw him demon-

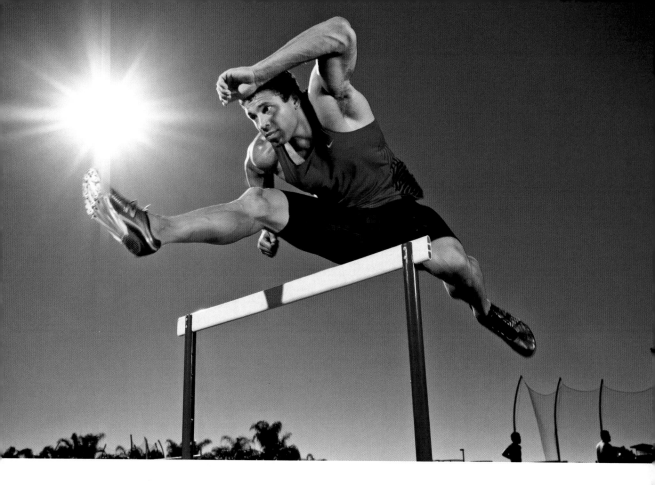

strating it. It was more of a relaxed motion."

We know what you're thinking: There's no shortage of creative types making unusual claims about the best paths to fitness. And it can be tempting to place Weck into that category. But if you look deeply enough into the biomechanics of running and the nature of connective tissue, eventually you'll want to start learning how to spiral.

First, some qualifiers: Gay spiraled only now and then against Bolt. (He was already pretty busy running his ass off.)

"I tried it, but because it was new, my body didn't adapt too fast," he explains. "My right wrist would break but the left wrist didn't do it as well." Plus, it goes without saying that no exercise innovation can take credit for a 9.84 in the 100-meter dash. If it could, we would all be doing that exercise and becoming much, much faster. Finally, Bolt has run a blistering 9.58 in the 100 and will surely dominate the event again on another day.

That said, learning to rotate his hands didn't hurt Gay's season in 2010. Weck notes that since Gay learned to spiral that year, he's run his fastest 200-meter and his fastest 400-meter races, and beaten Usain Bolt in a head-to-head competition. In fact, he ran his best when he was spiraling the most.

"The one race I know for sure he used it was the Great City Games [in May 2010] in Manchester [UK]," says Chase Kough, Gay's strength trainer. "He said he focused on it the second half of the race." In that race, Gay ran a 19.41, breaking a 44-year-old world record for a 200 race with no turns.

By taking up spiraling, Gay bought into something larger than a biomechanical tuneup for the world's fastest men. He joined a small handful of loosely affiliated test subjects hailing from mixed martial arts, Olympic high jumping, the NFL, and Major League Baseball, all working either with Weck or at training sites he has influenced. They share little more than a common willingness to add circular and spiral patterns of the hands, arms, and shoulders to their regimens.

"He's deep, man," says Todd Durkin, CSCS, the owner of Fitness Quest 10 in San Diego and one of the trainers using Weck's ideas. Durkin has trained Drew Brees, Aaron Rodgers, and a dozen MLB pitchers with Weck-designed cross-patterning tasks, rope-tossing tasks, and club-swinging movements. "Dave's always 10 steps ahead of where most people are. You talk about spiraling and he goes back to Michelangelo. It's not just strength training; it's training in three dimensions."

Setting Michelangelo aside for the moment, the value of spiral movement has been recognized in a variety of movement disciplines; it's an idea dating back decades, if not centuries. A well-regarded physical-therapy technique known as proprioceptive neuromuscular facilitation, for instance, first developed by neurophysiologists in the 1940s to treat polio-ravaged muscles, specifically singles out three-dimensional movements of the arms for fostering better integration of large and small muscles. Neurologically, something about the spiral appears to be hardwired into our internal gyroscopes as well, if a 100-year-old insight can be taken as evidence: Tell a blindfolded man to head out in a straight line and he will invariably move in a spiral toward one direction or the other, whether he's walking, running, driving, or swimming. It may be why we "go around in circles" when we're lost in the woods, and it is a trait we share with every moving creature.

Spiral movements were the basis of the club-swinging drills used by the U.S. Army in the early 20th century, an ancient warrior practice that hones primal battle skills and is currently gaining new devotees on the functional-training circuit. Today the drills are promoted as a way to increase integrity of the shoulder girdle and address postural deformities created by our forward-facing, slouching lifestyle. But they are also thought to affect the body the way playing a musical instrument affects the brain; they help write new code in your motor memory.

Spiraling movements are recognized both in tai chi chuan and in native dance

If you look deeply enough into the **biomechanics of running and the nature of connective tissue,** eventually you'll want to start learning how to spiral.

traditions from the South Pacific for their promotion of body harmony and for their mesmerizing aesthetic qualities. They have roots in the sports-science world as well: Biomechanics research suggests that athleticism is a function of passive muscle activation—an energy-harnessing, springlike stiffness in your muscles that occurs before you strike a ball, an object, or the ground—in addition to brute muscular force.

The tendency of muscle to spiral may be rooted in our anatomy. It can be seen in the twisted strands of protein that slide together at the cellular level so muscles can contract and in the way muscles are twisted to attach to and move bones. It's also seen in the way some of the largest muscles wind in pathways connecting the front of your body to your back and even your opposite side.

"There's always a relationship in biomechanics between one shoulder and the opposite-side hip," says Michol Dalcourt, an adjunct professor of sports science at the University of San Francisco. "The anatomy of the human lower body spirals as well. For example, my dog doesn't have a talus bone in his foot, but I do. With every step, the talus rotates down and in; it's there to allow a spiral action to take place in my lower limbs. It does that because rotating your bones is the most energy-efficient way to move while upright on two legs."

A 40-year-old fitness entrepreneur and student of movement, Weck believes spiraling movements "tell us the truth" about our proprioceptive and essential movement skills, especially when you use them to manipulate simple "feedback tools," as he calls them. (You or I would call them balls, ropes, and sticks.) In this view, learning to anchor your body while moving a heavy rope in a "weaponizing" pattern, for instance—a rhythmic figure 8 not unlike the movement required of early man using a strap and a rock to take down prey—is just one of many essential object-manipulation tasks we have evolved to carry out. This is why you can include Weck among proponents of an emerging, loosely knit fitness movement that's turning its focus away from the cardio/muscle dichotomy and toward "primal movements" and body control. This movement includes the callused-foot enthusiasts promoting barefoot running; the back-to-nature programs like Erwin Le Corre's Methode Naturelle or Frank Forencich's Exuberant Animal; and even establishment organizations like NASA and the U.S. military, who design physical training around movement. Spiraling fits into the emerging fitness idea of our time: Our bodies have built-in strengths and tendencies. Exercise should take advantage of them.

We probably wouldn't be talking about any of this, however, were it not for the fact that Weck invented something seemingly nonessential—the Bosu ball, that blue half-orb you'll find mounted on plastic at your gym. It has become the go-to tool for proprioceptive training. It took the risk out of vertical "core" stabilization work using physio balls (a Bosu ball can't go squirting out from under your feet) and opened the door for widespread balance training while upright on two

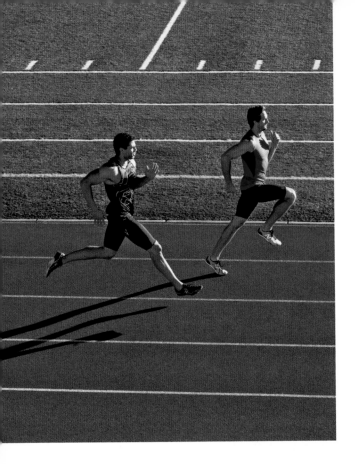

feet. But its inventor hardly fits the mold of the million-selling training-gizmo titan—you know, the guy hawking his wares on QVC. For one thing, Weck's product came about by accident.

As a struggling actor and fitness trainer during the early 1990s, Weck spent 3 years scooting around New York on inline skates—and doing no other form of exercise. Weck believes this weakened his feet. Research has shown that the greater the barrier between your foot and the ground, the less your body must work to reduce impact forces—through midfoot striking, hip/knee/ankle coordination, and so-called "eccentric" or force-absorbing muscular lengthening.

"One day I took off my shoes for a walk on a rocky shore in France," he remembers. "The pain was so bad I had to crawl off the beach." Obsessed with strengthening his feet, Weck took to standing on physio balls, then jumping on them. You can imagine how this story ends: Our hero crashes into the coffee table. But where you and I would break out an ice pack and tear open a bag of Combos, Weck stared at his ceiling and had a million-dollar idea.

"That night I lay in bed and thought, *What if I cut the ball in half?*" he says.

Ten years and more than a million Bosu balls later, Weck is renting an elegant but slightly tattered turn-of-the-century Tudor on a hill overlooking San Diego Harbor. His success has given him the gift of time, and he has used that freedom to experiment with new takes on some very old ideas about the body. His home has Arts and Crafts details and a chapel-like dining room, but at this stage in his life he appears to have little interest in dinner parties. The place is a monastery for the study of movement in the vertical position.

He has furnished his home with only a standing desk, assorted piles of anatomical reference books, and a bust of Michelangelo's *David*—and everywhere else you'll find only mats, ropes, athletic sticks and balls, and other smooth spheres. Except for a small kitchen set, he appears to own no couches, chairs, or benches, and he didn't sit, lean, or so much as shift his weight to one leg.

He is given to nonstop movement and enthusiastic statements about movement, gripping the ground with his toes while extrapolating on efficiency in staccato bursts. He often bounds across a room to demonstrate. He is enamored with the feeling of being upright—he wears "barefoot shoes," and for fun he takes those off and works while standing in a pan filled with river rocks. (He likes to turn his feet around the pan in slow, counterclockwise circles, engaging the far corners of his metatarsals.)

"Being vertical is a very good thing," he says. "As a kid, I once fell asleep standing up."

Weck believes in an arm swing that turns outward as the arm moves forward, and inward as the arm moves back. The arms stay close to your sides, and the fingers wrap tightly at the top—and then unwrap and extend at the bottom. His explanation for this seemingly trivial instruction—after all, how could cork-screwing your hands and fingers have any effect on your running speed?—is based on the supposed downstream effects of tightening one long network of connective tissue known as fascia. One example of fascia is the opaque membrane covering a chicken breast when you peel back the skin. You probably don't give it much thought when you eat meat, and early anatomists ignored it as well. But if anything is clear about physiology, it is that the body doesn't waste materials.

"Bending and internally rotating your wrist with your fingers spread uncoils the spring," says Weck. "Your connective tissue is a unitary structure spanning the body, so what happens at your hands impacts what happens everywhere else."

You can imagine the fascia, in this view, like a chain-link fence. If it's loose, a pull on one end has to take up the slack before that pull causes movement at the farthest point. If that chain-link fence is purposely pulled tight, however, as fascia is with spiraling, movement on one end will be transmitted through its entire length without delay.

"It is absolutely true that movement of the arms when you run will have an effect on the fascial bag, and it's all one fascial bag," says Thomas Myers, author of *Anatomy Trains,* a book dedicated to the subject. Myers calls fascia a "bag" because he has dissected enough of the stuff to view the interlocking bands of tissue as nothing more than the sack that holds us together. Like Weck, he believes subtle movements of our fingers may play a role in how precisely our legs move, because of the networks of fascia and nerves that link them.

"Just look at someone punting a football," says Myers. "You will see the person's fingers usually in very precise positions. Splinting two fingers together could change how the foot strikes the ball, and that could change the direction of a punt." To understand this strange connection, try running with your hands open. "Fascia absorbs and distributes biomechanical

Athleticism is a function of passive muscle activation— a springlike stiffness in your muscles that occurs before you strike a ball, an object, or the ground.

forces," Myers says. So even though your hands are far removed from your hips and legs, he says, running with them open will tire out your legs and back sooner than running with them closed will.

But you don't have to be a fervent believer in the all-powerful actions of fascia to see a potential biomechanical benefit in spiraling your arms. The movements also seem capable of translating to changes in what is happening in your back and hips. "If you pronate your hand while it's back, you help your hip flex on that side, which is what is happening when your arm is at the back of the swing," says Weck. "It will lead to the internal rotation of the upper arm, and the 'recoil,' for lack of a better term, of your lats, biceps, and pecs as they prepare to help bring the arm forward again."

Here Weck has some supporters in his argument. "Rotating your arm outward at the top of your swing is in fact going to stretch your lats," says the University of San Francisco's Dalcourt. "Your lats are on your back, but they connect to the front of your arm. Why are we set up this way? One reason is that lifting and externally rotating your palm stretches the muscle and helps create potential energy. Also, your lats blend in with and lift your pelvis." All of which is why Weck believes supinating your arm enables your opposite-side hip to rise more easily, while pronating your arm enables your near-side hip to rise more easily.

To understand why any of that would matter, it helps to break down some surprising new findings about the biomechanics of running. As the Dutch speed coach Frans Bosch explains, running is primarily an up-and-down event. "The direct force of the push-off is mainly vertical," he says. "It is seven times greater than the force propelling the runner forward." But don't take that as an endorsement of spiraling. "Arm rotation probably has no influence on whether the hip rises," Bosch says. "There is a relationship between arm swing and leg motion, but it is not as rigid as proposed in this particular argument."

The jury may be out on the science of spiraling, but after countless slow-motion viewings of the tapes of Tyson Gay running, Weck can only tell you what he sees with his own two eyes. While Gay's right hand is supinating, his left foot hits the ground "square and plumb," says Weck. "His foot is not traveling backward in the air before it strikes the ground," he says. "It hits the ground, and boom!"

If you like the idea of spiraling but find the thought of honing your sprint technique less than urgent, you might like this next part. You don't have to sprint to spiral. Spiraling movements with simple tools—a basketball, a heavy jump rope, or

Subtle movements of our fingers may play a role in how precisely our legs move, because of the networks of fascia and nerves that link them.

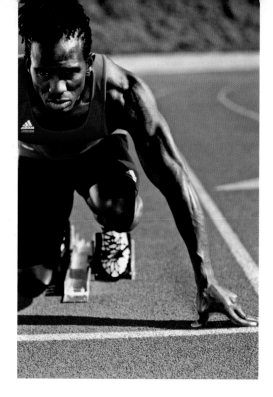

a hockey stick—are some of the most deceptively challenging tasks. If you add these movements to your workout, you'll learn to maintain your gravitational center while moving loads with your shoulders, arms, and hands—tasks we have evolved to master.

Sporting goods today—balls, sticks, and ropes—can reconnect us with our ancestors' success as bipedal beings. They treat your shoulder, elbow, and wrist in a way that seems closer to their intended purpose—as an integrated object-manipulation system. Simultaneous spiral movements in three joints makes the way we normally train our arms (triceps kickbacks, anyone?) seem uninspired, almost small-minded. In the gym we tend to use our arms as simple levers. Spiral movements work our limbs in three dimensions, fluidly flexing, extending, and rotating.

Moreover, these movements inevitably promote efficiency, by returning your hands to where they started without ever once having to reverse course. At the top-out of a bench press, for example, you are required to stop producing force and begin reducing force as you lower the bar. With spirals—figure 8 patterns with balls and ropes and sticks that return to their starting point with every cycle—the moment when you stop "pushing the bar" never arrives.

Weck first took to his passion for the spiral after thinking about the biblical David. "He beat a guy who was unbeatable," Weck says. He's talking about using a simple sling to take down a giant, but he could have been talking about Tyson Gay. Maybe he was. "He did it in a very unconventional manner, and it's an emotional toehold on that story."

"Sticks, stones, and rope—things you can find in a pure form in nature without having to machine their parts—are the quintessential tools that enabled us to harness our bodies so we could succeed on two feet," says Weck. "The human strategy is to create vertical potential. We stand upright and erect. When we let go of the branch, we freed our hands to manipulate our environment, and it was object manipulations that educated our bodies, and it was hunting and tools that passed our genes forward. We are the most effective large predator on the planet, all because of our tools."

But to use these tools, you have to use the movement, infinite, primal, and timeless, that gives them their power. It gives you your power as well—spiraling upward.

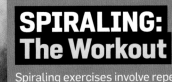

SPIRALING:
The Workout

Spiraling exercises involve repeatedly moving a simple object through space in a rotating trajectory—in other words, some form of corkscrewing, figure 8, or loop-the-loop pattern. They sharpen the capacity of your shoulders, elbows, and wrists to supinate and pronate i n coordinated succession. They also help you gain a greater sense of your gravitational center and enhance your ability to fluidly manipulate objects at arm's length. These exercises have no loads, so you can do them every day, intermittently during a workout. You may be surprised to discover that your body can become smarter at these tasks after you take a break to do something else.

"This isn't the meat and potatoes of a workout," says motion visionary David Weck. "It's more like the salt and pepper that gives it flavor." Sprinkle these in as "breaks" in your routine.

Single-Hand Figure 8

Stand tall and bend your right arm 90 degrees while making a tight fist. Moving from left to right, draw a horizontal figure 8, keeping your elbow slightly bent and your hands between your waist and shoulders. As you move your hand across your body to the left, your palm should be slightly rotated and facing the ground. When you change direction to the right, rotate your palm so it's facing up. When this pattern feels comfortable, hold both handles of a jump rope in one hand and perform the movement. The rope should hit with the ground between your feet. Do all reps, then switch sides.

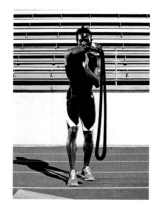 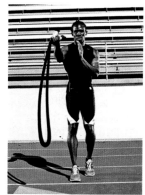

Race and Chase

Stand tall with your feet shoulder-width apart. Grab a jump-rope handle in each hand, and cross your right wrist over your left. Perform the same movement as the single-hand figure 8, but alternate snapping the rope about 6 to 12 inches in front of and outside your left and right foot (instead of between your feet). Make sure you keep your wrists crossed at all times. As the rope moves in front of your right foot, your right wrist should be turned outward and your left wrist facing inward. As you change direction, the angle of your wrists should alternate. Continue this pattern and try to establish a rhythm.

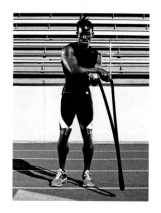 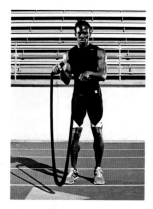

Swim Pattern

Perform the same movement used with race and chase. But after the rope makes contact with the ground in front of your left foot, change your hand positioning so that your left hand is on top of your right hand. Then, when you strike the ground in front of your right foot, change your hand positioning so your right wrist is on top again. The idea is that by alternating your hands, your wrists and forearms take turns rotating upward and downward on both sides of your body. (Rope strikes can hurt for all rope drills you might do. Keep the rope away from your toes and the exercise area clear of other people.)

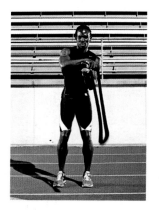 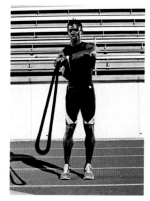

Heaven's Twirl

Hold a 4-foot pole horizontally with an overhand grip in front of your body. Your arms should be bent at 90 degrees, with your hands about 6 inches apart. Rotate your torso to the right and then press down with your left hand so that the right end of the stick rises up slightly, toward your right shoulder. Then cross your right arm over your left as your left arm remains in place. Push down slightly on the right end of the stick so that the left end rises up slightly behind your right shoulder. Twist to the left and press the left end down, and rotate back to the starting position. Repeat this in a fluid motion.

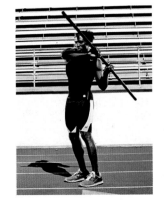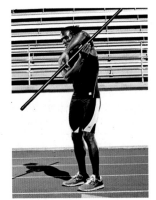

Earth's Twirl

Hold the pole as you did with the heaven's twirl. As you rotate your torso to the right, press upward with your left hand so that the right end points slightly down toward the ground. Then cross your right arm underneath your left, and press upward with the right end of the stick. Immediately rotate to the left, and raise the left end of the stick and bring the right end of the stick diagonally to your torso. Repeat the movement, this time moving from left to right. Continue this pattern to create a fluid motion.

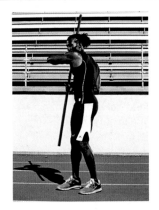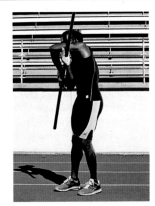

Vertical Ball Spiral

Stand tall with your arms at your sides and hold a basketball in your right hand with your palm facing backward. Pull the ball up toward your armpit by raising your elbow. Continue this movement until your shoulder nearly touches your ear. Then rotate your wrist clockwise so that your fingers are pointing forward. Continue to lift the ball and press it overhead while continuing to rotate your wrist. When your arm is extended, the ball should sit in the palm of your hand with your fingers pointing backward. Reverse the movement and return to the starting position. Do all your reps, then switch arms.

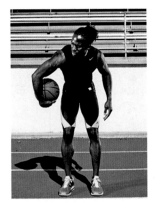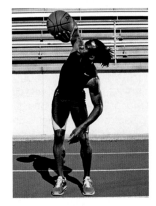

Lateral Ball-Control Drill

Hold a basketball in your right hand with your palm facing up and your arm extended out to your side. In one fast movement, slightly dip your hips and rotate your palm and shoulder counterclockwise. Your palm should remain underneath the ball throughout the movement. Finish the movement with your arm still straight, your hand rotated, and your palm facing upward. Then repeat the motion in reverse. Once you become comfortable performing the drill with one arm, try it with both arms at the same time. Work on speeding up the movement and challenging your body with heavier balls.

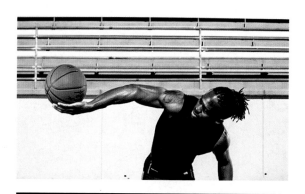 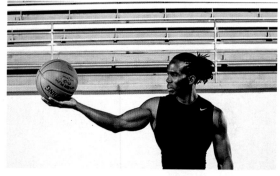

If you add these movements to your workout, you'll learn to maintain your gravitational center while moving loads with your shoulders, arms, and hands—tasks we have evolved to master.

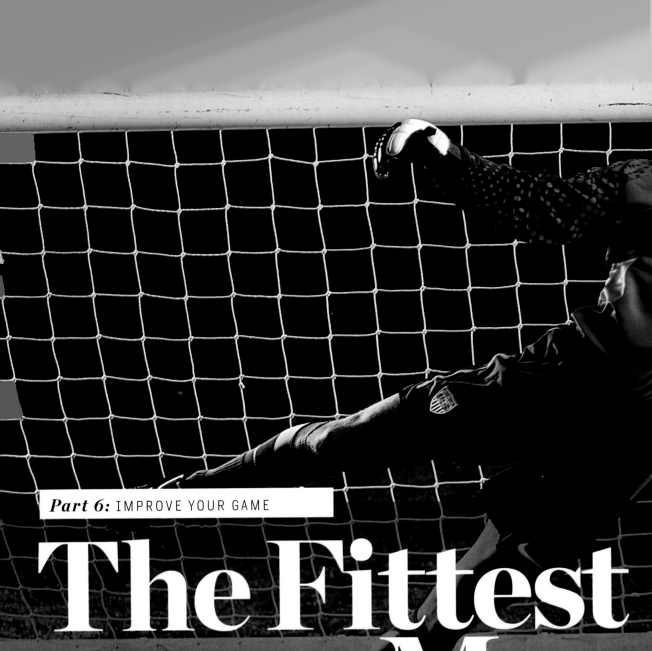

The Fittest Men

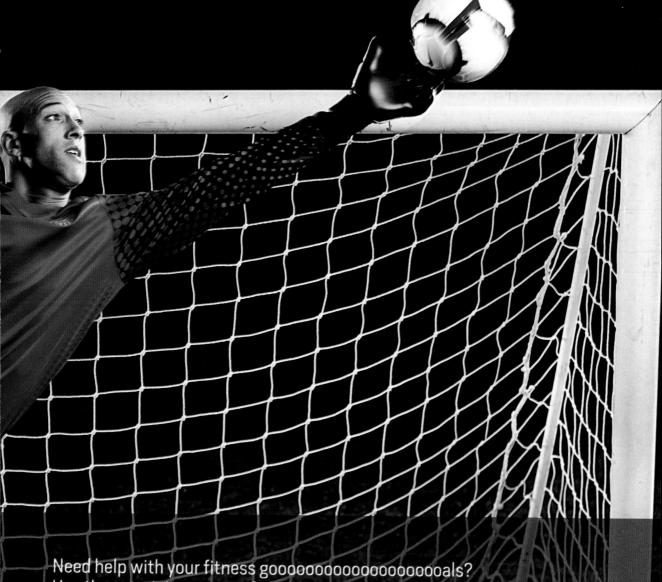

Need help with your fitness gooooooooooooooooooooals?
Use these training secrets from elite soccer players to build strength,
speed, endurance, and agility

on Earth

The World Cup is, for 95 percent of the globe, something like the Super Bowl, the Summer Olympics, and Mardi Gras rolled into one giant foot-stomping, hand-clapping, flag-waving fiesta. For the better part of a month, this quadrennial tournament fuels parties and clears cubicles as fans of the 32 participant nations sing, dance, and get day-drunk in the name of national pride. We in the United States are late to the party. We were raised to dismiss soccer as some foreign trifle that encourages tie scores and rewards theatrical turf dives at a whisper of contact. But a funny thing happened as the U.S. national team started to gain international respect. In 2009, it beat the world's number-one squad, Spain, and has since risen in the world rankings. By the 2010 Cup, in South Africa, the team had developed into a power that deserved to share the field with England, its first opponent that summer.

With success, more Americans began to pay attention. And they began to see soccer players at this level for what they are: arguably the best all-around athletes on the planet. First consider the talent pool, says Pierre Barrieu, fitness coach for the U.S. men's national team.

"In most countries, soccer is the number-one sport. Imagine if all the athletes in the NFL, the NBA, the NHL, and MLB played soccer. That's who we're competing against—the best of the best from around the world."

And then there's this: In no other sport do men run for so long, at such intensity, with so little rest, all the while being asked to excel at so many things: sprinting, jumping, cutting, tackling, and, of course, dribbling a slippery round ball with such skill that it seems to be teth-ered to their feet by a string.

"Soccer players are the world champions of intermittent exercise," says Peter Krustrup, PhD, an associate professor of exercise and sport sciences at the University of Copenhagen. "It's the combination of intense interval exercise with various activities requiring cardiovascular fitness and muscle strength. Elite soccer players have extraordinary intermittent exercise ability, high sprinting and jumping ability, and high endurance." They're strong, too: Norwegian research reveals that top soccer players can typically squat 440 pounds.

Dr. Krustrup says he and his colleagues have observed a 20 to 40 percent drop-off in performance between the first 15 minutes of a game and the final 15 minutes. "Soccer players become

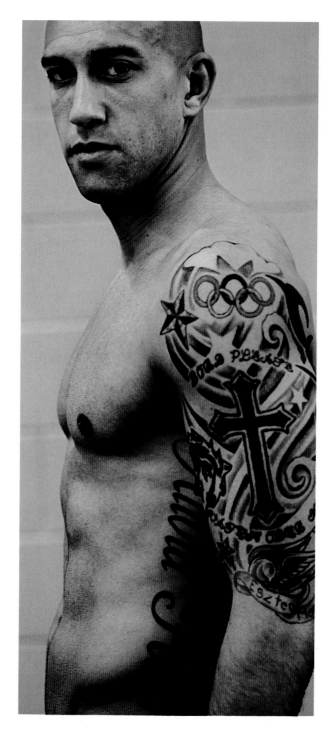

"Adding boxing to my workouts has made me a better, more confident athlete."
—Tim Howard, national team goalkeeper

fatigued," he says, which means that often the fitter team wins. That's good news for the United States. Our national team might not be the world's most talented (that's Brazil, Argentina, or Spain), but you'd be hard-pressed to find any team in better shape, according to various trainers interviewed for this story. On the following pages, take a closer look at four U.S. team members who will make us all proud to wear red, white, and blue. Each personifies a component of fitness—agility, endurance, speed, and strength—that can be systematically improved. Use their strategies to work yourself into world-class shape.

AGILITY
The Game Changer: Tim Howard

A sweetly hit free kick in soccer can hurtle through the air at 80 miles an hour. At that speed, the 16-ounce leather projectile strikes with about 5,000 pounds of force.

"It's like supporting an SUV on your abs for a thousandth of a second," says Louis Bloomfield, PhD, a professor of physics at the University of Virginia. Tim Howard's job as goalkeeper is to react instantly to catch or block these cannonballs. The 6'3", 210-pound Howard plays in England's Premier League. The 32-year-old is on top of his game. "I'm constantly strengthening my core, because that's what gives me the ability to react faster and the stability to control my body better."

Howard's training focuses on speed, balance, and range of motion. "Tim has to be able to shift his body weight and throw himself in any direction, without any preparation," says Steve Tashjian, fitness coach for Everton FC, Howard's club team. His agility workouts combine explosive lifting, core exercises, jumping drills (with a tether device called a Verti-Max, which allows him to jump against resistance), and boxing. "Sparring accelerates my hand speed, improves my footwork, and makes my punching more powerful," says Howard. (The goalkeeper often has to punch the ball away on corner and free kicks.) Howard alternates 60-second rounds of throwing jabs and combinations with

defensive drills, during which he blocks punches with hand pads. Agility training speeds up your reaction time and fine-tunes body control, says Tashjian, skills that give you an advantage in any sport.

ACHIEVE WORLD-CLASS AGILITY

Jump-start power. Howard can bang out 30-inch box jumps, but Tashjian recommends starting with a 12-inch box. Stand behind and to the right of the box, jump laterally to your left, and then jump straight onto the box. Step down and return to the starting position. Do a total of 5 reps from the right side, then 5 reps from the left. That's 1 set; do 3 sets with 30 seconds rest between each. Do this just after your warmup, 3 times a week.

Chop your core into shape. Howard uses chops to train his core, including the 4-way x-chop. Start in a split-squat stance, with your right leg forward and right knee slightly bent. Hold a dumbbell with both hands to your left side. Explode out of the squat, and rotate to lift the weight up to your right shoulder. Then reverse the movement and return to the starting position. Do 8 reps. Now switch sides with the dumbbell but keep your right leg forward and do 8 more reps. Then put your left leg forward and do 8 reps on each side. That's 1 set. Use a weight that allows you to complete 2 sets without losing form.

Fancy up your footwork. Mark off five 2-foot squares, like a ladder. Then…

1. With both feet, jump as fast as you can sideways into every square.
2. Jump as fast as you can sideways 2 squares left, then 2 squares right.

AGILITY: The Self-Test

The men's national team relies on a seven-part functional-movement exam, but you can use the simple T-test, says Steve Tashjian, fitness coach for Everton FC, Howard's club team. Set up markers in a T configuration, 10 yards for the stem and 5 yards out to each side. Ask a friend to time you. Start at the base of the T, sprint to the top, side-shuffle to the left, side-shuffle all the way (10 yards) to the right, side-shuffle back to the middle, and backpedal to the start. Howard does it in 9.6 seconds.

AVERAGE GUY: 12+ seconds

GREAT: 10 to 12 seconds

WORLD CLASS: Under 10 seconds

Peak Performance Tip

PADDLE YOUR WAY TO A POWERFUL CORE. In the off-season, Howard rows in the gym or kayaks on lakes near his home in Memphis, Tennessee. "It's a great aerobic workout," he says. "Plus it works my core. My goal is to always strengthen my core." When kayaking, keep your arms straight and twist your torso to generate maximum power.

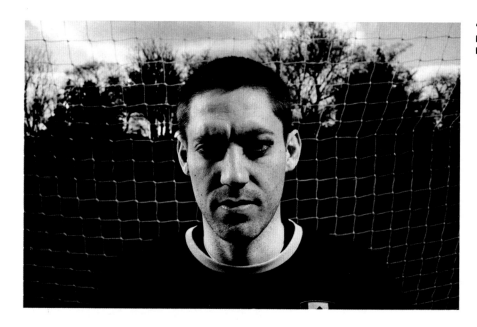

3. Slalom: Jump into a square from the side, jump forward 2 squares, and then jump out. Then reverse: Jump in, back 2 squares, and out.

4. Crossovers: From the left of the ladder's base, cross your left foot over your right as you step into square 1. Step to the right with your right foot and follow with your left out of square 1. Cross your right foot over the left and step into square 2, repeating the sequence up the ladder and then down the ladder.

Do 3 to 5 reps of each drill, with 30 seconds rest between each set.

ENDURANCE

The Deciding Factor: Clint Dempsey

After the first round of the 2009 Confederations Cup, which gathered eight of the world's top teams in South Africa, the U.S. team's trainers pulled the results of video tracking that followed every footstep of every player. One result stood out: Out of nearly 200 players, the top three runners who covered the most ground were all Americans. In a typical game, the data showed, they ran almost 8 miles. They were also all midfielders. Number two on that list, just behind his teammate Michael Bradley, was Clint Dempsey, who stars on Fulham FC, a team in the English Premier League.

"Stats don't lie," says the 28-year-old Dempsey. "That gives you an idea of the work going into every game."

Midfielders occupy the central portion of a soccer team's formation; they play both offense and defense, so their territory is the entire field. In truth, a tireless midfielder like the 6'1", 170-pound Dempsey isn't really ever at rest.

Running in soccer is interval-based,

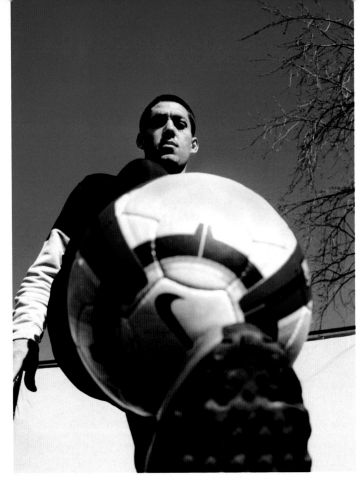

says Scott Piri, director of soccer for Athletes' Performance, which oversees fitness for the U.S. men's team, the German national team, and several pro teams. "Midfielders mix jogging, running, high-speed running, and sprinting," says Piri. Jogging is 40 to 60 percent of your maximum effort, running is 60 to 80 percent, high-intensity running is 80 to 95 percent, and sprinting is all-out.

What's more, elite players typically perform 1,000 to 1,400 short activities per game, changing every 4 to 6 seconds, according to a review in *Sports Medicine*. Along with running, this includes about 50 activities with the ball, 30 passes, 15 tackles, and 10 headers. Players also sustain forceful contractions to maintain balance and control against defensive pressure. To achieve this level of fitness requires a combination of running drills and body-strength exercises to build muscular endurance.

"My competitiveness pushes me," says Dempsey. "That's where I gain my edge—the willingness to push myself. If you're not doing it, someone else will." Dempsey has made it a priority to improve his endurance.

"Clint's not a freak born with incredible running ability," says Barrieu, the national team fitness coach. "He's worked a lot on his running because he knows he needs it to play at his best." There's a special payoff to having gas left in the tank. "You see most goals scored in the final 15 minutes of a game," says Piri. "You've been running for 75 minutes, and the question is, Can you still run hard?"

BUILD WORLD-CLASS ENDURANCE

Forge speed stamina. Doing four 4-minute incline-running intervals twice a week at 90 to 95 percent of maximum heart rate—with 3 minutes easy jogging between each interval—improves cardiovascular fitness by half a percent each session, according to Norwegian research.

(Think of the cumulative effect!) A recreational athlete can benefit from similar training, but at lesser intensity. Piri recommends starting out with five 15-second, 110-meter sprints with 30 seconds active recovery, twice a week. As you become fitter, gradually extend the number of reps and the length of the sprint, and reduce the recovery time.

Extend muscle endurance. Piri recommends adding this mini-circuit to your workout three times a week. Do 1 set of each exercise with 30 seconds rest. For complete descriptions, see MensHealth.com/worldcup.

Plank with arm lift: Assume a pushup position but with your forearms firmly on the ground. Lift your right arm up and slightly to the right and hold for 2 seconds. Return to the starting position and repeat with your left arm. Complete 5 to 10 reps on each side.

Marching lateral plank: Lie on your left side with your legs straight and your body in a straight line propped on your left foream. Lift your bottom knee to your chest, hold for 2 seconds, and return. Lift your top knee to your chest, hold for 2 seconds, and return. That's 1 rep. Do 5 to 10 reps. Switch sides.

Marching hip raise: Lie faceup with your arms at your sides, knees bent, and heels on the ground. Lift your hips until your knees, hips, and shoulders form a straight line. Hold the position while lifting your right knee to your chest. Return your foot to the ground and repeat with your left knee. That's 1 rep. Complete 5 to 10 reps on each side.

Build your foundation. To make running more interesting and to quicken your gains, do a fartlek workout once a week, says Piri. *Fartlek* is Swedish for "speed play" and involves 30 minutes of running. Within that session, you sprint when you feel great, run when you feel good, and jog when you're panting. The key is to listen to your body and push yourself by creating your own impromptu interval workout.

SPEED

The Secret Edge: Jozy Altidore

U.S. soccer doesn't have many defining moments, but one transpired in 2009 when the men's team faced top-ranked Spain. The score was tied 0-0 when a U.S. player passed the ball to his teammate, striker Jozy Altidore, who was near the top of Spain's penalty area. First Altidore used his leg strength and body control to hold off his defender. Then as the ball

---

ENDURANCE: The Self-Test

You can run around a track or use a treadmill for this test from German national team fitness coach Shad Forsythe. Run at the fastest pace you can maintain for 4 minutes; note your distance. Jog slowly for 3 minutes. Do this a total of three times. The average distance you cover at your fastest is your score.

AVERAGE: 0.4 mile

GREAT: 0.6 mile

WORLD CLASS: 0.8 mile

Peak Performance Tip

SWIM. "I try to swim for 30 minutes the day after every game," says Dempsey. "It's a great way to exercise and boost circulation without putting pressure on your joints."

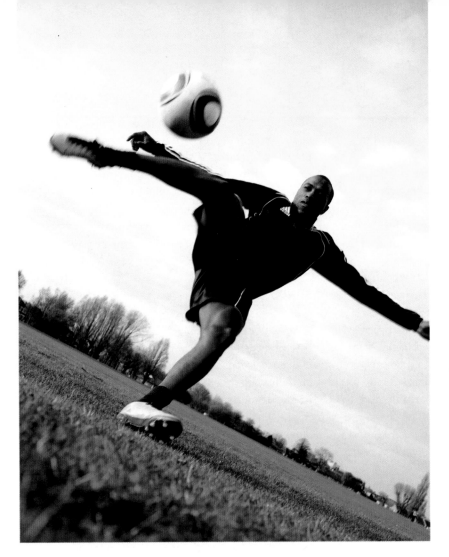

to contain, whether it's on the ground or through the air."

It's the 6'2", 190-pound Altidore's bursts of speed that give him an edge. He followed a strict strength program to reach that level, Barrieu says. To develop greater explosiveness, Altidore does sprinting exercises while wearing a Bullet Belt, a harness that allows him to run with resistance.

"By doing drills that overload the acceleration phase, you train the muscles to be stronger and the nerves to fire faster," says Piri. The aim is not necessarily bigger muscles, but faster-reacting ones. It's the difference between brute strength and explosive power.

"I need only one step," says Altidore. "One step—that yard of space—and bang!"

HONE WORLD-CLASS SPEED

Ignite your thrusters. "If a muscle is tight, it functions on only half its length, so you're producing half the force," says Barrieu. "If you become more flexible and

rolled past, he turned and, with only that slightest gap, exploded into the box and drilled the ball past the keeper for a goal that helped the Americans pull off what was dubbed the Miracle on Grass.

"That goal was just a sign of what's to come," says Altidore, who plays for the Villarreal club in the Spanish League.

This was certainly evidence that the 20-year-old New Jersey phenom, whose nickname is Juice, has the potential to become America's first world-class striker. Piri says Altidore "can run through you, past you, and around you. Jozy's a monster use 100 percent of your leg muscles, then your thrust will be better." The U.S. team's warmup consists of 20 exercises performed consecutively, down and back over 15 yards. Barrieu streamlined it to serve as a warmup for any sport: high knees, butt kicks, single-leg hops, back-pedals, carioca, dynamic and reverse lunges, A and B skips, dynamic abductions and adductions, forward and backward jumps, and lateral bounds. To watch a video of this warmup, visit MensHealth.com/worldcup.

Accelerate and brake faster. Doing intervals with 180-degree turns works muscle harder than doing regular intervals, according to a French study in the

Journal of Strength and Conditioning Research. Pros do 30-second intervals, but Piri recommends shorter ones. Set up three cones 5 yards apart. Sprint to the second cone, touch it, and sprint back to the starting cone and touch it; repeat the sequence to the third cone, and then to the second one again. That's 1 rep. Start with 5 reps with 30 seconds rest, and work up to 10 reps. Add this into all your workouts, says Piri. "As long as you do it as fast as you can, this is going to help first-step quickness and speed."

Push your speed. If you don't have a trainer handy to hold a Bullet Belt harness, you can achieve the same results while pushing against a wall, says German fitness coach Shad Forsythe. With your hands flat against a wall, straighten your arms so your body is 45 degrees to the wall. Raise your right knee to your chest in an explosive marchlike movement, then your left knee. Do 2 sets of 20 reps on each side. Next connect three steps in a running motion—right, left, right—as fast as you can. (You should end up standing on your left foot with your right knee raised.) Aim for 3 to 5 reps on each side. Do this exercise three times a week.

STRENGTH

The Essential Force: Oguchi Onyewu

No American player has a more stressful time in a game than Oguchi Onyewu, the U.S. team's central defender, who goes by the nickname Gooch. Every game, the 6'4", 210-pounder is responsible for muzzling the opposing team's best scorer.

SPEED: The Self-Test

Although some soccer teams still test speed using 5-to-15-yard sprints, a repeated sprint test is better, says Ermanno Rampinini, head of Italy's Mapei Human Performance Lab. This is a modified version of the speed test he uses on pros. (You'll need a stopwatch.) Mark out 20 yards on a field. Sprint to that line, bend down to touch it, turn, and sprint back. Rest for 20 seconds. Do 6 sprints total. The average of your sprint times is your score.

AVERAGE GUY: 8+ seconds

GREAT: Between 7 and 8 seconds

WORLD CLASS: Less than 7 seconds

Peak Performance Tip

TAKE SMALL STEPS FOR GIANT GAINS. Altidore says he's on a constant quest to feel lighter on his feet. One drill that helps instill this ephemeral quality is the rapid-response 2-inch run, says Barrieu. Start in an athletic stance and move your feet as fast as you can in microsteps—2 inches up and forward—for 5 seconds. Swing your arms and stay on the balls of your feet. Repeat twice, with 30 seconds of rest in between. Add this to your workouts three times a week to build acceleration.

"Strikers get the fame, but as a defender you do just as much work and you don't have the luxury of making so many mistakes," says Onyewu, 28, who plays for Sporting Clube de Portugal. "I like that adrenaline, that responsibility."

In Onyewu's case, with great responsibility comes great power. And the source of that power is his strength.

"Gooch has to anchor himself, hold off contact, and withstand bumping," says Barrieu. Plus, he needs to be quick and nimble, be strong in tackles, and jump the highest on corners and free kicks so he can head the ball away. Soccer players tend to focus on heavy lifts to develop maximum strength so they can generate greater explosiveness. They also use single-leg whole-body exercises, because most athletic movements in a game take place on one leg.

Norwegian soccer research reveals that doing squats with maximal loads dramatically improves jumping ability, sprinting speed over 10 meters, and running economy. Here's why: "Because of the high resistance, the movement speed is slow, but the muscular contraction when you push with your quads is fast," says Jan Hoff, PhD, a professor of medicine at the Norwegian University of Science and Technology. In other words, you're teaching your muscles to activate faster. In Dr. Hoff's 2008 study, participants who did three squat sessions a week for 8 weeks saw a 5 percent increase in running economy, which means they used less energy to move on the field. That translates to over half a mile more covered in a match. Another benefit to strength training: It reduces your risk of soccer injury by 50 percent, according to a University of Maine study. Use these tips to sculpt a strong body like Onyewu's.

BUILD WORLD-CLASS STRENGTH

Detonate your big muscles. To strengthen your quads and activate your glutes, hamstrings, calves, and core, Barrieu recommends barbell squats: 3 sets of 5 reps at 85 percent of your 1-rep max, with 90 seconds of rest between sets. "Descend in a slow, controlled way, and then accelerate as you push the bar back up." Do them twice a week.

STRENGTH: The Self-Test

The best strength test for soccer is your 1-rep maximum (1RM) for a barbell squat, says Barrieu, the national team fitness coach. The safest way to test your 1-rep max is to recruit a couple of spotters and load the bar with the heaviest weight you think you can squat at least 8 times. Lower your body until the tops of your thighs are parallel to the floor, and push up. To calculate your 1-rep max, multiply the weight used by one of these numbers:

10 REPS: 1.3 [If you lifted 150 pounds, your 1RM is 195 pounds (150 x 1.3)]

8 REPS: 1.27 [If you lifted 150 pounds, your 1RM is 190 pounds (150 x 1.27)]

6 REPS: 1.2 [If you lifted 150 pounds, your 1RM is 180 pounds (150 x 1.2)]

AVERAGE GUY: 1 to 1½ times your body weight

GREAT: 1½ to 2 times your body weight

WORLD CLASS: More than double your body weight

Peak Performance Tip

TRAIN USING THE TRX. To build strength without adding bulk, Onyewu uses the TRX, a suspension training system of nylon straps that anchor to a fixed object so that you can do a wide range of body-weight exercises. "It helps with power, flexibility, and balance," he says. See MensHealth.com/trx for TRX video workouts.

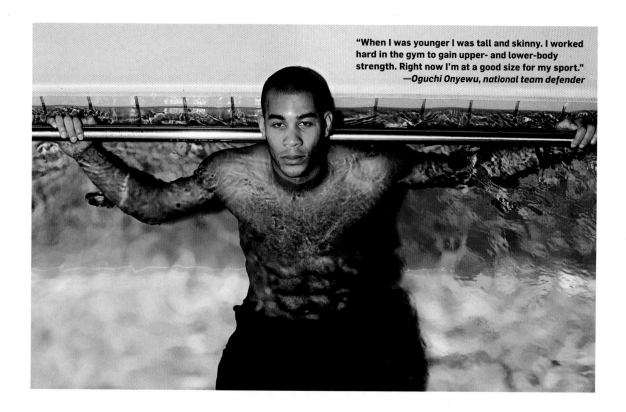

"When I was younger I was tall and skinny. I worked hard in the gym to gain upper- and lower-body strength. Right now I'm at a good size for my sport."
—Oguchi Onyewu, national team defender

Steal Olympic thunder. Many soccer players do single-leg Olympic-style lifts because these exercises build whole-body strength. But they're difficult to do without a trainer, so Barrieu recommends starting with the dumbbell high pull. Grab the dumbbells using an overhand grip and squat so the dumbbells are on the ground and your lower back is naturally arched. Raise your chest and hips until your arms are straight. Then pull the dumbbells as high as you can by explosively standing up as you bend your elbows and raise your upper arms. The dumbbells should be at chin height, and you should rise up onto your toes. Reverse the movement and return to the start. Use a weight that allows you to complete 12 to 15 reps and aim for 3 sets with 30 seconds rest in between.

Single out weaknesses. Barrieu has his players do single-leg squats to reveal differences in leg strength and range of motion. "The aim is to look the same on both sides," he says. On a bench or box that's knee height, balance on your left leg and hold your arms straight out in front of you. Bend your left knee and lower your body until your right heel almost touches the floor. Push yourself back to the starting position. Onyewu does 3 sets of 15 reps with 30-pound weights in each hand. You should start with no weight and do 3 sets of 5 for each leg. Aim to do them 3 days a week.

The Winner's Edge

Runner-up, sister kisser, loser . . . whatever you're competing for in life—promotions, women, ringers—no one will ever put you and those descriptions in the same sentence again

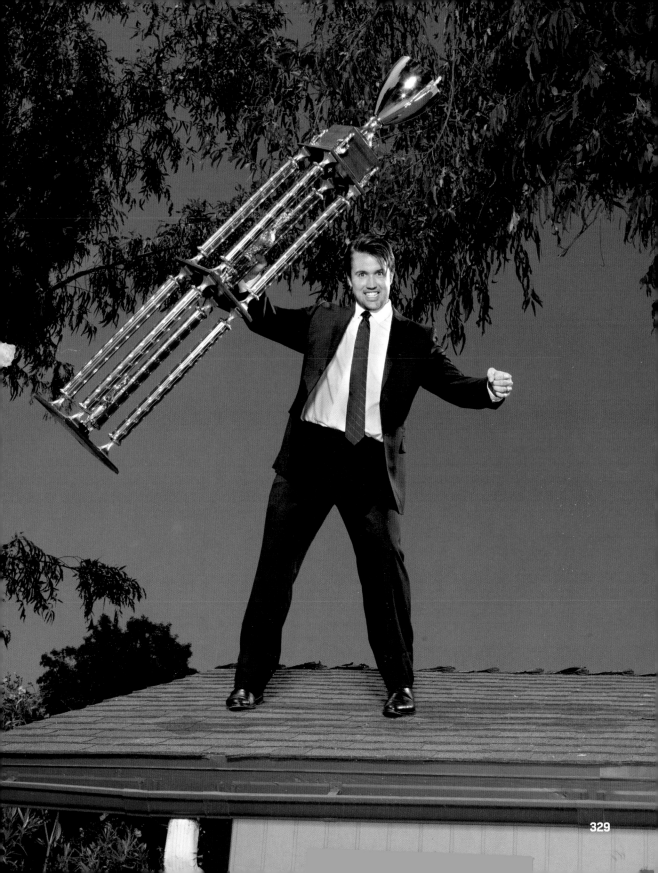

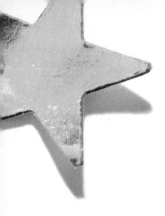

Think about it: What do you want? Here's how to get it!

LAND A PROMOTION

Here's the script for your review: "I love it here. I love working for you. But I want to know what I have to do for you and the organization to rise to the next level."

According to Donald Asher, author of *Who Gets Promoted, Who Doesn't, and Why,* "Bosses assume that any employee who doesn't ask for more is satisfied with his job."

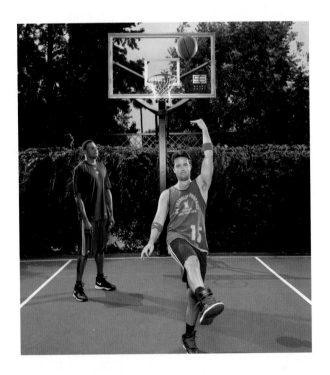

DESTROY ANYONE AT H-O-R-S-E

You might dream of playing against an NBA star, but Mark Selig actually did that. The 5'8" sports reporter at the *Daily News-Record,* in Harrisonburg, Virginia, challenged 6'6" Greivis Vasquez, a first-round pick of the Memphis Grizzlies, to a game of H-O-R-S-E, and he actually led for a while before losing by two letters.

How do you stay competitive against an opponent with superior skill? Unveil shots he's never practiced.

Selig shot from a sitting position, from his knees, and over his back, and even banked one in off the shot clock.

"The goal isn't to hit as many shots as possible. It's to get your opponent to miss shots you make," he says. Know your hot spot. "If you're money from the baseline, find ways to keep going back to the baseline, whether you're shooting with your eyes closed or left-handed," he says.

MASTER *MADDEN NFL*

Here are three key tricks, courtesy of Ian Cummings, creative director of *Madden NFL 11.*

1. If a defender is about to tackle you from behind on a long run, pull back on the right stick and you'll have a better chance of kicking out.
2. When using the new "shoulder lean" feature, make sure to shield the ball and turn away from contact to increase your chance of falling forward and breaking the tackle.
3. If an opponent is constantly sending heat up the middle, keep a running back in the backfield and "hot route" him to block using the new strategy pad.

EARN YOUR MOTHER-IN-LAW'S RESPECT (AND LOVE)

The problem is, you're both competing for the same girl. So turn that competition into collaboration, says Terri Apter, PhD, a Cambridge University psychologist and the author of *What Do You Want from Me? Learning to Get Along with In-laws.* Follow this three-step process.

1. The next time Mom calls, don't just hand the phone to your wife. Ask her about work, her favorite TV show, or any new recipes she's cooked. Show an interest in her life.
2. The following week, e-mail, text, or (gulp) phone her directly. Say something like, "I saw this and thought of you," or simply share some good news. Before long, you'll have a rapport.
3. At the next family gathering, compliment Mom by saying, "I see my wife learned how to…[cook, design interiors, climb the corporate ladder] from you." Make sure as many people as possible hear you, including your father-in-law. There—now you're as good as in the will.

SPELL SUCCESS AT SCRABBLE

Learn the words "za" and "qi," says John D. Williams, executive director of the National Scrabble Association. *Za* is slang for "pizza," and *qi* is a variant of "chi," the Asian life force. They're legal words. You can score big by using them around a triple-letter square, and your opponent might challenge them, and lose his turn.

WIN AT FLIP CUP

Rob McElhenney, creator of the FX comedy *It's Always Sunny in Philadelphia*, knows this drinking game and even wrapped an entire episode around it. Here's how to emerge victorious every time.

1. Pour a bit of beer on the exact spot you're flipping the cup onto.
2. Wet the cup's rim.
3. Flip it: The moisture will create a suction, helping the upturned cup adhere to the table.
4. Pump fist, repeat.

TROUNCE EVERYONE AT JENGA!

Here's a little-known fact about this classic tower-building game, and it'll allow you to consistently destroy your family and crush your children's confidence. (Hey, it builds character!) All Jenga blocks are not the same, according to Matt Donie, a manager of design and development for Hasbro Games.

"I can't reveal the exact measurements, but the blocks are actually made in three subtly different thicknesses," he says, "and these tolerances are carefully monitored."

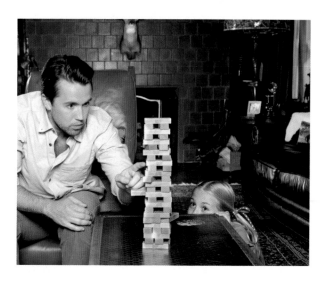

By tapping different blocks with your fingertip, he says, you can eventually identify the thinner (and looser) blocks. Remove them from the tower to lower your chances of knocking it over.

CLEAN UP AT POKER

Forget about wearing dark glasses, bluffing, and trying to read subtle tells. To gain the edge in a friendly game, just bring the beer, says Michael Craig, editor of *The Full Tilt Poker Strategy Guide*.

"Most guys play too many hands, and they keep drawing as long as they have even a whisper of a chance," he says. "It's smarter to play fewer hands and fold more often." Bringing the beer gives you something to do while watching the action, and keeps you from being called a party pooper for folding so much.

BED A WOMAN WHO'S WAY OUT OF YOUR LEAGUE

It's possible to make even the most beautiful woman quiver in less than 5 seconds.

"The trick is to look very deeply into her eyes," says Leil Lowndes, author of *How to Make Anyone Fall in Love with You*,

"almost as if you're searching for her optic nerve." Biological anthropologists call it the "copulatory gaze," and it can trigger a fight-or-flight response. It could make her heart race, her palms dampen, and her body tingle, and she'll think it's because she likes you. "Love, lust, and fear are closely intertwined," Lowndes says.

RULE AT TENNIS

To significantly improve every aspect of your game, hit the bottom inside quarter of the ball, says Steve Mallory, a teaching pro in La Costa, California. This will make you focus more precisely on the ball and produce more consistent and effective shots.

"This part of the ball is always on the side that's closest to your body, and it's usually your optimal strike point."

RING UP A VICTORY AT HORSESHOES

Despite how heavy a standard 2½-pound shoe might feel, strength has nothing to do with throwing it accurately. The key is letting the shoe do the work, says Bobby White, a nationally ranked player. Master the mechanics using these tips.

1. Use a pendulum-style swing, letting the momentum of the shoe carry it forward.
2. Stand with your pitching arm closest to the stake so your swing lines up with the target. Your forward step should stay parallel to your swing so everything remains in line.
3. Step slightly ahead of the swing, timing it so your weight shifts onto your lead foot just prior to releasing the shoe. The release is lower than most

MY RULE FOR WINNING: Passion

"The common denominator among every great athlete I've ever known is passion. 'Luck' and 'talent' are often used to describe winners. Luck can be manufactured through determination, and there is nothing natural about talent. If you do everything by the book, you'll be beat by those who write their own. The talent and luck it takes to win starts with passion." —*TRAVIS PASTRANA, who has won 11 gold medals at the X Games in rally and motocross*

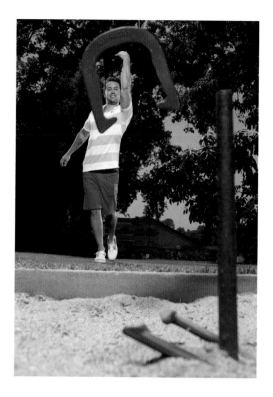

training," he says. "Making it harder on yourself in practice will make competition easier. The 16-ounce cups will look like trash cans."

ZOOM AWAY IN A CYCLING SPRINT

Practice this sound: *PsssSSSsssSSSsss*.

"The trick is to modulate the hiss so that it sounds exactly like a puncture spinning out of a bike tire," says Don Cuerdon, a former racer and *Bicycling* magazine editor. By making the sound precisely when you jump out of the saddle to sprint, you'll momentarily freeze the competition as they check to see if it's their tire that's flatted. This is all the time you'll need to break away.

TRIUMPH AT FLAG FOOTBALL

You need to learn two moves, says Michael Cihon, a 16-time flag football national champion. On offense, it's the spin move. Instead of trying to fool a tackler with a cutback or head fake, plant your lead foot and spin 360 degrees. This spins the flags as well, making them tougher to grab.

On defense, Cihon recommends keeping your eyes on the midsection of the ball carrier. "That's the only part of his body that never moves," he says.

PICK UP A FIRST DOWN

If it's fourth and long, "send 'em deep," says Drew Brees, Saints QB and a former Super Bowl MVP. Have your receivers set up on both sides and send all of them deep except one.

"The inside guy runs an option route," says Brees. "He can hook it up, run right,

people think; it's generally just as your hand clears your lead leg.

4. Complete the upward circle of your swing after the shoe has left your hand. Follow-through is the most critical element. Clang!

ACE BEER PONG

If you're expecting heated competition, find some time to practice, but on a longer table, and with smaller cups.

"You will be an animal," promises Duncan Carroll, cofounder of the annual World Series of Beer Pong. Specifically, he suggests using a 9-foot Ping-Pong table (rather than the 8-foot beer pong standard) and 8-ounce cups (instead of the regulation 16-ouncers). "It's like altitude run left." Hopefully the D will be looking downfield at the deep threats and at worst you'll gain the first down.

NEVER LOSE AT ROCK, PAPER, SCISSORS

Pound, slice, and wrap up your average opponent with these tips from Graham Walker, coauthor of *The Official Rock Paper Scissors Strategy Guide*. Rock is for rookies. Men tend to throw Rock first. So if you're matched against another guy (and he's no expert), throw Paper, and then gloat. If it's a woman you're squared off against, throw Scissors, since she's less inclined to throw Rock, and Scissors trumps Paper. When in doubt, go with Paper. Walker has observed that Scissors is thrown slightly less often than the statistical average (29.6 percent versus 33.33 percent).

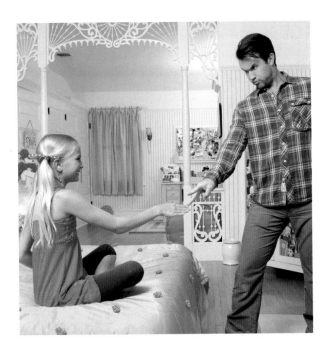

PREVAIL IN AN ARGUMENT

Whether it's your boss, your spouse, customer support, or the kids you're facing off against, try to keep your voice deep, like James Earl Jones's. This sound advice comes from Aaron Sell, PhD, of the Center for Evolutionary Psychology at the University of California at Santa Barbara. His recent study found that people are capable of accurately predicting a man's physical strength based on the timbre of his voice alone.

"So if you lower your voice, you'll sound stronger and should win more conflicts."

BE THE BEST AT BOWLING

If your bowling knowledge is limited to what you've gleaned from *The Flintstones,* don't worry. Walter Ray Williams Jr., the Professional Bowlers Association career title leader, advises keeping it simple. Choose a 14-to-16-pound ball and focus on throwing it dead straight down the middle of the lane. As you deliver the ball, keep it an inch or two from your body, and remember to follow through.

"My arm goes straight up, like it's reaching for the ceiling, and that's where a lot of my accuracy comes from." Nice shot, Fred.

KILL IT AT DARTS

The biggest mistake novice throwers make is holding the dart like a pencil, according to Karl Remick, vice president of the American Darters Association. But as with any throwing sport, the weaker your grip, the less control you have over it.

"Get as many fingers as you comfortably can on the dart," says Remick. "I use every one of mine except the pinky. I have my index and middle fingers on top, my ring finger slightly underneath the tip, and my thumb as the base." When it's time to launch, try throwing the dart *through* the board rather than at it. This subtle shift in mind set helps you throw more naturally and accurately.

STAND OUT IN A FOOTBALL-THROWING CONTEST

The following technique isn't easy to master, but it's unmatched for launching a football long distances. It's also how Terry Bradshaw did it. Grip the ball so your index finger rests directly on its nose and as many other fingertips as possible are on the laces, says Timothy Gay, PhD, a professor of physics at the University of Nebraska at Lincoln. When you release the ball, let your fingertips impart the all-important rotation (try for at least 10 revolutions per second) that stabilizes flight and reduces air drag. But—here's the Bradshaw booster—just before it leaves your hand, push off with that index finger.

"You'll be applying force over greater distance, which will give the ball more speed and distance," says Gay.

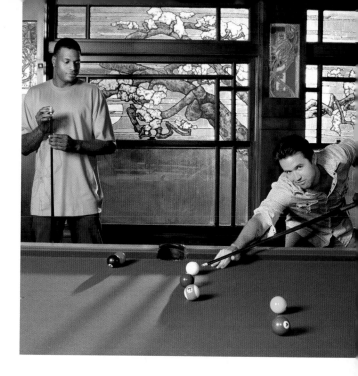

PUT AN EIGHT-BALL GAME IN YOUR POCKET

Reverse your usual strategy, says Jeanette "the Black Widow" Lee, who has won more than 30 pool titles. Instead of going for the easiest shots first, do the opposite. That's right, go for the challenging ones. By leaving your tap-ins next to the pockets, you'll reduce your opponent's targets while increasing your chances of having him drop a ball for you.

"This strategy will give you the best chance of winning," the Black Widow says.

DOMINATE PICKUP HOOPS

Chris Ballard visited 1,000 courts while researching his book *Hoops Nation*. Along the way, he witnessed all manner of sneaky moves. This is one anyone can execute: When you grab an offensive rebound, don't immediately take it up. Instead, push your butt into the guy on your back. The space you create will prevent him from blocking your shot.

MY RULE FOR WINNING: Trust

"My coach, Chuck Noll, always put an emphasis on fundamentals. Champions are champions not because they do extraordinary things, but because they do the ordinary things better than everyone else. I always believed in concentrating on your job and trusting your philosophy, not worrying about how your opponents did things: Do what you do."

—*TONY DUNGY, who coached the Indianapolis Colts to victory in Super Bowl XLI and is an analyst on* Football Night in America

ATTRACT INFLUENTIAL FOLLOWERS ON TWITTER

The key is emphasizing quality over quantity, says Laura Fitton, coauthor of *Twitter for Dummies*.

"Any hack can cheat his way to thousands of followers," she says. "Remember that 'Be yourself' crap from your mom, or the Palinese variant, 'Be a maverick'? Being absolutely you wins on Twitter," says Fitton. "Take a position, make wisecracks, and link to stuff—funny, smart, harsh, controversial—that you feel strongly about."

GAIN MORE FRIENDS

We're not talking the Facebook kind, but true-blue, backslapping buds. The first step, says Geoffrey Greif, MSW, DSW, the author of *Buddy System: Understanding Male Friendships*, is determining where you rank on the masculinity scale.

Mano a mano: You're a macho weekend warrior who talks sports and hangs out in the locker room. You're capable of dealing with some feelings, but you generally lack an interest in doing so.

> ### MY RULE FOR WINNING: Practice
>
> "Take a recreational tennis player who misses a backhand volley. Play will resume, and later he could make the same mistake again. Contrast this experience with a coach practicing volley drills. In a few hours the player's volleys will improve more than after hundreds of hours of recreational tennis. Identifying weaknesses and designing deliberate practice lies at the core of the development of excellence. Research suggests that it takes over 10,000 hours of deliberate practice to win at an international level." —*K. ANDERS ERICSSON, PHD, a psychology professor at Florida State University*

Guy to guy: You have plenty of interests but nothing extreme. You're reasonably fit, feel comfortable in locker rooms, and follow and play sports—but not obsessively. You're okay with feelings (others and your own).

Person to person: You edge toward androgyny and might feel ill at ease in locker rooms. You follow sports peripherally and play them only for fun or with women. You favor books over TV, and initiate discussions about emotions.

Now that you know what kind of guy you are, concentrate on seeking the same type of friends. Do this by being the organizer, says Greif, a professor at the University of Maryland. "Guys like guys who reach out and start things. Simply think about what you like doing and enlarge it by inviting similar guys."

WIN A PUSHUP CONTEST

We reached out to 36-year-old Cybele Forbes, a 5'2", 134-pound mother of two. Don't laugh. This TNT camera operator prevailed over NBA veteran Charles Barkley in two pushup tests, banging out 28 and 32. Use her advice to kiss the floor and humble giants.

Go second or at the same time. Going first puts you at a disadvantage.

Take a wide stance. "I position my feet and hands a little wider than shoulder-width apart so I'm evenly balanced," says Forbes.

Align your back, butt, and legs. Check yourself in a mirror; your body should form a straight line from ankles to head.

Concentrate more on breathing than on the actual pushups. Inhale up, exhale down,

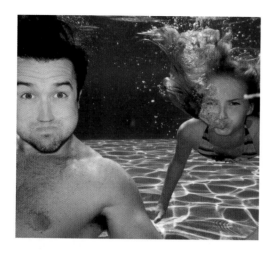

slowly and deliberately in rhythm with the movement. When your muscles start to burn, focus on your breathing.

When all else fails, wear a baggy shirt. Forbes went with form-fitting Spandex while Sir Charles went the opposite route—and reaped the benefit. "His shirt was so loose you couldn't even see if he was touching the ground," she says.

HOLD YOUR BREATH THE LONGEST

Endurance artist David Blaine lasted 17 minutes and 4 seconds without air using a technique called glossopharyngeal insufflation, or lung packing. He trained for months, but this simplified version can give you an instant boost, says Ralph Potkin, MD, Blaine's advisor and the US Freediving team's physician.

Inhale and exhale deeply four times; then inhale deeply again, and when your lungs are full, inhale sharply three times, gulping down air. Hold it! Distract yourself by working from A to Z in your head, matching celebrities' names to each

letter. You'll be thinking "Shakira" while your buddy flounders.

FINISH FIRST IN A 5-K CHALLENGE

So you made a wager with a buddy and now it's decision day. Assuming you've trained properly (speed work once a week and a slow, long run every weekend), here's the strategy that will earn you bragging rights.

"During the race, take a 20-second walk break at the 2- and 4-kilometer marks," says Olympian Jeff Galloway, who has coached more than 250,000 runners to their goals at jeffgalloway.com. Although that might sound counterintuitive, giving your leg muscles a break even in a short race helps them perform at a higher level overall.

WIN AN UPHILL FOOTRACE

So the same buddy, distraught at losing the 5-K, has now challenged you to a hill climb, double or nothing. Once again, assuming you've done the necessary conditioning, you can win. Follow this advice, courtesy of John Stifler, who has run the Mt. Washington Road Race course six times.

Shorten your stride. Running uphill is no different from bicycling uphill. As the grade steepens, you need to shift to lower gears so that you can maintain your rpm's, or leg turnover.

Look down. Your focus should be anywhere from just in front of the tip of each shoe to the road 20 feet in front of you. This puts your body in a more efficient forward lean—and keeps you from focusing on how far from the top you are.

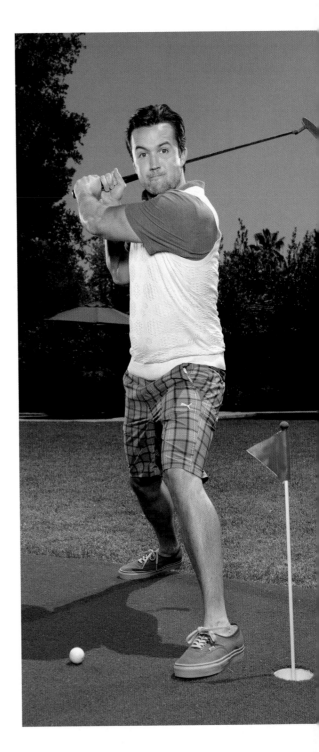

MY RULE FOR WINNING: Reach

"My rule for winning: Dream, plan, reach. It started with a dream: to do something that nobody had ever done before. To turn that into reality, I needed a plan. Yes, the plan was tough to follow and I made many sacrifices along the way, but it was my commitment to the plan that kept my dream alive. All of which enabled me to reach for it—literally!"

—*MICHAEL PHELPS,*
who has won 14 Olympic gold medals in swimming
and founded the Michael Phelps Foundation

WIN IN AN ALL-OUT SPRINT

So the same buddy challenges you to a 40-yard sprint on a football field, triple or nothing. You don't even need to train for this one. Just follow the advice of Mark Sisson, a former elite runner and the author of *The Primal Blueprint.*

Take off your shoes. Your opponent will think you're nuts, but going barefoot accomplishes two things: (1) It lightens your feet to boost leg turnover, and (2) it involves more of the small muscles in the feet to add to your propulsion.

Pump your arms. Focus on raising your elbows when they're behind your body, because this will cause them to pop up to shoulder level in the front, which speeds your stride.

Be the hunted or the hunter. "Adopt a kill-or-be-killed mind set," says Sisson. If he springs to a quick lead, hunt him. If you're out front, imagine you're being hunted by a lion. Roar.

CONQUER THE GOLF COURSE

Gio Valiante, PhD, a sports psychologist, gives a bottle of shampoo to all his athletes, including Vijay Singh and Camilo Villegas, and has them repeat what's on the label. Use his crazy scheme to wash frustration out of your game.

Wash = Pick a precise target. Be decisive about where you're hitting the ball, and focus on it. The human brain is wired to react to targets.

Rinse = Take a fearless swing. Don't try to steer the ball. Be aggressive.

Repeat = Forget about it.

Whether it's a good shot or a bad shot, accept it and move on. Whether you're 5 under or 5 over, keep cycling through this routine: "Pick the target, take a fearless swing, accept the outcome. Wash. Rinse. Repeat."

On the driving range: To be a bigger hitter, you need to increase your clubhead speed. For every 10 miles per hour you add to your swing, you'll put 25 more yards on the ball, says Steve Griffith, 60, a world long-drive champ who can still whack 'em nearly 400 yards. Besides just swinging harder, the key is making a full shoulder turn. Rotate so your back is to the target when you're at the top of your backswing. "Do this with a smooth, slow motion that allows your body to turn but keeps your head still," says Griffith. Then let your torso lead your shoulders, arms, and hands as you uncoil. Boom!

On the putting green: When you sign your name on a check, you do it fast and fluidly. If you tried to slowly copy your signature letter by letter, it would be a mess. That's the simple secret to successful putting, says Dave Stockton, who has 25 PGA wins, including five majors. He recommends cutting the time you spend with a putt by at least 50 percent. "Just line it up from the low side, go back to the ball, look at your line, and let it go," he explains. "Roll the ball across the green as if your putter were a paintbrush."

OUTSMART THE CARNIVAL SPEED PITCH

You've always suspected that these games were rigged, but you've never been able to figure out how. Until now. Tom Mody sells radar guns and speed-pitch booths, so he knows all the tricks. A radar gun is most accurate when (1) it's aligned with the delivery (either directly behind or in front of the pitcher) and (2) it "sees" the release (since that's when a thrown ball has the highest velocity). But—surprise—a lot of carneys don't position their units this way. Usually they're off to the side, meaning they miss the release and see only a portion of the ball's flight, which results in lower readings.

To circumvent this, Mody recommends aligning your release and pitch as much as possible with the eye of the gun. This might mean standing more to one side or even throwing the pitch to an off-center part of the backstop. Just remember that the more it sees, the faster you'll be. Choose the giant panda.

MY RULE FOR WINNING: Innovation

"The key is to distinguish between official rules and self-imposed rules. I won a kickboxing championship by throwing my opponents off the platform for TKOs. The crowd booed, but it worked. Think of high jumper Dick Fosbury at the '68 Olympics. People laughed at his approach, but he won gold. Now everyone uses the Fosbury Flop."
—*TIMOTHY FERRISS, former Chinese kickboxing champ and the author of* The 4-Hour Workweek

PROVE IT

"Great athletes are defined by their agility—their ability to change speed and direction instantly," says Todd Durkin, CSCS. And according to researchers in Tunisia, the modified agility T-test, which tests sprinting and lateral movement, is the best assessment of agility in sports like basketball and tennis. Try to improve your time on this test to improve your agility on the court.

How to do it: Sprint from cone A to cone B. Immediately shuffle left to cone C, and then shuffle right, passing B, to cone D. Shuffle as quickly as possible to cone B, and then run backward to cone A.

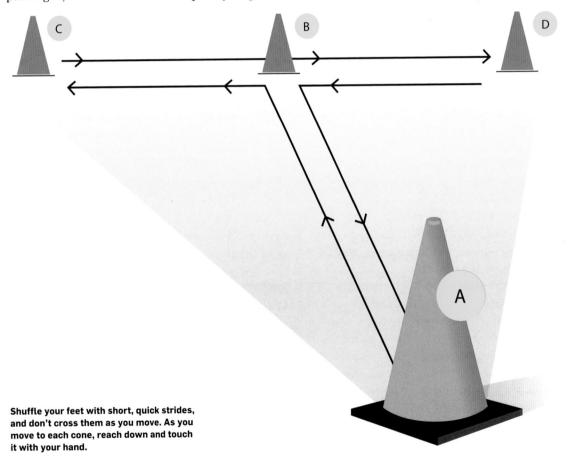

Shuffle your feet with short, quick strides, and don't cross them as you move. As you move to each cone, reach down and touch it with your hand.

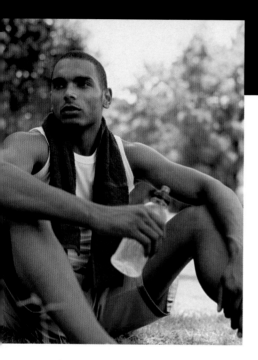

DRINK UP

A lunchtime workout can leave you dragging instead of energized if you don't stay hydrated. In a recent Tufts University study, athletes who didn't drink water during workouts felt angrier and more depressed afterward than those who did. Researchers calculated that the dehydrated group's "global negative mood"—including confusion, fatigue, and decreased vigor, none of which help a career—was one-third higher than the hydrated group's.

Simple thirst partially explains this, says study coauthor Kristen D'Anci, PhD. "But you're also seeing slight shrinkage of brain cells," she says. This may upset your brain's chemical balance, making you irritable or triggering a headache. Even if you're not thirsty, down 8 to 10 ounces of water every 30 minutes during your workout, she says.

Rehydrating is also critical when you're exercising. Water helps your body—and brain—work properly. Dehydration alters a runner's perceptions and affects his pacing, a new *Journal of Strength and Conditioning Research* study suggests. During a 12-K race, dried-out runners felt they were hotter and working harder than hydrated runners did. Also, the time variance between fastest and slowest laps was twice as long for the dehydrated group. A lack of water might affect your ability to gauge work ahead, says study author Rebecca Stearns, MD, ATC. During a long run, drink at least 7 ounces of water every 20 minutes, she says.

PHONE A FRIEND

No wonder boot camps are popular. Researchers at the University of Oxford found that people who train in groups can boost their pain tolerance more than those who work out alone. The scientists aren't sure why, but they think group exercise may contribute to an underlying endorphin surge. No training partners? Pop in a pair of earphones. Music can also make strenuous exercise seem easier.

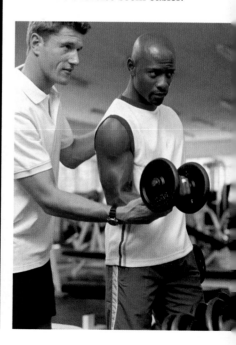

PROVE IT

TAKE IT OUTSIDE

Feeling fried? Nature wakes up your brain and your body, say University of Rochester scientists. They found that people who spent at least 20 minutes a day outdoors felt up to 20 percent more physical and mental energy than those who stayed inside. More research is needed to determine why, but the study authors ruled out the effects of exercise and socialization, which people do more of when they're outdoors. Can't finagle some fresh air? Open the blinds: Just eyeballing nature can recharge you.

Better yet, exercise outdoors. It means a lungful of fresh air—and a more satisfying workout for your body and brain. Science proves it.

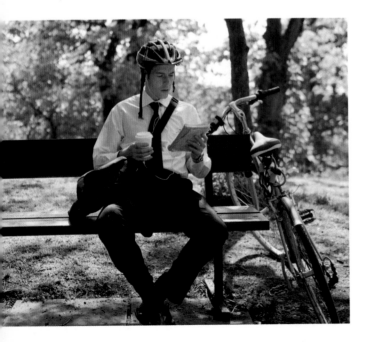

RUNNING

The sport: Treadmill vs. outdoors
Mental benefit: Runners who took it outside reported feeling 225 percent more satisfied than those who ran on indoor treadmills, a Utah State study found.
Physical benefit: In the same study, outdoor runners completed a 5-K run 4 minutes faster than treadmill runners did.

BICYCLING

The sport: Stationary bike vs. road ride
Mental benefit: In a recent French study, men who used bike trainers perceived a higher level of exertion than those who rode outdoors at the same pace.
Physical benefit: Road riding requires 5 percent more propulsive force than pedaling a stationary bike at the same speed does, the French researchers say.

ROWING

The sport: Ergometer vs. scull
Mental benefit: Team rowing on the water creates a greater sense of euphoria than solo indoor rowing, a recent British study found.
Physical benefit: In a Brazilian study, outdoor rowers burned 26 percent more calories during a mock race than those on sliding rowing ergometers did.

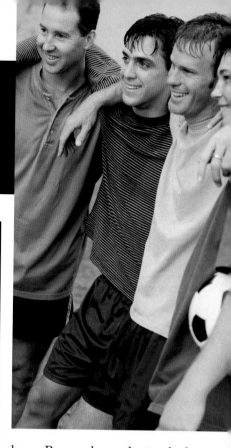

RUN LESS, GO FASTER

Running less can make you faster. In a University of Copenhagen study, runners slashed an average of 1 full minute off their 10-K times by switching to a "speed endurance" regimen of fewer miles combined with intense intervals. The runners cut their weekly mileage from 34.2 to 20.6 miles. Plus, two or three times a week, they ran eight to 12 intervals lasting 30 seconds each at 95 percent effort, taking 3 minutes of rest between them. After 9 weeks, the speed group fared better on most performance tests—half of the group members set personal records—than runners who continued with their usual routines.

The intense training elevates levels of a protein that regulates the potassium that can accumulate around muscle fibers and cause fatigue, says study author Jens Bangsbo, PhD.

PREVENT RUNNER'S KNEE

You might be able to ward off the soreness known as runner's knee by following a smart lifting plan. According to new research, strengthening your quadriceps and hamstrings may help prevent this condition, which is caused by abnormal movement of the patella on the thigh-bone. Researchers who tracked some 1,600 midshipmen at the US Naval Academy found that those with weak hamstrings were nearly 3 times more likely to develop the syndrome, while those with weak quadriceps were 5½ times more likely, says lead study author Michelle Boling, PhD. Hip raises and lunges can help build those muscles.

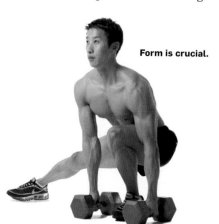

Form is crucial.

TALK IT UP!

You've heard it from coaches; now listen to the science: Talk among teammates is the sign of a winner, at least in tennis. In a Florida State University study, winning doubles teams

343

PROVE IT

talked strategy twice as much as losing teams did, and the teammates vocally encouraged each other nearly three times as frequently.

"Emotional exchanges help teams feel more capable," explains study coauthor Gershon Tenenbaum, PhD. Whatever team game you're playing, try to discuss strategy and express encouragement between plays.

POWER THROUGH THE SNOW

Cross-country skiers are more than just lungs on legs. Upper-body power is crucial in cross-country ski racing to help maintain momentum, a new *European Journal of Applied Physiology* study suggests. The researchers found that trained XC skiers with the greatest upper-body power had the fastest race speeds. Why? Not only does upper-body power encourage the efficient use of oxygen, it's also essential for generating the bursts that are needed when starting and

finishing a race, cresting hills, and carrying speed through corners, says study coauthor Dan Heil, PhD. In addition to upper-body exercises like the bench press, lat pulldown, and shoulder press, he recommends plenty of core work, like the cable chop.

FINISH FAST

Carry extra stamina in your pocket in the form of menthol, which can boost your aerobic endurance. In a recent British study, men who gargled a menthol solution for 10 seconds every 10 minutes while bicycling in 93°F heat lasted 9 percent longer than a placebo group did—but felt as if they were breathing with 15 percent less effort. Menthol might activate pleasure centers in the brain, improving motivation, says study coauthor Toby Mundel, PhD. It also helps breathing by making your airways feel clearer and cooler, he says.

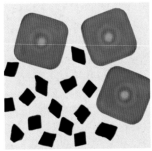

Sucking on a mentholated lozenge before a workout or race may give a weekend athlete an aerobic boost, according to a new study. One possibility: Fisherman's Friend.

HIT THE TURBO

Sometimes looking back can propel you forward. In South Africa, researchers found that cyclists who completed five 40-K time trials performed more aggressively when they were told at intervals how far they'd ridden. Study author Jeroen Swart, MBChB, says knowing the distance you've already covered can give you the confidence to release energy reserves rather than saving and perhaps never using them.

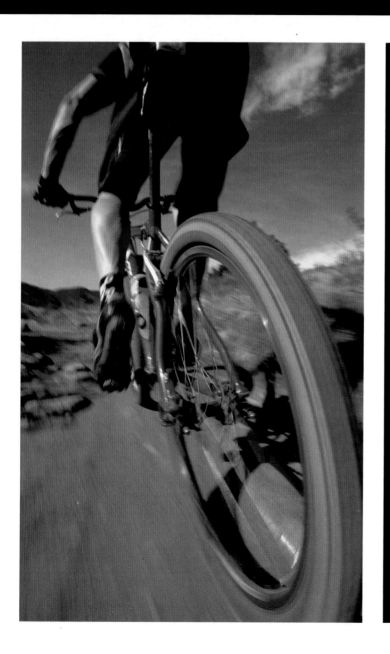

PUSH HARDER

For cyclists, doing low-cadence intervals might be the best way to build strength, say New Zealand researchers. In the study, well-trained cyclists performed 3 sets of five 30-second intervals (twice weekly for 4 weeks) at either 60 to 70 rpm or 110 to 120 rpm. The slower, harder-gear group saw a 97 percent increase in testosterone and a 5 percent increase in fitness and performance, versus gains of 62 percent and 3 percent, respectively, for the faster pedalers. Even for recreational riders, lower-cadence training is better because of the muscle-building boost in testosterone, says study author Carl Paton, PhD.

BENCH BACK PAIN

Inspired by the World Cup? Play soccer to protect your back. Recreational soccer can reduce your risk of lower-back injury, according to a new study in the *Journal of Strength and Conditioning Research*.

YOU ASKED

Q: I hate stretching before I exercise. What's the least I can get away with?

1. Walking High-Knee Hug

Stretches your glutes and requires more than 90 degrees of hip flexion, a range of motion that challenges most desk jockeys.

Do it: Stand with your feet shoulder-width apart and your arms at your sides. Raise your left knee toward your chest, grasping it with both hands just below your kneecap. Pull it to the middle of your chest as you stand tall. Release it and step into the offset lunge.

2. Offset Lunge

Stretches your groin area and legs.

Do it: Step forward with your left leg toward about 11 o'clock. Slowly lower your body until your left thigh is parallel to the floor. (Your right knee should nearly touch the floor.) Keeping your lower back straight, bend forward, and touch both hands to the floor just by the inside of your left foot. You're now in position for stretch #3.

3. Overhead Reach

Targets the middle of your back, stretches your chest, and activates your core.

Do it: Keeping your left hand on the floor, reach overhead with your right arm as you rotate your torso upward. Both arms should form a straight line. Bring your right hand back down to the floor so that you're in the offset lunge position again.

4. Hip Lift

Stretches your hamstrings.

Do it: Keeping your hands on the floor, rock your hips back and straighten both legs. Step forward with your right leg and stand up straight.

Now repeat this four-stretch sequence, but use the opposite leg or arm for each move.

Q: I can't do even one single-leg squat. Am I weak, or uncoordinated?

A: Neither. Single-leg squats are really hard. In fact, they're probably the most challenging leg exercise, says Mike Robertson, CSCS, a strength coach in Indianapolis and the author of *The Single-Leg Solution*. "They demand mobility, strength, and balance. That makes doing them difficult but also rewarding, because they strengthen your glutes, quads, and hamstrings."

To train your body to do a single-leg squat, Robertson suggests starting off with 3 sets of 10 split squats and 10 lunges three times a week until you can bang them out easily. (For more instruction, visit MensHealth.com/singlelegsquat.) Then try a single-leg squat on a 12-inch-high box. Stand on the box holding your arms straight out in front of you. Balancing on your right foot, bend your right knee and lower your body until your left heel touches the floor. Pause, then push yourself up. Three sets of 5 reps on each side twice a week is all you need, says Robertson. When you improve, switch to a 6-inch box, and when you can do them perfectly, try a flat surface.

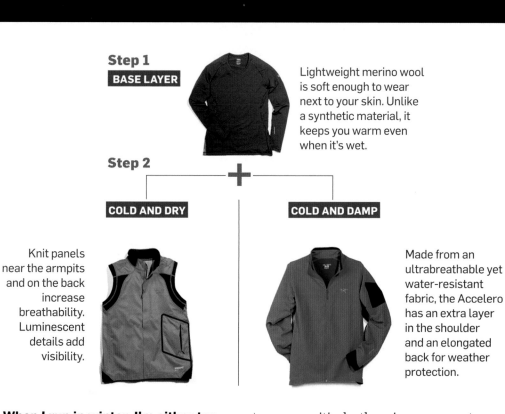

Step 1
BASE LAYER

Lightweight merino wool is soft enough to wear next to your skin. Unlike a synthetic material, it keeps you warm even when it's wet.

Step 2

COLD AND DRY

COLD AND DAMP

Knit panels near the armpits and on the back increase breathability. Luminescent details add visibility.

Made from an ultrabreathable yet water-resistant fabric, the Accelero has an extra layer in the shoulder and an elongated back for weather protection.

Q: **When I run in winter, I'm either too hot or too cold. What should I look for in a cold-weather running jacket?**

A: Your body temperature can rise 1 degree as you pound the pavement over a 45-minute run, so you should dress as if it's 20 degrees warmer than it actually is. To let some body heat escape, you need to layer yourself with garments that breathe yet also shield you from the chill, says Lisa Jhung, a gear tester for *Runner's World* magazine.

"Breathable materials or ventilation fea-tures are critical; otherwise your sweat can accumulate and dampen your base layer, and you'll feel cold," she says. If it's cold and dry out, wear a long-sleeved merino wool base layer, like Icebreaker's GT Baselayer Sprint Crew ($90, icebreaker.com), with a wind-blocking soft-shell vest, like Mountain Hard-wear's Transition ($90, mountainhardwear.com). If it's cold and damp out, throw on the same base layer but zip up a more protective shell, like the Arc'teryx Accelero ($130, arc-teryx.com). It weighs about the same as a dress shirt, yet repels wind and water.

Q: I see more guys at the gym wearing mouth guards. What's the point?

A: They're pumping up by chomping down. That's because wearing a mouth guard allows you to safely clench your teeth, which can help you heft more iron, says William P. Ebben, PhD, an exercise scientist at the University of Wisconsin at Parkside. "It's a concept called 'concurrent activation potentiation': When your brain signals your jaw to clench, it may also cause a little more activation of the other muscles." The result: You might lift as much as 15 percent more weight, according to Dr. Ebben's research. If you want to give it a try, pick up the Cramer dental vinyl mouth guard ($1.50 for the basic model, sportsunlimitedinc.com); it's the same gym bit used in Dr. Ebben's study.

Q: What are the benefits of barefoot-style shoes?

A: They provide the potential for greater explosiveness, improved coordination, and less musculoskeletal pain, says Jay Dicharry, MPT, CSCS, director of the motion analysis lab at the University of Virginia's Center for Endurance Sport.

Here's why: Because they have thin and flexible soles, barefoot-style shoes boost proprioception, which is the feedback that travels from your feet to your brain with every step. And the more data you deliver to your brain, the more efficiently and powerfully the brain's signals can move your body. "Your muscles fire faster and you have improved stability," says Dicharry. But don't toss your current kicks and jump into a pair of Vibram FiveFingers without first testing your wheels: Close your eyes and stand barefoot on one leg

for 30 seconds. Repeat with the other leg. If either foot rolls outward, it's too weak to train in barefoot shoes. The best way to improve: Balance on each leg for 30 seconds, 15 times a day.

1. Terra Plana Evo: With a 4 millimeter (mm) outsole and no midsole, these 8-ouncers offer minimal support, like the Vibram FiveFingers. However, their more conservative design doesn't scream ninja-in-training. $160, *terraplana.com*

2. Nike Free 5.0: The 8.2-ounce Free's foam midsole, which is 20 mm thick at the heel and 10 mm thick at the forefoot, provides moderate support. But strategically placed grooves make it superflexible. It's an ideal first step in the transition to minimalism. $85, *nikestore.com*

3. Vibram FiveFingers Bikila: These 6-ounce foot gloves have a barely there 4 mm outsole and no midsole, so they replicate the barefoot experience more closely than any other shoes. Wear them with Injinji toe socks if you need a bit more comfort. $100, *vibramfivefingers.com*

4. Mizuno Wave Ronin 2: The midsole of a regular running shoe is about 30 mm thick in the heel. This 8-ounce shoe's midsole is half as chunky, which makes it a good choice for people who can't give up cushioning completely. $95, *mizunousa.com*

Q: Are there any yoga moves every man (even men who hate yoga) should do?

A: Guys need to get over their yoga phobia; there are simply too many benefits to becoming pretzel flexible. For instance, recent research reveals that yoga can help reduce stress, lower blood pressure, and even boost levels of the mood-enhancing neurotransmitter GABA.

"Every guy should do the pigeon pose 3 days a week," says Tara Stiles, the author of *Slim Calm Sexy Yoga*. "It will release tension in your hips, back, glutes, and quads. And the emphasis on breathing helps you stay in the moment, which is a great skill to develop to intensify sex." How intense? Men who practiced yoga an hour a day for 12 weeks not only had erections that remained harder longer, but also had better staying power in the sack and a 25 percent increase in overall sexual satisfaction, according to a study in the *Journal of Sexual Medicine*. Tell that to your buddies when they start chortling at your contortions.

Pigeon: Start on all fours with your palms flat on the ground. Slide your left knee forward to your left wrist and move your left foot in front of your right knee. The outside of your left shin will now rest on the floor. Slowly slide your right leg back and lower your thigh to the floor. (If your hip doesn't reach the floor, put a folded blanket under you.) Press your butt down and adjust your hips to face forward. Push off with your fingertips and lift your torso. Move your hands to your sides, pull your shoulders back, and puff out your chest. Take 10 deep breaths.

Relaxed Pigeon: From the Pigeon, walk your fingertips about a foot squarely in front of you. Press your elbows to the floor, keeping your forearms parallel to each other. Stay here for a breath. Then stretch your arms out in front of you and lower your head to the floor. Take 10 deep breaths, and revert to the Pigeon position.

Full Pigeon: From the Pigeon, lift your left leg and put that foot out in front of you so you're on one knee. With your left hand resting on your thigh, shift your weight forward slightly. At the same time, raise your right shin and reach back with your right hand to grab the top of that foot. Gently pull it closer to your right glute. Take 10 deep breaths. Then switch sides and repeat the entire sequence.

Q: The pros take ice baths after workouts. Should I?

A: "Ice baths reduce inflammation caused by intense, repetitive exercise, and they also speed recovery. Proper workouts shouldn't cause that kind of damage. I do advise ice baths for runners with tendinitis, and spot icing for guys rehabbing—for example, a man lifting after a rotator-cuff injury," says Andrew J. Feldman, MD, a sports-medicine adviser for *Men's Health*.

Q: After a game, I feel wiped out for days. How can I recover more quickly?

A: A hard workout requires a smart recovery plan. First, rehydrate, eat some protein and carbs, and try these.

After a hard ride...

Do this: Put your feet up, at least as high as your heart.

Why: Gravity will move fluids from your legs to the rest of your body, says Sam Callan, USA Cycling's coaching education manager. Pro cyclists receive massages, but researchers in Canada discovered that massaging muscles after a tough workout can actually inhibit blood flow.

After a long swim...

Do this: Press your palms and forearms against each side of a door frame, elbows bent 90 degrees. Take a step forward to stretch your chest. Hold for 20 seconds.

Why: Swimmers' anterior muscles tend to tighten. This stretch can combat stiffness.

Credits

Index

Boldface page references indicate illustrations.
<u>Underscored</u> references indicate boxed text.

Migraines, 230–31
Milk
for breakfast, 4
chocolate reduced fat, 11
whole, 109
Mizuno Wave Ronin 2, 348
Mocktail, 73
Moisturizer
after shower, 222
in hand sanitizers, 241
Mother-in-law, earning respect
of, 331
Mouth
bad breath, 174
best products for, 174
chapped lips, 175
yellow teeth, 174–75
Mouth guard, 348
Mouthwash, 280
Muscle
building in your twenties,
183–85
calories burned by, 125
loss after ceasing workouts,
155
loss with age, 188, 192
Muscle spasm, 228, 230
Mushrooms
most nutritious, 106
Mushroom-Blue Cheese
Sliders, 82
Music, 341
MVP training, 284–89

N

Nachos, 55
NEAT, 127, **131**
Negative chinup/pullup, 148, **148**
Negative pushup, 148, **148**
Neurogenesis, 191–92
Nightcap, drinks for, 12–13
Nike Free 5.0, 348
Nitrates, in meat, 280
NMR lipoprofile test, 247
Nonexercise-activity, 36–37
Nonexercise-activity
thermogenesis (NEAT),
127, **131**
Norepinephrine, 236
Norovirus, 110

O

Obesity, alcohol and, 12
Odor, body, 170
Office coffee mug, germs in,
240
Offset dumbbell reverse lunge,
120, **120**
Oily skin, 165
Olive oil, 77
Omega-3 fatty acids
anti-inflammatory properties,
192
in fish oil, 104
Onyewu, Oguchi (soccer player),
325–26, 326, **327**
Orgasm, female, 261
Osteoporosis, 192
Overheader's walk, 135, **135**
Oxidation, 50

P

Pants, 197
Paper cuts, 281
Passion, 332
Pasta
Linguine with Clams, **78**, 80
Paxil, for premature ejaculation,
261–62
PCBs, 237
Peaches, 77
Peanut butter, 74, 76
Peanuts, curried, 77
Pecan pie, 76
Pec deck, 152
Pelvis, tilted, 144
Pepper hash, 93
Peppermint, 278, **279**
Peppers, 102
Peptide YY, 235
Periodontitis, 215, 280
Personality, five dimensions of,
161–62
Pesticides, 109–10, 234–35
Pizza
eat this, not that, 107
Pesto-Goat Cheese Mini
Pizzas, 72
Plank with arm lift, 323

Plank with opposite arm and leg
lift, 149, **149**
Plants, office, 278, **279**
Plyometrics, 184
Pocket square, 198
Poker, cleaning up at, 332
Polychlorinated biphenyls
(PCBs), 237
Pool, 335
Popcorn, 71
Pork
Backyard Baby Backs, 66
Dr Pepper Ribs, 83, **83**
pot stickers, 77
prosciutto, 72, 73
shoulder, 99
Portobello, 106
Postworkout drinks, 10–11
Potassium
muscle fatigue and, 343
sodium-potassium ratio, 55
Potato chips, 76
Potato skins, 75
Practice, as rule for winning,
336
Premature ejaculation, 256–63,
260
Priligy, for premature
ejaculation, 258, 261–63
Probiotics, 280
Promotion, landing, 330
Prone arm lift, 139
Propecia, 222–23
Proprioceptive neuromuscular
facilitation, 306
Prosciutto, 72, 73
Prostate cancer, 276–77
Protein
satiety and, 32
in your twenties, 183–85
Proton-pump inhibitors, 274
Prozac, for premature
ejaculation, 261–62
PSA test, 276–77
Pullup, **152**, 152–53
Pumpkin seeds, 74
Push press, 26, **26**
Pushup, 114–15, 119, **119**, 189,
286
challenge, 114–15
contest, winning, 336–37
self-test, 189
Pushup and row, 137, **137**

Pushup-position row, 135, **135**
Pushup Pro, <u>45</u>

Q

Quads, weak, 230
Quinoa, <u>17</u>

R

Radiation, from cell phones,
    264–73, <u>269</u>
Rapid eye movement (REM)
    sleep, 281
Razor burn, 169, 220
Recipes, barbecue, 65–69
Recovery from workout, 349
Red Robin, <u>84</u>
Remote control, germs on, 243
Repetitions, number to increase
    fat-burning hormones, <u>119</u>
Rest, between exercises, <u>121</u>,
    150
Restaurants
    buffet, 43
    calorie postings at, 41
    dishes, 78–85
        Beer-Can Chicken, 84, **85**
        Dr Pepper Ribs, 83, **83**
        fast-food fixes, <u>84</u>
        Linguine with Clams, **78**, 80
        Salmon with Ginger-Soy
            Butter, 81, **81**
        Sliders Two Ways, 82, **82**
Reverse lunge and swing, 28, **28**
Reverse lunge with a reachover,
    288
Rhinovirus, 243
Righetti, Amanda (actress), **159**,
    160, <u>163</u>
Rock, paper, scissors (game), 334
Rogaine, 223
Rowing, 342
Runner's knee, 343
Running
    fartlek, 323
    5-K, winning, 337
    incline-running intervals,
        322–23

intervals with 180-degree turn,
    325
speed, 343
sprint, winning all-out, 338
treadmill *versus* outdoor,
    342
uphill footrace, winning, 337
winter clothing, 347, **347**
Rye bread, 40–41

S

Salad
    muscle-building, 110–11, **111**
    ready-to-eat, 110
    seaweed, 77
Salmon
    Salmon with Ginger-Soy
        Butter, 81, **81**
Salsa, 279
Salt, 52–55
    eat this, not that, <u>107</u>
    positive attributes of, 54
    reducing intake of, 54, 107
    saltiest foods, <u>55</u>
    use in cooking, 55
Satiety, 32–33, <u>33</u>
Scallops, 72
Scapular wall slide, <u>39</u>
Scoville heat scale, 102, <u>102</u>
Scrabble (board game), 331
Seafood
    Crab Cakes, 73
    Linguine with Clams, **78**, 80
    Sautéed Calamari, 77
    scallops, 72
Seated calf raise, 154–55
Seaweed salad, 77
Selective serotonin reuptake
    inhibitors (SSRIs), 261,
    263, 275
Self-test
    agility, <u>320</u>
    body fat percentage, <u>186</u>
    endurance, <u>323</u>
    pushup, <u>189</u>
    sit-and-reach, <u>191</u>
    speed, <u>325</u>
    strength, <u>326</u>
    vertical jump, <u>183</u>
Serotonin, 261, 274

Sets
    giant, 288
    number to increase fat-burning
        hormones, <u>119</u>
    supersets, 151
Sex hormones, 236
Sexual health
    grooming products, effects of,
        218–19
    premature ejaculation, 256–63,
        <u>260</u>
    sex drive, 236
Shake
    TD's Preworkout Shake, <u>289</u>
Shake Weight For Men, <u>44</u>
Shaving
    best products for, <u>168–69</u>
    body hair, 169
    close shave, 168–69
    razor burn, 169, 220
    razors, 180–81
    soothing face after, 221
Sheets, germs on, 240
Shirts, <u>196</u>, <u>197</u>, 199, <u>199</u>, 204,
    212
Shoes, 202, 203, 213, 348
Shoulders, exercise for pain
    relief, 151
Sideburns, styling tips, 179
Single-arm dumbbell row, 27, **27**
Single-arm overhead dumbbell
    press, 21, **21**
Single-leg squat, 326, 346
Sit-and-reach (self-test), <u>191</u>
Sitting, health risks and, 34–39,
    275
Skater hops, <u>286</u>
Skiing, cross-country, 344
Skin, grooming products for,
    165–67, <u>166–67</u>
Skin cancer, 214
Skin elasticity, 43–44
Skirt steak, <u>99</u>
Sleep
    diabetes risk increase with
        poor, 277
    extra pillow, <u>175</u>
    melatonin and, 237
    remembering dreams, 281
    valerian as enhancer of, 281
Sleep hormone, 237
Slushie, 155
Smoking, 276